# Human Dignity and Bioethics

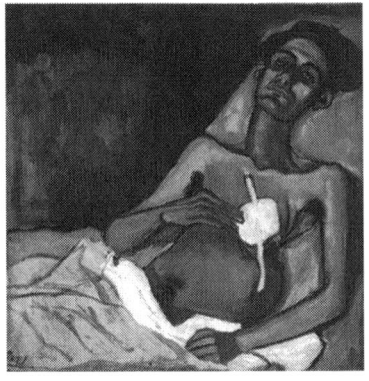

**Alice Neel** (1900-1984), *T.B. Harlem,* 1940, American. Oil on Canvas. 76.2 x 76.2 cm.

Courtesy of the National Museum of Women in the Arts, Washington, D.C.; gift of Wallace and Wilhelmina Holladay. © Estate of Alice Neel.

WHILE MOST OF THE ART WORLD TURNED TO ABSTRACTION TOWARDS THE middle of the twentieth century, Philadelphia-born Alice Neel (1900-1984) courageously chose to remain a figure painter. Occasionally she painted the rich and famous—artists, playwrights, scientists, even a papal nuncio—but mostly her subjects were the unnoticed, the overlooked, the difficult. They were her neighbors in Spanish Harlem: stay-at-home mothers, pregnant mothers, door-to-door salesmen, restaurant workers, tradesmen. Nor did she shy away from those most would rather not confront—a dying, querulous old woman, a middle-aged man in the late stages of cancer, a young man ravaged by tuberculosis. But whether her subjects are young, old, famous, unknown, nude or clothed, Neel's gift was to reveal their common denominator: an ineffable, undefinable, invisible human quality we call dignity.

*T.B. Harlem,* completed in 1940, is one of the most well-known of Neel's paintings. Gaunt and resigned, the subject could have been a young man dying on a battlefield of World War II pinned with a medal of honor. Instead he is a young man in a Harlem hospital fighting an all too prevalent disease to the death. His badge of honor covers the wound of thoracoplasty, or surgically induced lung collapse, then a radical treatment of last resort for tuberculosis. Neel also accurately portrays the side-effects of both the treatment and the disease: owing to the loss of several ribs on the affected side, compensatory thoracic and cervical curvatures of the spine pull it into the opposite directions of an S-curve. Atrophied muscles of the arms and hands and the lax abdominal muscles suggest that the battle has been a long one; the atrophy is the result of disuse, the protuberant abdomen indicative of a long-standing lack of proper nutrition. But Neel's painting is not a medical treatise on tuberculosis. It is rather an eloquent essay on the inherent dignity of human beings that exists quite independently of exterior circumstances.

M. Therese Southgate, MD

# Human Dignity and Bioethics

**Essays Commissioned
by the President's Council
on Bioethics**

Washington, D.C.
WWW.BIOETHICS.GOV

March 2008

# Contents

Letter of Transmittal to The President of The United States..... xi

Members of The President's Council on Bioethics........... xi

Council Staff.................................... xvii

Acknowledgements............................... xix

## Introduction

1  Bioethics and the Question of Human Dignity
   Adam Schulman ................................3

2  Human Dignity and Respect for Persons: A Historical Perspective on Public Bioethics
   F. Daniel Davis ...............................19

## Part I. Dignity and Modern Science

3  How to Protect Human Dignity from Science
   Daniel C. Dennett .............................39

4  Human Dignity and the Mystery of the Human Soul
   Robert P. Kraynak.............................61
      Commentary on Kraynak
         Daniel C. Dennett .........................83
      Commentary on Dennett
         Robert P. Kraynak.........................89

| Table of Contents

    Commentary on Dennett
        Alfonso Gómez-Lobo . . . . . . . . . . . . . . . . . . . . . . .95

5  Human Dignity from a Neurophilosophical Perspective
    Patricia S. Churchland. . . . . . . . . . . . . . . . . . . . . . . . . . . . .99
    Commentary on Churchland
        Gilbert Meilaender . . . . . . . . . . . . . . . . . . . . . . . .122

## Part II. Human Nature and the Future of Man

6  Human Uniqueness and Human Dignity: Persons
    in Nature and the Nature of Persons
    Holmes Rolston III . . . . . . . . . . . . . . . . . . . . . . . . . . . . .129

7  Human Dignity and the Future of Man
    Charles Rubin . . . . . . . . . . . . . . . . . . . . . . . . . . . . . . . . .155

8  Dignity and Enhancement
    Nick Bostrom . . . . . . . . . . . . . . . . . . . . . . . . . . . . . . . . .173
    Commentary on Bostrom
        Charles Rubin . . . . . . . . . . . . . . . . . . . . . . . . . . . .207

## Part III. Dignity and Modern Culture

9  Human Dignity and Public Discourse
    Richard John Neuhaus . . . . . . . . . . . . . . . . . . . . . . . . . .215

10  Modern and American Dignity
    Peter Augustine Lawler . . . . . . . . . . . . . . . . . . . . . . . . . .229

11  Human Dignity: Exploring and Explicating the
    Council's Vision
    Gilbert Meilaender . . . . . . . . . . . . . . . . . . . . . . . . . . . . .253
    Commentary on Meilaender and Dennett
        Peter Augustine Lawler . . . . . . . . . . . . . . . . . . . . .278
    Commentary on Meilaender and Lawler
        Diana Schaub . . . . . . . . . . . . . . . . . . . . . . . . . . . .284

TABLE OF CONTENTS

## Part IV. The Sources and Meaning of Dignity

12  Defending Human Dignity
    Leon R. Kass . . . . . . . . . . . . . . . . . . . . . . . . . . . . . . . .297

13  Kant's Concept of Human Dignity as a Resource for
    Bioethics
    Susan M. Shell . . . . . . . . . . . . . . . . . . . . . . . . . . . . . . .333

14  Human Dignity and Political Entitlements
    Martha Nussbaum . . . . . . . . . . . . . . . . . . . . . . . . . . . .351
        Commentary on Nussbaum, Shell, and Kass
            Diana Schaub . . . . . . . . . . . . . . . . . . . . . . . . . . .381

15  The Irreducibly Religious Character of Human Dignity
    David Gelernter . . . . . . . . . . . . . . . . . . . . . . . . . . . . . .387

## Part V. Theories of Human Dignity

16  The Nature and Basis of Human Dignity
    Patrick Lee and Robert P. George . . . . . . . . . . . . . . . . .409

17  Two Arguments from Human Dignity
    Paul Weithman . . . . . . . . . . . . . . . . . . . . . . . . . . . . . .435

18  Dignity and Bioethics: History, Theory, and Selected
    Applications
    Daniel P. Sulmasy, O.F.M. . . . . . . . . . . . . . . . . . . . . . .469

## Part VI. Human Dignity and the Practice of Medicine

19  Human Dignity and the Seriously Ill Patient
    Rebecca Dresser . . . . . . . . . . . . . . . . . . . . . . . . . . . . .505

20  The Lived Experience of Human Dignity
    Edmund D. Pellegrino . . . . . . . . . . . . . . . . . . . . . . . . .513

Contributors . . . . . . . . . . . . . . . . . . . . . . . . . . . . . . . . . . . .541

Index . . . . . . . . . . . . . . . . . . . . . . . . . . . . . . . . . . . . . . . . .545

# Letter of Transmittal to The President of The United States

The President's Council on Bioethics
1425 New York Avenue, NW, Suite C100
Washington, D.C. 20005
March 1, 2008

The President
The White House
Washington, D.C.

Dear Mr. President,

With this letter I am pleased to send you *Human Dignity and Bioethics: Essays Commissioned by the President's Council on Bioethics.* Like the Council's earlier volume, *Being Human: Readings from the President's Council on Bioethics*, this book is an anthology, in this case a collection of essays exploring a fundamental concept crucial to today's discourse in law and ethics in general and in bioethics in particular.

Since the Council's establishment in 2001, the concept of human dignity has figured frequently in many of the Council's reports. As a result, there have been repeated requests for clarification of the meaning of the term. The Council has decided to respond by putting the question to a diverse group of scholars, including members of the Council, the better to provide a sense of the breadth of opinions on what has become a controversial subject.

These essays make it clear that there is no universal agreement on the meaning of the term, human dignity. Some argue that human

| LETTER OF TRANSMITTAL

dignity has lost its traditional meaning. Others, by contrast, hold firmly to the view that dignity is an essential identifying and irreducible element of human nature. Still others take a more biological than philosophical or theological viewpoint on the question of the meaning of human dignity. An appreciation of the variety of these views is critical, if we are to understand the divergences in how we think and act in response to the challenges posed by contemporary bioethics.

Ultimately, the fundamental questions in law and ethics will be shaped by what we think it means to be human and what we understand to be the ethical obligations owed to the human person. We believe that the two volumes—*Being Human* and *Human Dignity and Bioethics*—provide the public and policymakers with the materials for a deeper understanding of the foundations upon which we build our answers to life's most challenging questions.

Sincerely,

Edmund D. Pellegrino, M.D.
Chairman

# Members of The President's Council on Bioethics

EDMUND D. PELLEGRINO, M.D., CHAIRMAN
Professor Emeritus of Medicine and Medical Ethics and Adjunct Professor of Philosophy, Georgetown University.

FLOYD E. BLOOM, M.D.
Professor Emeritus in the Molecular and Integrative Neurosciences at The Scripps Research Institute, and the founding CEO and board chairman of Neurome, Inc.

BENJAMIN S. CARSON, SR., M.D.
Professor and Director of Pediatric Neurosurgery, Johns Hopkins Medical Institutions.

REBECCA S. DRESSER, J.D., M.S.
Daniel Noyes Kirby Professor of Law and Professor of Ethics in Medicine, Washington University, St. Louis.

NICHOLAS N. EBERSTADT, PH.D.
Henry Wendt Chair in Political Economy and Government, American Enterprise Institute.

| MEMBERS OF THE PRESIDENT'S COUNCIL ON BIOETHICS

**DANIEL W. FOSTER, M.D.**
John Denis McGarry, Ph.D. Distinguished Chair in Diabetes and Metabolic Research, University of Texas Southwestern Medical School.

**MICHAEL S. GAZZANIGA, PH.D.**
Director of Sage Center for the Study of Mind, University of California, Santa Barbara.

**ROBERT P. GEORGE, J.D., D.PHIL.**
McCormick Professor of Jurisprudence and Director of the James Madison Program in American Ideals and Institutions, Princeton University.

**ALFONSO GÓMEZ-LOBO, DR. PHIL.**
Ryan Family Professor of Metaphysics and Moral Philosophy, Georgetown University.

**WILLIAM B. HURLBUT, M.D.**
Consulting Professor, Neurology and Neurological Sciences, Stanford Medical Center, Stanford University.

**LEON R. KASS, M.D., PH.D.**
Addie Clark Harding Professor in the Committee on Social Thought and the College at the University of Chicago and Hertog Fellow in Social Thought, American Enterprise Institute.

**PETER A. LAWLER, PH.D.**
Dana Professor and Chair of the Department of Government and International Studies, Berry College.

**PAUL MCHUGH, M.D.**
University Distinguished Service Professor of Psychiatry, Johns Hopkins School of Medicine.

**GILBERT C. MEILAENDER, PH.D.**
Richard and Phyllis Duesenberg Professor of Christian Ethics, Valparaiso University.

MEMBERS OF THE PRESIDENT'S COUNCIL ON BIOETHICS |

*JANET D. ROWLEY, M.D.*
   Blum-Riese Distinguished Service Professor of Medicine, Molecular Genetics and Cell Biology, and of Human Genetics, Pritzker School of Medicine, University of Chicago.

*DIANA J. SCHAUB, PH.D.*
   Professor of Political Science, Loyola College.

*CARL E. SCHNEIDER, J.D.*
   Chauncey Stillman Professor of Ethics, Morality, and the Practice of Law, and Professor of Internal Medicine, University of Michigan.

# Council Staff

*F. Daniel Davis, Ph.D.*
Executive Director

*Judith E. Crawford*
Administrative Director

*Sam Crowe, Ph.D.*
Policy Analyst

*Diane M. Gianelli*
Director of Communications

*Ginger Gruters*
Research Assistant

*Emily L. Jones*
Executive Administrator

*Audrea R. Medina*
Information Technology Specialist

*Thomas W. Merrill, Ph.D.*
Research Analyst

*David G. Miller, Ph.D.*
Research Analyst

*Marti Patchell*
Special Assistant to the Chairman

*Joseph A. Raho*
Research Assistant

*Alan Rubenstein*
Research Analyst

*Adam Schulman, Ph.D.*
Senior Research Consultant

This collection of essays on human dignity, like previous reports of the Council, is the result of a collaborative effort. Customarily, the Council has not singled out individual staff members who have contributed to the reports. However, in the case of this volume on human dignity, I would like to express our gratitude for the singular efforts of Adam Schulman and Thomas W. Merrill for their excellent editing and coordinating of the collection.

Edmund D. Pellegrino, M.D.
Chairman

# Introduction

# 1
# Bioethics and the Question of Human Dignity

## Adam Schulman

Human dignity—is it a useful concept in bioethics, one that sheds important light on the whole range of bioethical issues, from embryo research and assisted reproduction, to biomedical enhancement, to care of the disabled and the dying? Or is it, on the contrary, a useless concept—at best a vague substitute for other, more precise notions, at worst a mere slogan that camouflages unconvincing arguments and unarticulated biases?

Although the President's Council on Bioethics has itself made frequent use of this notion in its writings, it has not, until now, undertaken a thematic exploration of human dignity, its meanings, its foundations, and its relevance for bioethics. In the meantime, at least one critic, noting that "appeals to human dignity populate the landscape of medical ethics," has recently called into question whether human dignity has any place in bioethical discourse at all.[1] It would seem timely, then, for the Council to take up the question of human dignity squarely, with the aim of clarifying whether and how it might be a useful concept in bioethics. That is the purpose of the present volume of essays, some contributed by Council Members, others by guest authors at the invitation of the Council.

The task of this introduction is to illuminate, in a preliminary way, *the question of human dignity* and its proper place in bioethics. To that end, it will first give some examples of how human dignity can be a difficult concept to apply in bioethical controversies. It will then explore some of the complex roots of the modern notion of human dignity, in order to shed light on why its application to bioethics is so problematic. Finally, it will suggest, tentatively, that a certain conception of human dignity—dignity understood as *humanity*— has an important role to play in bioethics, both now and especially in the future.

## The Problem of Human Dignity in Bioethics: Some Examples

That human dignity might be at least problematic as a bioethical concept is suggested by the many ways it gets invoked in bioethical debates, often on different sides of the same issue. Consider, for example, a question raised in the fourth chapter of *Taking Care,* the Council's recent exploration of ethical caregiving at the end of life:[2] Is it morally acceptable for an elderly patient, diagnosed with early Alzheimer's disease and facing an inexorable decline into dementia and dependency, to stop taking his heart medicine in the hope of a quicker exit, one less distressing to himself and his family? One possible answer discussed in our report is that it is morally permissible (and perhaps even admirable) for such a patient, who finds the prospect of years of dementia humiliating or repellent and who is reluctant to become a burden to his family, to forgo medication and allow heart disease to carry him off in a more *dignified and humane* way. Another possible answer is that it is morally impermissible, because deliberately hastening the end of one's life, even by an act of omission, is incompatible with the *equal dignity and respect owed to all human life*. A third answer is that respect for the *dignity and autonomy* of all persons requires us to defer to the personal choice of a competent individual in such intimate matters, regardless of how he or she might decide. Note that all three answers (and perhaps others that could be given) are grounded in part in some appeal to human dignity, though they reach quite different conclusions.

Or, to take an example from the beginning of human life, consider a question that might arise in a neonatal intensive care unit: What medical interventions are appropriate to save the life of a critically ill premature infant who is likely to survive, if at all, only with severe mental defects? One possible answer is that, because *human dignity rests on our higher mental capacities,* it is wrong to bring a person into the world burdened with a devastating lifelong mental incapacity. Another answer might be that every reasonable measure should be taken, because the *equal dignity of all human life* forbids us to declare some lives "not worth living." Yet a third answer might be that, out of respect for their *dignity and autonomy,* the parents must be left free to resolve this moral dilemma for themselves.

Or, again, consider an example of biomedical "enhancement" examined in the fifth chapter of the Council's *Beyond Therapy*:[3] If science were to develop memory-blunting drugs that could free us from the emotional burdens of intrusive and painful memories, would it be ethically permissible to give such drugs freely to people who have suffered grievous disappointments or witnessed horrifying events? One answer might be that such an invention, with its promise of liberating miserable people from the emotional tyranny of past misfortunes, ought to be embraced as an unqualified enhancement to *human freedom, autonomy, and dignity.* But another answer might be that *human integrity and dignity* require of us that we confront our painful memories and learn to deal with them (if possible) and not just "flush" them away by taking a pill. A third answer would be that this decision is properly left to the individual, whose *dignity and autonomy* entail the right of voluntary, informed consent.\*

In each of these examples, a variety of strong convictions can be derived from powerful but conflicting intuitions about what human dignity demands of us. Little wonder, then, that some bioethicists are inclined to wash their hands of "dignity" entirely, in favor of clearer and less ambiguous ethical concepts.

---

\* On "human dignity" as used in the Council's writings, see Gilbert Meilaender's essay in this volume. For a defense of the equal dignity of all human life, see the essay in this volume by Patrick Lee and Robert P. George.

6 | ADAM SCHULMAN

## The Tangled Sources of Human Dignity

If human dignity seems a malleable concept of uncertain application in bioethics, that is partly because the idea of human dignity comes to bioethics from several disparate sources. Each of these sources contributes something of value for bioethics; yet each source also brings its own peculiar difficulties to the application of the concept of human dignity to bioethical controversies. At least four such sources of human dignity seem worth mentioning:

a. *Classical antiquity:* The word "dignity" comes to us, via the Latin *dignus* and *dignitas*, from Greek and Roman antiquity, in whose literature it means something like "worthiness for honor and esteem." This classical notion of dignity as something rare and exceptional retains some of its power even in our egalitarian age: witness the admiration we bestow on outstanding athletic and musical performance, on heroism in war, on courageous statesmanship, or on the selflessness of those who make sacrifices or undergo hardships for the sake of their young children, or their aging parents, or their neighbors stricken by misfortune or tragedy. But if dignity implies excellence and distinction, then to speak of "human dignity" raises the question, what is it about human beings as such that we find distinctive and admirable, that raises them in our estimation above other animals? Is there some one attribute or capacity that makes man worthy of respect, such as reason, or conscience, or freedom? Or is it a complex of traits, no one of which is sufficient to earn our esteem? These are not easy questions to answer; yet most would acknowledge that there must be *something* about humankind that entitles us to the special regard implicit in this sense of human dignity.\*

One problem with the classical notion of dignity that has only grown more acute in our age of rapid biomedical progress is the complicated relationship between technology and human dignity

---

\* Of course there are some sophisticated thinkers who, in the name of animal rights, assail the very idea of a special status for man as an expression of naïvely anthropocentric "speciesism," a word coined by analogy with racism and sexism. See Peter Singer, *Animal Liberation*, 2nd ed. (New York: Avon, 1990); for a different perspective, see Bernard Williams, *Ethics and the Limits of Philosophy* (Cambridge, Massachusetts: Harvard University Press, 1985). On human uniqueness see Holmes Rolston's essay in this volume.

(understood as grounded in excellence). Is the dignity of the soldier enhanced by the invention of modern weapons? Is the dignity of the athlete enhanced by drugs that improve his performance, or even by his reliance on trainers, nutritionists, and other experts? Some might argue that new technologies ("bio" and otherwise) serve human dignity by augmenting those traits that make human beings worthy of esteem; yet others might view such inventions as undermining human dignity, by making our excellence depend too much on the artifice of others.

A second problem with dignity in its classical sense is that it lends itself to invidious distinctions between one human being and another; it is not fully at home in democratic times, where it keeps uneasy company with the more characteristic democratic ideals of equality, freedom, easygoingness, and tolerance.* Now for that very reason one might argue that human dignity is especially vulnerable and worth defending in democratic times. But to make the case for human dignity as a robust bioethical concept for our age, one would have to show that dignity can be something universal and accessible to all human beings as such.

There was in fact a school of philosophy in ancient Greece and Rome, the Stoics, who believed in dignity as a genuine possibility for all human beings, regardless of their circumstances, social standing, or accomplishments. For the Stoics, human beings have dignity because they possess reason, and the best life, the life according to nature, is available to anyone who chooses to live in a thoughtful or reflective way. And what our reason dictates, above all, is that everything necessary for our happiness and peace of mind is within our control; despite poverty, illness, or oppression it is always possible to live in a dignified way. Nothing that anyone can say or do to you can rob you of your dignity and integrity. For the Stoics, dignity is a profoundly democratic idea, in that it is just as likely to be found among the wretched as among the lofty: as possible for the slave Epictetus as for the emperor Marcus Aurelius.†

---

\* That "dignity" retains an aura of Roman exclusivity even in modern times is suggested by a quotation attributed to humorist James Thurber: "Human Dignity has gleamed only now and then and here and there, in lonely splendor, throughout the ages, a hope of the better men, never an achievement of the majority."
† That the Stoic conception of human dignity might not be entirely incompat-

Yet while dignity as the Stoics conceived it is a universal possibility for all human beings everywhere, it nonetheless sets a rigorous and exacting standard that few of us, in practice, manage to attain. And while the Stoic teaching of indifference to bodily suffering might well prove to be a valuable discipline for those who have to live with pain, illness, or infirmity, the Stoic attitude of detachment from the things of this world—embodied in the principle that "nothing that can be taken from you is good"—means that particular bioethical questions are ultimately of little significance from the Stoic point of view.*

b. *Biblical religion:* Another powerful source of a broader, shared notion of human dignity is the Biblical account of man as "made in the image of God." This teaching, together with its further elaborations in Jewish and Christian scripture, has been interpreted in many different ways, but the central implication seems to be that human beings, because they are in some respects godlike, possess an inherent and inalienable dignity. One part of that dignity, suggested by the Book of Genesis, has to do with the special position of man in the natural world: within that realm man is like God not only in having stewardship or dominion over all things, but also because he alone can comprehend the whole and he alone concerns himself with the good of the whole.[4] In light of this suggestion, "being made in God's image" could even be taken to imply a special responsibility on our part to perfect nature in order to finish God's creation. Interpreted in this way, the idea of human dignity could lend support not only to the practice of healing and medicine in general, but also, some might argue, to a defense of such activities as *in vitro* fertilization or even cloning, here understood as fixing nature in a godlike way.

Yet if man's mastery of nature has some sanction in the Biblical teaching on human dignity, that teaching also points in another, humbler direction: for although made in God's image, we are not ourselves divine; we are creatures, not creators. In this sense, "made

---

ible with our easygoing American culture is suggested by the recent popularity of the movie *Gladiator* (directed by Ridley Scott, DreamWorks SKG, 2000) and of the Tom Wolfe novel *A Man in Full* (New York: Farrar, Straus & Giroux, 1998), both of which explore Stoic responses to misfortune. Consider also the example of Admiral James Stockdale, whose education in Stoic principles helped him survive with dignity through seven harrowing years as a prisoner of war in Vietnam.

* For problems with the Stoic notion of dignity, and for an Aristotelian alternative, see Martha Nussbaum's essay in this volume.

in God's image" has the implication that all human beings, not only those healthy and upright but also those broken in body or soul, have a share in this God-given dignity. Dignity in this sense would give ethical guidance to us in answering the question of what we owe to those at the very beginning of life, to those at the end, to those with severe disability or dementia, and even to tiny embryos. Seeing human beings as created in the image of God means, in some sense, valuing other human beings in the way a loving God would value them. It means seeing dignity where some might see only disability, and perhaps seeing human life where others might see only a clump of cells.

Yet because the Biblical account of human dignity points in different directions, its implications for bioethics are not always clear and unambiguous. In the controversy over stem cell research, for example, would the inherent dignity of man mean that human life at every stage is sacred, and that the destruction of human embryos is therefore forbidden? Or would it mean that healing and preserving human life is our preeminent duty, justifying all kinds of otherwise morally questionable research?

Some will argue that a concept of human dignity derived from the Bible (or other religious texts) is inherently unreliable, a mask for religious dogmas that have no legitimate place in secular bioethics.* Thus Ruth Macklin, who advocates banishing the term "dignity" from medical ethics entirely, suspects that religious sources, especially Roman Catholic writings on human dignity, may explain why so many articles and reports appeal to human dignity "as if it means something over and above respect for persons or for their autonomy."[5] More recently, Dieter Birnbacher has suggested that the idea of human dignity, when invoked (as it has been in the cloning debate) to defend the natural order of human procreation against biotechnical manipulation, is nothing more than camouflage for a theological tradition that sees "the order of nature as divinely sanctioned."[6] Yet, while it might be problematic to rely on religious texts for *authoritative guidance* on bioethical questions, such texts may still be quite valuable in helping

---

* See the essays by Daniel C. Dennett and Patricia S. Churchland in this volume. Of course, others argue that religious sources of ethics are both legitimate and necessary. In this volume, see the essays by David Gelernter, Robert P. Kraynak, and Richard John Neuhaus.

all of us—whether believers or not—to articulate and think through our deepest intuitions about human beings, their distinctive powers and activities, and the rights and responsibilities we believe them to possess.* Furthermore, those who would dismiss all religious grounds for the belief in human dignity have the burden of showing, in purely secular terms, what it is about human beings that obliges us to treat them with respect. If not because they are "endowed by their Creator with certain unalienable rights," then why *can* men rightfully defend their "life, liberty, and pursuit of happiness"?†

c. *Kantian moral philosophy:* A daring attempt to set universal human dignity on a strictly rational foundation was made in the 18th century by the German philosopher Immanuel Kant. Kant's primary purpose was to show how moral freedom and responsibility could still be possible in a world governed by the laws of mathematical physics. For Kant, in agreement with the Stoics, dignity is the intrinsic worth that belongs to all human beings and to no other beings in the natural world. All men possess dignity because of their rational autonomy, i.e., their capacity for free obedience to the moral law of which they themselves are the authors. Kant's doctrine of human dignity demands equal respect for all persons and forbids the use of another person merely as a means to one's own ends. Kant's celebration of autonomy and his prohibition of the "instrumentalization" of human subjects have certainly had a lasting impact on modern ethical thought and on bioethics in particular (especially in the ethics of human experimentation and in the principle of voluntary, informed consent). And it cannot be denied that Kant's account of what the moral law demands of us (his various formulations of the "categorical imperative") has a certain austere majesty and logical economy that compel grudging respect if not wholehearted allegiance. Yet the application of Kant's moral theory to bioethics remains problematic for a number of reasons.

First, Kant's achievement in reconciling morality with mathematical physics was won at a great price: in locating human dignity

---

* See the essay by Leon R. Kass in this volume.
† Whether the rights proclaimed in the Declaration of Independence rest ultimately on a religious or a secular foundation is, of course, a complex question that cannot be settled here. On dignity in the context of modern—and especially American—thought, see Peter Lawler's essay in this volume.

entirely in rational autonomy, Kant was forced to deny any moral significance to other aspects of our humanity, including our family life, our loves, loyalties, and other emotions, as well as our way of coming into the world and all other merely biological facts about the human organism.* His exclusive focus on rational autonomy leaves Kant with a rather narrow and constricted account of our moral life, one that has precious little to say about the moral significance of a whole range of biomedical interventions that currently arouse ethical controversy.† If the rational will alone is the seat of human dignity, why should it matter if we are born of cloned embryos, or if we enhance our muscles and control our moods with drugs, or if we sell our organs on the open market?

Second, the doctrine of rational autonomy itself, clear and unambiguous though it may be in theory, can be difficult to apply in practice, especially in a biomedical context. Consider these examples: If dignity depends on the rational will, must we conclude that those human beings who do not yet have the powers of rational autonomy (infants), or who have lost them (those with dementia), or who never had them (those with congenital mental impairment) are beneath human dignity? How far can a person go in the use of mood- and mind-altering drugs before rational autonomy is compromised? Are choices made under the influence of such drugs less than free? On such basic questions in bioethics Kant's account of human dignity does not offer clear moral guidance.

Third, Kant's moral philosophy has bequeathed to later ethical thought a deplorable legacy in the form of the rigid distinction between deontology and consequentialism, i.e., between a morality (such as Kant's) of absolute imperatives and one (such as utilitarianism) that considers only the good and bad results of our actions. Nowadays, if human dignity is invoked in the discussion of some

---

* One will not, for example, find much hint of human dignity in Kant's definition of marriage as "the association of two persons of different sex for the lifelong reciprocal possession of their sexual faculties" (*die verbindung zweier Personen verschiedenen Geschlechts zum lebenswierigen wechselseitigen Besitz ihrer Geschlechtseigenschaften*); my own translation from Immanuel Kant, *The Metaphysics of Morals* [*Die Metaphysik der Sitten*] (Königsberg: Nicolovius, 1797), Part I, Metaphysical Elements of the Doctrine of Right, §24.

† For an alternative view of the resources Kant can bring to bear on controversies in bioethics, see Susan M. Shell's essay in this volume.

bioethical issue, the first question that is usually raised is whether the term is being used as a categorical moral principle (e.g., "human cloning is wrong in principle, because it violates some inalienable right of the child") or as an argument based on consequences (e.g., "human cloning is wrong because of the degrading effects it is likely to have on the child, the family, and society at large"). Bioethics in practice requires a healthy measure of old-fashioned *prudence* and is not well served by a dogmatic adherence to the artificial division between an ethics of principles and an ethics of consequences.

d. *20th-century constitutions and international declarations:* Finally, another prominent yet problematic source for the introduction of "human dignity" into contemporary bioethical discussions is the frequent use of that phrase in national constitutions and international declarations ratified in the aftermath of the Second World War. By proclaiming a belief in "human dignity," such documents would seem, at first blush, to point beyond the prosaic safeguarding of "rights" advocated in the American founding ("life, liberty, and the pursuit of happiness") or in the writings of John Locke ("life, liberty, and property") and other modern natural right theorists.

The preamble to the *Charter of the United Nations* (1945) begins:

> We the people of the United Nations, determined to save succeeding generations from the scourge of war, which twice in our lifetime has brought untold sorrow to mankind, and to reaffirm faith in fundamental human rights, in the *dignity and worth of the human person*, in the rights of men and women and of nations large and small.... [emphasis added]

In the *Universal Declaration of Human Rights* (1948), recognition "of the inherent dignity and of the equal and inalienable rights of all members of the human family" is said to be "the foundation of freedom, justice, and peace in the world."* At least thirty-seven national constitutions ratified since 1945 refer explicitly to human dignity, including the *Basic Law* (*Grundgesetz*) *of Germany* (1949), which begins: "Human dignity is inviolable. To respect and protect it is the

---

* On human dignity as a source of political entitlements, see the essays by Paul Weithman and Martha Nussbaum in this volume.

duty of all state authority."[7]

As Doron Shultziner has emphasized,[8] while human dignity in these documents plays the role of a supreme value on which all human rights and duties are said to depend, the meaning, content, and foundations of human dignity are never explicitly defined. Instead, their affirmations of human dignity reflect a political consensus among groups that may well have quite different beliefs about what human dignity means, where it comes from, and what it entails. In effect, "human dignity" serves here as a placeholder for "whatever it is about human beings that entitles them to basic human rights and freedoms." This practice makes a good deal of sense. After all, what mattered most after 1945 was not reaching agreement as to the *theoretical* foundations of human dignity but ensuring, as a *practical* matter, that the worst atrocities inflicted on large populations during the war (i.e., concentration camps, mass murder, slave labor) would not be repeated. In short, "the inviolability of human dignity" was enshrined in at least some of these documents chiefly in order to prevent a second Holocaust.

Yet because of its formal and indeterminate character, the notion of human dignity espoused in these constitutions and international declarations does not offer clear and unambiguous guidance in bioethical controversies.* Certainly the fact that human dignity is mentioned prominently in these documents is to be welcomed as an invitation to explore the question, "What is the ground of human dignity?" And the sensible idea of invoking universal human dignity in order to establish a baseline of inviolable rights—in effect, a floor of decency beneath which no treatment of human beings should ever sink—may well prove to be of some value in holding the line against the most egregious abuses of the new biotechnologies (e.g., the deliberate creation of animal-human chimeras). Yet if we are content

---

* UNESCO's recently adopted (though still provisional) *Universal Declaration on Bioethics and Human Rights* refers to "human dignity" or "the dignity of the human person" (in close conjunction with "human rights" and "fundamental freedoms") eleven times but does not spell out what that dignity is or why human beings have it. Reflecting its status as a consensus statement among many nations, the draft suggests that "due regard" should be paid to "cultural diversity and pluralism," but not so as to infringe upon or limit the scope of "human dignity, human rights and fundamental freedoms." The text of the Declaration may be found online at www.unesco.org/ibc.

to regard human dignity as nothing more than an unspecified "Factor X"[9] in virtue of which we are obliged to treat all persons with respect, then some bioethicists have wondered why we should bother invoking it at all. Why not dispense with dignity and simply spell out precisely what "respect for persons" demands of us? Ruth Macklin adopts this viewpoint, arguing that respect for persons is a sufficient principle for bioethics, one that entails "the need to obtain voluntary, informed consent; the requirement to protect confidentiality; and the need to avoid discrimination and abusive practices."[10] Her approach may have the virtue of simplicity, but it does not explain *why* all persons are entitled to respect;\* and it is far from clear that all present and future controversies in bioethics can be resolved merely by providing informed consent, honoring confidentiality, avoiding discrimination, and refraining from abuse.†

e. *Summary:* To recapitulate the findings of this section: Important notions of human dignity are to be found both in classical antiquity and in Biblical scripture, each with lasting influence on modern thought. Yet the classical conception of dignity (in the general sense of human worth, grounded in excellence) is of problematic relevance to present-day bioethics, in part because of its ambiguous relationship to technological progress and in part because of its aristocratic and inegalitarian tendencies; while the specifically Stoic notion of human dignity is of limited use in bioethics both because of the severe and exacting standard it sets and because of the basic Stoic attitude of indifference to the external world, including the suffering of the body. And although the Biblical teachings on human dignity are rich and evocative, they have ambiguous implications for bioethics, pointing both toward godlike mastery of nature and toward humble acknowledgment of the sanctity of human life in all its forms. Turning to the modern era, both the moral philosophy of Kant and various constitutions and international declarations of the 20th century appear to

---

\* One recognizes, in the various principles of autonomy or "respect for persons" that populate contemporary bioethics, the remote and enfeebled descendants of Kant's categorical moral imperative; yet the devotees of autonomy today are seldom willing to embrace anything like the metaphysical system Kant felt obliged to supply as the ground for his moral principles.

† For responses to Macklin's critique of "dignity" see the essays by Daniel P. Sulmasy, O.F.M., and Rebecca Dresser in this volume.

provide support for a belief in the equal dignity of all human beings. Yet Kant's idea of human dignity carries certain theoretical baggage that limits its utility for bioethics, while the recently ratified constitutions and declarations tend to invoke dignity without clearly specifying either its ground or its content, suggesting that the concept itself might well be superfluous. On the other hand, it is hard to see how ethical standards for the treatment of human beings can be maintained without relying on *some* conception of what human beings are and what they therefore deserve.

## Dignity Understood as Humanity—An Indispensable Concept for Bioethics?

Having disentangled some of the roots of the modern concept of human dignity, can we make a compelling case for the usefulness of this concept in present-day and future bioethics? Only a tentative answer to this question can be hazarded here.

There is a strong temptation to say no, for the following reason. The fundamental question we have alluded to several times in this paper—the question of the specific excellence or dignity of man—has proved sufficiently daunting that a long line of great modern thinkers, from Hobbes and Locke to the American founders, have found it prudent, for political purposes, to assert that all human beings have rights and freedoms that must be respected equally, without spelling out too clearly the ground of that assertion.* And such deliberate reticence as to the foundation and content of human dignity has arguably served liberal democracy well, fostering tolerance, freedom, equality, and peace. In the particular context of medical ethics, it must be acknowledged that for a long time the liberal principle of "respect for persons"—including the rights of voluntary, informed consent and confidentiality, as well as protection from discrimination and abuse—has proved serviceable in resolving many (though

---

* Hobbes, however, was somewhat less reserved than the others: in chapter 13 of *Leviathan* (1651) he indicates that our equal rights are derived ultimately from our roughly equal vulnerability to being killed by one another. Note that, for Hobbes, dignity is not intrinsic to human beings but is merely "the public worth of a man, which is the value set on him by the Commonwealth" (*Leviathan*, chapter 10).

by no means all) ethical problems.

But in this extraordinary and unprecedented era of biotechnological progress, whose fruits we have scarcely begun to harvest, the campaign to conquer nature has at long last begun to turn inward toward human nature itself. In the coming decades we will increasingly acquire the power to isolate and modify the biological determinants of human attributes that hitherto have been all but immune to manipulation. For example, we are learning to control the development of human embryos *in vitro*, and this may one day make possible the cloning of human beings, the creation of animal-human chimeras, and the gestation of human fetuses in animal or artificial wombs. We are assembling a growing arsenal of psychoactive drugs that modulate not only behavior but also attention, memory, cognition, emotion, mood, personality, and other aspects of our inner life. We are acquiring the ability to screen out unwanted gene combinations in preimplantation embryos and may in the future be capable of direct germ-line genetic modification. We may one day be able to modify the human genome so as to increase resistance to diseases, optimize height and weight, augment muscle strength, extend the lifespan, sharpen the senses, boost intelligence, adjust personality, and who knows what else. Some of these changes may amount to unobjectionable enhancements to our imperfect nature; but surely not all forms of biomedical engineering are equally benign and acceptable.*

Our ever-increasing facility at altering human nature itself poses an acute challenge to any easygoing agnosticism on the question of the ground and content of human dignity. As we become more and more adept at modifying human nature at will, it may well prove impossible to avoid a direct confrontation with the question posed by the Psalmist, "What is man that thou art mindful of him?" That is, among all the features of human nature susceptible to biotechnological enhancement, modification, or elimination, which ones are so essential to our humanity that they are rightly considered inviolable? For example, if gestation of fetuses in artificial wombs should become feasible, would it not be a severe distortion of our humanity and an affront to our dignity to develop assembly lines for the mass

---

* On biomedical enhancement, see the essays by Nick Bostrom and Charles Rubin in this volume.

production of cloned human beings without mothers or fathers? Would it not be degrading to our humanity and an affront to human dignity to produce animal-human chimeras with some human features and some features of lower animals? Would it not be a corruption of our humanity and an affront to human dignity to modify the brain so as to make a person incapable of love, or of sympathy, or of curiosity, or even of selfishness?*

In short, the march of scientific progress that now promises to give us manipulative power over human nature itself—a coercive power mostly exercised, as C. S. Lewis presciently noted, by some men over other men, and especially by one generation over future generations†—will eventually compel us to take a stand on the meaning of human dignity, understood as the essential and inviolable core of our *humanity*. If the necessity of taking that stand is today not yet widely appreciated, there will come a time when it surely will be. With luck, it will not be too late.

---

\* In the novel *White Noise* (New York: Viking Penguin, 1985) by Don DeLillo, a drug is invented whose specific effect on the human brain is apparently to suppress the fear of death. Would it be compatible with human dignity for all of us to start taking such a drug?

† C. S. Lewis, *The Abolition of Man* (Oxford: Oxford University Press, 1943), chapter 3: "From this point of view, what we call Man's power over Nature turns out to be a power exercised by some men over other men with Nature as its instrument.... There neither is nor can be any simple increase of power on Man's side. Each new power won by man is a power over man as well. Each advance leaves him weaker as well as stronger. In every victory, besides being the general who triumphs, he is also the prisoner who follows the triumphal car."

## Notes

[1] Ruth Macklin, "Dignity is a Useless Concept," *BMJ* 327 (2003): 1419-1420, available online at www.bmj.com/cgi/content/full/327/7429/1419?etoc. Dieter Birnbacher, another skeptic on the usefulness of human dignity as a bioethical concept, acknowledges that there is a "nearly worldwide consensus that reproductive cloning is incompatible with human dignity and should be prohibited by law." See his "Human cloning and human dignity," *Reproductive BioMedicine Online* 10, Supplement 1 (2005): 50-55.
[2] The President's Council on Bioethics, *Taking Care: Ethical Caregiving in Our Aging Society* (Washington, D.C.: Government Printing Office, 2005), chapter 4, pp. 154ff.
[3] The President's Council on Bioethics, *Beyond Therapy: Biotechnology and the Pursuit of Happiness* (Washington, D.C.: Government Printing Office, 2003), chapter 5, pp. 214ff.
[4] On the meaning of "in the image of God" in the Bible, see Leon R. Kass, *The Beginning of Wisdom: Reading Genesis* (New York: The Free Press, 2003), pp. 36-40, as well as the essays by Kass and by Robert P. Kraynak in this volume.
[5] Ruth Macklin, op. cit.
[6] Dieter Birnbacher, op. cit.
[7] See Teresa Iglesias, "Bedrock Truths and the Dignity of the Individual," *Logos* 4 (2001): 114-134.
[8] See Shultziner's helpful review article, "Human dignity—functions and meanings," *Global Jurist Topics* 3 (2003): 1-21.
[9] See Francis Fukuyama, *Our Posthuman Future: Consequences of the Biotechnology Revolution* (New York: Farrar, Straus & Giroux, 2002), chapter 9, "Human Dignity."
[10] Ruth Macklin, op. cit.

# 2

# Human Dignity and Respect for Persons: A Historical Perspective on Public Bioethics

## F. Daniel Davis

Several aims converge in this volume of essays on the significance of human dignity for bioethics, commissioned and published by the President's Council on Bioethics.* One aim is to take up the challenge implicitly issued by American medical ethicist Ruth Macklin, who bluntly asserted four years ago that "dignity is a useless concept in medical ethics and can be eliminated without any loss of content."[1] In her critique of human dignity as a bioethical concept, Macklin singled out the work of the President's Council on Bioethics, claiming that the concept functions as "a mere slogan" in such Council reports as *Human Cloning and Human Dignity*.[2]

Macklin goes on to compare the Council's allegedly indistinct use of dignity with the more precise meaning that the concept is given in *Genetics and Human Behavior: the Ethical Context,* a report published in 2002 by the Nuffield Council on Bioethics in the United Kingdom.[3] In that report, she notes, dignity refers to the idea that "one is a person whose actions, thoughts and concerns are worthy

---
* Hereinafter, "the President's Council."

of intrinsic respect because they have been chosen, organized and guided in a way that makes sense from a distinctly individual point of view."[4] Macklin's favorable comparison of this sense of dignity with the Council's "hopelessly vague" usage of the concept is but a Trojan horse for the central contention of her critique: namely, that dignity is a poor, blurred substitute for what she describes as *the* principle of medical ethics, *respect for persons*—or, as she later says, *respect for autonomy*. Even in the Nuffield report, she argues, the truth of the matter emerges: dignity adds nothing to, and in fact casts a confusing haze over, the ideas clearly conveyed by the principle of respect for autonomy.[5]

Macklin's critique of human dignity is, to say the least, open to question; and many of the respondents who were moved to submit rejoinders to her article did raise pointed questions:[6] In what sense is respect for persons *the* principle of medical ethics? Does respect for persons mean the same as respect for autonomy? Does either principle fully exhaust the meaning of human dignity? Is dignity really reducible to autonomy? In what follows I will merely touch on possible responses to these questions, for what intrigues me here is the provocation implicit in Macklin's critique: her comparison of human dignity and respect for persons (or autonomy) invites historical analysis and reflection on the role that concepts of this sort have played in the work of national forums in public bioethics.

Respect for persons is one of three principles enunciated in the 1979 *Belmont Report,* the final report issued by the National Commission for the Protection of Human Subjects of Biomedical and Behavioral Research\*, the *first* major national forum in public bioethics in the United States. A quarter of a century later, human dignity has been a pivotal concept in some (albeit not all) of the reports of the President's Council on Bioethics, the country's *current* national forum in public bioethics. How does the principle of respect for persons (as well as the other two principles, beneficence and justice) function in the deliberations and reports of the National Commission? What is the meaning of the principle, what are its origins, and what has been its fate since 1979? Likewise, how does the present Council appeal to and ground its arguments in the concept of human dignity, and what does the Council mean by human dignity, which, like respect for

---

\* Hereinafter, "the National Commission."

persons, has a history that begins long before the establishment of the President's Council? What, if anything, comes to light when the differing historical contexts in which the two national forums were created are compared? To address these questions, I turn first to the context in which the National Commission was conceived and established.

## Respect for Persons, the *Belmont Report,* and the National Commission

On July 12, 1974, then President Richard M. Nixon signed into law Public Law 93-348, the National Research Act, which created the National Commission and charged its members with several tasks. One task was to identify the ethical principles that should govern the conduct of biomedical and behavioral research with human subjects. Another was to develop guidelines to ensure that specific investigations would be designed and conducted in accordance with these principles. The events that led to Congressional passage of the National Research Act of 1974 are well known but merit explicit remembrance here. Two years before, in the midst of the civil rights movement, the now-notorious Tuskegee Syphilis Study was brought to light in a series of newspaper investigations. Funded and conducted by the U.S. Public Health Service, the Study began in 1932 in Macon County, Alabama, and enrolled 399 poor African-American men suffering from syphilis. While its purpose was to track the natural history of the disease, researchers from the Public Health Service told the participants that they were subjects in an investigation of "bad blood," an umbrella term encompassing several conditions including syphilis, anemia, and fatigue.[7] In 1947, fifteen years into the study, penicillin was established as an effective cure for syphilis, but the Tuskegee researchers withheld the antibiotic from the subjects, whose participation was enticed and sustained with offers of free meals, physical examinations, and burial insurance. In the course of the 40-year study, 28 of the men died of the disease, 100 died of related complications, and at least 40 wives and 19 children became infected.[8]

The public outrage sparked by the Tuskegee revelations was unprecedented, though similar abuses in human subjects research had been reported. The preceding decade of the 1960s was marked by repeated disclosures of unethical conduct in clinical research. From 1963 to 1966, for example, the Willowbrook State School for "mentally defective persons" in New York was the site of a study of the natural history of infectious hepatitis and of the effectiveness of gamma globulin in its prevention and treatment. Researchers at Willowbrook deliberately infected children with the hepatitis virus, later arguing in their own defense that infection was inevitable due to the poor hygienic conditions at the school. Willowbrook was closed to new admissions during the study, but space remained available in the institution's hepatitis program—and parents who wished to admit their children to the school had little choice but to agree to their enrollment in the study. The year 1963 also marked the initiation of a study of cancer immunology at New York City's Jewish Chronic Disease Hospital, where clinical investigators injected live cancer cells into patients hospitalized for various chronic diseases—without the patients' knowledge (although the researchers did claim that oral consent had been sought but not documented). And in 1966, in the *New England Journal of Medicine,* Harvard's Henry K. Beecher (who chaired the Harvard ad hoc committee that proposed a neurological standard for determining death) described his analysis of 22 ongoing clinical studies involving unethical practices in human subjects research.[9] Concluding that such practices were far from uncommon, Beecher ended his controversial exposé with a broadside against the utilitarian defense of their legitimacy: "An experiment is ethical or not at its inception; it does not become ethical post hoc—ends do not justify the means."[10] Thus, with the uproar over Tuskegee, a steadily mounting concern, fueled by one revelation of abuse after another, reached such a crescendo that in 1973 Congress began a series of hearings, aiming both to prevent further abuses and to grapple with the paradoxical challenge of harvesting the fruits of biomedical science and technology while mitigating their dangers. The National Commission was born of this resolve.

Over the next four years, the Commission issued seven reports.[11] Several were in fulfillment of the Commission's legislative mandate: *Research Involving the Fetus* (1975), *Research Involving Prisoners* (1976), *Research Involving Children* (1977), *Psychosurgery: Report and Recommendations* (1977), *Disclosure of Research Information under the*

*Freedom of Information Act* (1977), *Research Involving Those Institutionalized as Mentally Infirm* (1978). Only at the very end—one is tempted to say as the culmination—of its work did the Commission issue its famed *Belmont Report*.[12]

In the *Belmont Report,* the National Commission began by citing the "troubling ethical questions" raised, not by the Tuskegee Syphilis Study, but rather by the 1946 Nuremberg War Crime Trials, and the prosecution, there and then, of Nazi physicians for their conduct of often horrific experiments involving inmates from the concentration camps. The Nuremberg tribunal ended its written judgment of these physicians and their "crimes against humanity" with the declaration of a ten-point code of ethics for the conduct of research with human subjects, the first element of which reads "the voluntary consent of the human subject is absolutely essential."[13] In the *Belmont Report,* the National Commission acknowledges the Nuremberg Code as the progenitor of "many later codes," but it contends that the general as well as specific rules set forth in these codes often prove to be inadequate in the complicated circumstances of human subjects research—for example, when subjects are incapable of providing voluntary consent. With the conviction that "broader ethical principles will provide a basis on which specific rules may be formulated, criticized, and interpreted,"[14] the National Commission asserts that three such principles are "relevant" to human subjects research: respect for persons, beneficence, and justice.[15]

In the *Belmont Report,* the National Commission describes these principles as "comprehensive": they are "stated at a level of generalization" that should prove helpful to investigators, human subjects, and interested citizens, and together they "provide an analytical framework that will guide the resolution of ethical problems."[16] Principles, in the National Commission's view, are "general prescriptive judgments" that offer "a basic justification for the many particular ethical prescriptions and evaluations of human actions."[17] In brief, these principles illuminate the focus for ethical evaluation, directing how we are to think about, and how we are to act to resolve, ethical problems in human subjects research. As for the source of these principles, they are neither the products of pure reason nor the dictates of natural law; nor are they the constructs of philosophers or of professional ethicists. Instead, according to the National Commission, the three principles are beliefs "generally accepted in our cultural tradition":[18] they are derived, that is, from what principlists call "the common morality." Such, in outline, is the National Commission's understanding of principles, as is evident in its treatment of the first of the three principles, viz., respect for persons.

The principle of respect for persons embraces two "ethical convictions," each of which has a correlative moral requirement. That is, embedded in each of the two convictions are directions for action or practice; these directions are moral requirements spelling out what is required in any action that seeks to be faithful to the conviction. One of the two convictions is that "individuals should be treated as autonomous agents," and its corresponding requirement is to "acknowledge autonomy." The other conviction is that "persons with diminished autonomy are entitled to protection,"[19] and its correlative requirement is to "protect those with diminished autonomy." Thus autonomy, the capacity to deliberate about one's personal goals and to act in accord with these deliberations and goals, looms large among those attributes of persons that merit respect—and respect is what leads us to "give weight to autonomous persons' considered opinions and choices while refraining from obstructing their actions unless they are clearly detrimental to others."[20] Recognizing that some persons have not yet acquired or never will fully acquire the developmental capacities critical to the exercise of autonomy, the National Commission asserts that such individuals need protection, to a degree or kind dependent upon the risks and benefits of participation in human subjects research. Finally, in concrete application, the principle of respect for persons makes it imperative to secure informed, voluntary consent when enrolling participants in human subjects research.[21]

How does the principle of respect for persons, along with the principles of beneficence and justice, figure in the work of the National Commission? One way of answering the question is, of course, to consult the Commission's published reports with an eye on the ethical reasoning that undergirds particular findings and recommendations. Although there are differences from report to report, their logic is consistent: they lay out the questions and issues engendered by the focal topic, summarize and describe current practices and thinking about the topic, and then proceed with ethical analysis. Other sources of insight into the National Commission's deliberations and ethical reasoning are the first-person accounts penned by such participants as Albert Jonsen, a commissioner, and by Tom Beauchamp, a staff philosopher during the Commission's waning days and the principal authorial force behind the ultimate form of the *Belmont Report*.

In his *Birth of Bioethics* and other writings, Jonsen hones in on the process of ethical reasoning used by the Commission: he says that the commissioners "believed as principlists" but "worked as casuists." They believed that broad norms exist; that these norms apply to human behavior *per se* and enjoy widespread acceptance as such, but have special relevance for such circumscribed areas of concern as human subjects research; and that such norms hold in general, though any one may admit of exceptions.[22] The commissioners did not, however, begin their deliberations on specific topics with an agreement about governing principles from which more directed guidance could be deduced. Their process was a thoroughly inductive one.

In his recollections, Beauchamp offers a more precise picture of how the National Commission's deliberative process joined principlist convictions with casuist methods:

> Casuistical reasoning more so than moral theory or universal abstraction often did function to forge agreement during National Commission deliberations. The commissioners appealed to particular cases and families of cases, and consensus was reached through agreement on cases and generalization from cases when agreement on an underlying theoretical rationale would have been impossible. Commissioners would never have been able to agree on a single ethical theory, nor did they even attempt to buttress the *Belmont* principles with a theory.[23]

Widely esteemed as an authoritative statement of ethical precepts, the *Belmont Report* is a landmark in the evolution of the ethics of clinical research and of principlism, a theory of ethical justification that has spread beyond the sphere of human subjects research and has, for several decades now, been dominant as well in the clinical sphere, i.e., in relations between physicians and patients.[24] One principle in particular has come to prominence, the principle of respect for autonomy, a conceptual offspring of the *Belmont* principle of respect for persons. While Ruth Macklin seems to treat respect for persons and respect for autonomy as identical principles, a careful reading of the intertwined histories of the ethical concepts of "respect," "persons," and "autonomy" suggests otherwise; indeed, none of these concepts has had or even now has a univocal meaning, though a particular meaning may be dominant at one time or another.

Consider the concept of a person: for the National Commission, that concept embraces every human being, regardless of the degree to which he or she is autonomous. In its breadth, the Commission's concept of a person mirrors the inclusive scope that it has, for example, in the work of theologian Paul Ramsey—although for Ramsey the ultimate source of every person's inviolable worth, regardless of his or her capacity for autonomous self-determination, is God; and the respect owed to every person is a duty that has its ultimate source in God's covenantal relationship with humankind.[25] At the time of the National Commission's deliberations, a stark alternative to this understanding of a person could be found in the work of Joseph Fletcher, also a theologian but one who radically circumscribed the concept, restricting it to human beings who have threshold levels of intelligence, self-awareness, self-control, and neocortical function, among other prerequisites.[26] For some critics and observers of recent and contemporary bioethics, this narrower sense of personhood—of which the Princeton bioethicist Peter Singer is a prominent exponent—has come to overshadow both discourse and practice, although the broader understanding has by no means been extinguished and survives, for example, in mainstream Catholic moral theology.[27] And what the narrower sense champions as essential to humanity is autonomy. Thus, it is not that the concept of a person has been attenuated in the intervening years: rather, the subject of respect has shifted from the person to autonomy,[28] in the restrictive sense this term has in the moral philosophy of Immanuel Kant. For Kant, human autonomy consists in submission to the moral law. The ultimate test of our moral decisions, choices, and actions is whether these expressions of the self can be universalized as law. The meaning of autonomy that finds assertive expression in contemporary bioethics, however, owes less to Kant than to John Stuart Mill, for whom "liberty" consists in "framing the plan of our life to suit our own character;...doing as we like, subject to such consequences as may follow: without impediment from our fellow creatures, so long as what we do does not harm them, even though they should think our conduct foolish, perverse or wrong."[29]

The concept of respect has undergone a similar process of evolution, with a tapering of its meaning over time. For Ramsey, respect is a duty, the fulfillment of which demands multiple interrelated modes of responsiveness to the unique, irreducible worth of the person, a worth affirmed not only in honoring the individual and deferring to his wishes, but also in tending to his needs and caring for him. Today, however, respect is often understood more narrowly, as a duty strictly correlative to the individual's rights to privacy and self-determination—a duty to refrain from interfering with the free, unfettered choice of the autonomous individual, a duty that can be set aside only in the interest of protecting another from harm. It is this sense of respect that seemingly animates the principle of respect for autonomy that Macklin champions as central to contemporary medical ethics. And as a description of medical ethics today, her assertion is reasonably accurate.

The critical question, which Macklin never fully explores in her essay, is whether this centrality of respect for autonomy as a bioethical principle should be embraced as an unqualified good for theory and practice in human subjects research, clinical medicine, and beyond. Nor does she note that interest in human dignity as a bioethical concept has been prompted, in part, by the growing sense that the prevalence of autonomy in bioethics and beyond, in American culture and society, reflects an incomplete and inadequate—even a *distorted*—grasp of humanity and thus of what is at stake in many of the controversies provoked by the advance of biomedicine and biotechnology.[30]

## Human Dignity, This Volume, and the President's Council

One such controversy was on the mind of President Bush when, on August 9, 2001, he addressed the nation in a televised speech devoted to articulating and justifying his policy on federal funding for embryonic stem cell research. In his speech, the President also announced his intent to establish, by executive order, a "president's council on bioethics" to advise him on this and other contentious issues engendered by the remarkable but sometimes morally troubling progress of biomedicine and biotechnology. As the establishment of the National Commission was spurred by ethical problems of broad, public significance, so too was the President's Council born of a serious bioethical problem—with implications not only for such moral questions as *What should or should not be done in the sphere of biomedical research?* but also for such arguably more fundamental questions as *What is a human being?* and *What are the implications of our humanity for how we pursue the growth of our knowledge and its applications in practice?* With the National Commission and the President's Council, these problems—the subject matter of an ever-expanding field of experts, specialized organizations, and journals—have been brought into the public square for analysis, discussion, reflection, and debate by policymakers, legislators, and the citizens to whom they are accountable. This is the rationale for any national forum in public bioethics.

As initiatives in public bioethics, the National Commission and the President's Council have a key feature in common: they are both creatures of the Federal Government, formed to pursue their missions in the full light of public observation and scrutiny and with public participation. The differences between the two bodies, however, are arguably more interesting and revealing; and this is also true of the *Belmont Report* when compared to this volume, and of the principle of respect for persons compared to the concept of human dignity. Consider, first, the agents of their respective formations. The National Commission was established through the legislative authority of the U.S. Congress, as was its immediate successor, the President's Commission for the Study of Ethical Problems in Medicine and Biomedical and Behavioral Research. By contrast, like its immediate predecessor, the National Bioethics Advisory Commission,* the President's Council was launched by executive authority and, strictly speaking, answers to the President and to the President alone.

The mandates of the two bodies reveal an even more striking difference. The U.S. Congress endowed the National Commission with

---
* Created by Executive Order 12975, signed by President Clinton in 1995.

an ambitious but precisely detailed agenda, along with a set of specified outcomes or required "deliverables"; with one exception, the "deliverables" were all inquiries involving human subjects research, anchored to the explicit expectation that their findings and recommendations would inform, or even decisively shape, the formation of federal law and regulation. Since its inception, the President's Council has labored under an altogether different mandate, as is clear in this passage from Executive Order 13237:

> The Council shall advise the President on bioethical issues that may emerge as a consequence of advances in biomedical science and technology. In connection with its advisory role, the mission of the Council includes the following functions: (1) to undertake fundamental inquiry into the human and moral significance of developments in biomedical and behavioral science and technology; (2) to explore specific ethical and policy questions related to these developments; (3) to provide a forum for a national discussion of bioethical issues; (4) to facilitate a greater understanding of bioethical issues; and (5) to explore the possibilities for useful international collaboration on bioethical issues.

The "deliverables" that the Council has been expected to produce are not specified reports on a prescribed list of topics: they are, instead, *advice* to the President; a *forum* for public discussion and to foster *understanding* of bioethical issues; and, by implication, the *fruits* of its "fundamental" inquiries and of its explorations of "specific ethical and policy questions." As I previously noted, particular problems in bioethics were important in the genesis of both the National Commission and the President's Council; and thus, in the creation of both there was, more or less, a degree of external compulsion or need. The agenda that the President's Council has pursued has not, however, been strictly tethered to the morality of embryonic stem cell research, the dilemma that attended its birth. On several different occasions, for varying lengths of time, the President's Council has explored this topic, as well as the related topic of human cloning, and issued reports on both; but it has also undertaken inquiries into biotechnology and human enhancement, assisted reproduction, organ transplantation, newborn screening, neuroethics, psychopharmacology and children, the determination of death, aging and end of life care, and nanotechnology.[31] And the President's Council has both formed and pursued this varied, wide-ranging agenda in complete freedom from any external constraint or pressure—including constraint or pressure from any quarter of the executive branch, including the White House.

The direct link between the deliberations of the National Commission, on the one hand, and policymaking at the federal level, on the other, demanded that the Commission seek and develop among its members a consensus: only agreement on the form and content of its findings and recommendations could provide a firm foundation for federal law and regulations in human subjects research. The U.S. Congress needed clear, unequivocal guidance, especially in addressing difficult, emergent questions about clinical research involving specific populations that are, by definition, vulnerable: fetuses, children, the mentally infirm, and prisoners. And as an ethical framework for all federally funded research involving human subjects, the U.S. Congress sought, as well, a set of norms distinguished, in part, by broad acceptance and endorsement, not only by the members of the National Commission but also by the American public. Although several reports by the President's Council do include recommendations for policymaking (or recommendations with clear implications for policymaking), its inquiries have not been structured or conducted with the overriding aim of agreement among its members; instead, in the words of President Bush's executive order, "the Council shall be guided by the need to articulate fully the complex and often competing moral positions on any given issue...and may therefore choose to proceed by offering a variety of views on a particular issue, rather than attempt to reach a single consensus position."

This particular contrast between the National Commission and the President's Council is not simply one of procedures and aims, for it offers a revealing window on striking differences between their respective historical contexts. The U.S. Congress established the National Commission in 1974, at a time of profound social change ignited by the civil rights and women's movements and one year after the U.S. Supreme Court's historic and, in the years since, increasingly divisive decision in *Roe v. Wade*. The ideological tensions generated by these events and forces were apparent but nascent in American society. The process of developing and exploiting the potential of biomedicine and biotechnology had been well underway for years, but the effort to reckon with the full (and still uncertain) implications of this potential was in its infancy, as was the field of bioethics itself. The issues that, by Congressional mandate, dominated the agenda of the National Commission were ones that could reasonably command public support and concern: what ethical precepts should guide clinical research, permitting it to go forward on a more secure moral footing? And in justifying its response to this question, in advocating the practical application of the *Belmont* principles, the National Commission could appeal to beliefs and perceptions that derive their normative authority from widespread acceptance in American society and—especially in the case of the principle of respect for persons, with its focus on autonomy—from deep roots in the American political tradition.

Thirty years later, it would be an understatement to say that much has changed, although many features of the present era were discernible in germinal form at the time of the National Commission. The ideological tensions that led to and were further aggravated by *Roe v. Wade* have evolved into the stark polarities of today's so-called culture wars, thereby frustrating if not precluding any facile appeal to a common, shared morality. Meanwhile, a steady stream of discoveries in biomedicine and novel applications of biotechnology have extended and strengthened our reach over human biology, equipping us with new tools, not only for curing and ameliorating human disease but also for enhancing certain traits and capacities, for conceiving and gestating human life, and for forestalling the fate that awaits us all, death itself. Today, more than ever before, we seem poised for mastery over many aspects of human life, including those that unite us with nonhuman animals and those that separate us from them. For some, these achievements of the ongoing revolution in biomedicine and biotechnology testify to the triumph of human ingenuity and to the efficacy of the human will to fashion our environment—and ourselves—as we wish. For others, the claim that all these impressive achievements make positive contributions to human flourishing is misguided and even dangerous, neglecting the sober lesson of Tuskegee: that the quest for new knowledge, and for new applications of that knowledge, can be perverted so as to inflict egregious harms on our fellow human beings—harms that go far beyond the failure to secure their voluntary informed consent.

In brief, in light of such deep-seated divisions in the American public, the chance for consensus seems slim, and the goal of agreement may even be ill-advised, at least at this time for a national forum in public bioethics. An alternative goal, challenging but achievable, is to bring broader and deeper insights to the public understanding of the issues of bioethics. In the service of *this* goal, the President's Council is to undertake, in the words of its charter, "fundamental inquiry into the human and moral significance of developments in biomedical and behavioral science and technology"; it is "to strive to develop a deep and comprehensive understanding of the issues that it considers"; and, it is "to articulate fully the complex and often competing moral positions on any given issue."

These passages from the charter of the President's Council implicitly suggest a *critical* view of contemporary academic bioethics, and of the way bioethical questions are debated in the public square. Today, for the most part, two justifications are advanced when bioethics seeks to shape policy: first, the utilitarian justification, that the good to be achieved for the many by X, Y, or Z (for example, by embryonic stem cell research or by the use of "net benefit" calculations in organ allocation) far outweighs the harm to the few; and second, the principlist argument that respect for autonomy—that tried-and-true American value—legitimates such controversial practices as unconstrained reproductive decision making, assisted suicide, and euthanasia. Now this depiction of contemporary bioethics is admittedly rendered only in broad strokes. In the decades since the National Commission, discourse in academic bioethics *has* been diversified by theoretical "voices" other than utilitarianism and principlism: by feminist bioethics, the ethics of care, and communitarianism, as well as by the resurgence of such traditions as virtue ethics and Kant-inspired theories of duty. Nonetheless, the tendency to seek ethical justification for our gathering powers over human nature either in the calculated good of the many or in the primacy of individual autonomy is undeniably prevalent and is mirrored, for example, in Macklin's essay. For some observers, including some members of the President's Council, this tendency is the mark of an impoverished bioethics—a bioethics in need of an account of humanity more probing and comprehensive than that which undergirds the now-prevalent theories of ethical justification. The work of the President's Council—and especially its explorations of human dignity, including the present volume—can be understood as a response to that need.

I shall conclude with a few more comparisons and a prediction. Previously, I highlighted the place of the *Belmont Report* in the work of the National Commission: it was the Commission's last report and was in part a retrospective endeavor, an effort to reflect back on and clarify the ethical reasoning, implicit and explicit, in the Commission's previously published, "problem-specific" reports. But *Belmont* was also a prospective endeavor, attempting to prescribe a needed ethical framework for future human subjects research. This volume exhibits a similarly bifocal perspective. Some of its essays look back to older sources of wisdom about human dignity or attempt to explicate invocations of human dignity in the published reports of the President's Council; while others have a more prospective trajectory, seeking to stimulate bioethical inquiry, and propelling it forward in relatively unexplored directions.

For an American readership, some of these explorations may seem rather novel. Unlike the principles enunciated in the *Belmont Report,* the concept of human dignity is not derived from a common morality of American vintage. The story of dignity's origins and evolution is a complex one, with roots in the Biblical account of human creation as well as in ancient Stoicism and the philosophy of Immanuel Kant, among other sources. To appreciate this complexity and the challenges it poses for dignity as a bioethical concept, one could do no better than read the introductory essay by Adam Schulman, the project director and co-editor of this volume. What is at issue here, however, is the significance of these facts about the origins and development of the concept of human dignity, especially about its distinctly un-American beginnings. Certainly, any national forum in public bioethics should be knowledgeable about and responsive to the unique intellectual and political traditions of the nation it serves. But if its inquiries are to be rigorously fundamental, it will necessarily also look beyond these traditions for an understanding of humanity that is as broad as it is deep. After all, the urgent and fundamental questions at the heart of bioethics do not respect geographical and cultural boundaries.

Finally, a prediction—and an acknowledgement of the partial truth of Ruth Macklin's complaint. Many of the essays in this volume do explore in depth the complex and divergent meanings of human dignity and thus fill a void left open by the published work of the President's Council—*until now*. I predict, however, that after carefully reading and reflecting on these essays, most readers will reject Macklin's conclusion that human dignity is a "useless" concept and will, instead, find their understanding of questions and issues in contemporary bioethics deepened and enriched. That is the hope and aim of the President's Council in publishing this volume of essays on the bioethical significance of human dignity.

# Notes

[1] Ruth Macklin, "Dignity Is A Useless Concept," *BMJ* 327 (2003): 1419-1420.
[2] Ibid., p. 1420.
[3] See chapter 12, "Genetics, freedom and human dignity," of the Nuffield Council report, available online at www.nuffieldbioethics.org/go/ourwork/behaviouralgenetics/publication_311.html.
[4] Macklin, loc. cit.
[5] Ibid.
[6] Rapid responses to Macklin's editorial are published online at www.bmj.com/cgi/eletters/327/7429/1419.
[7] See James H. Jones's *Bad Blood: The Tuskegee Syphilis Experiment* (New York: The Free Press, 1981).
[8] Resources on the history and sequelae of the Tuskegee study are numerous. A portal to internet-based resources is available online at www.gpc.edu/~shale/humanities/composition/assignments/experiment/tuskegee.html.
[9] Henry K. Beecher, "Ethics and Clinical Research," *New England Journal of Medicine* 274 (1966): 1354-1360.
[10] Ibid. p. 1360.
[11] Most of the reports of the National Commission are available online from the website of the President's Council on Bioethics at www.bioethics.gov/reports/past_commissions/index.html.
[12] The *Belmont Report* was approved by the National Commission at its 42nd meeting on June 10, 1978, and published in the *Federal Register* on April 18, 1979. Citations in this essay are to a reprint of the report included as an appendix (pp. 253-265) to *Belmont Revisited: Ethical Principles for Research with Human Subjects*, ed. James F. Childress, Eric M. Meslin, and Harold T. Shapiro (Washington, D.C.: Georgetown University Press, 2005).
[13] For discussion, see Evelyne Shuster, "Fifty years later: the significance of the Nuremberg Code," *New England Journal of Medicine* 337 (1999): 1436-1440. The Nuremberg Code is available online at: http://ohsr.od.nih.gov/guidelines/nuremberg.html.
[14] *Belmont Report*, p. 255.
[15] Ibid.
[16] Ibid.
[17] Ibid., p. 256.
[18] Ibid.
[19] Ibid., p. 257.
[20] Ibid.
[21] Ibid., p. 260.
[22] Albert Jonsen, "On the Origins and Future of the Belmont Report," in *Belmont Revisited*, p. 8.
[23] Tom L. Beauchamp, "The Origins and Evolution of the Belmont Report," in *Belmont Revisited*, p. 19.

[24] For an account of the influence of the Belmont principles on clinical practice, see Eric J. Cassell's "The Principles of the Belmont Report: How Have Respect for Persons, Beneficence, and Justice Been Applied in Clinical Medicine," in *Belmont Revisited*, pp. 77-95.

[25] Paul Ramsey, *The Patient as Person: Explorations in Medical Ethics*, 2nd ed. (New Haven, Connecticut: Yale University Press, 2002).

[26] Fletcher developed these views of personhood and humanity in a series of influential books and articles, including his *Morals and Medicine* (Princeton, New Jersey: Princeton University Press, 1954) and, later, his *Humanhood: Essays in Biomedical Ethics* (Buffalo, New York: Prometheus Books, 1979).

[27] See, for example, Singer's *Rethinking Life and Death: The Collapse of Our Traditional Ethics* (New York: St. Martin's, 1994). With respect to Catholic moral theology, see Pope John Paul II's encyclical, *Evangelium vitae* (1995), available online at www.vatican.va/edocs/eng0141/_index.htm.

[28] Two of the more compelling expositions of this argument about the relationship between the Belmont principle of respect for persons and the principle of respect for autonomy are made by M. Therese Lysaught (see her "Respect: Or, How Respect for Persons Became Respect for Autonomy," in *The Journal of Medicine and Philosophy* 29 [2004]: 665-680) and by Karen Lebacqz, a former member of the National Commission (see her "We Sure Are Older But Are We Wiser?" in *Belmont Revisited*, pp. 99-110).

[29] John Stuart Mill, *On Liberty*, in *Collected Works of John Stuart Mill*, ed. John M. Robson (Toronto: University of Toronto Press, 1977 [1859]), vol. XVIII.

[30] For a thorough, sustained critique of the prevalence of autonomy in American bioethics and society, see Willard Gaylin and Bruce Jennings, *The Perversion of Autonomy: Coercion and Constraints in a Liberal Society*, revised and expanded edition (Washington, D.C.: Georgetown University Press, 2003).

[31] All of the Council's published reports can be found online at www.bioethics.gov/reports/.

# Part I.
# Dignity and Modern Science

# 3

# How to Protect Human Dignity from Science

## Daniel C. Dennett

Many people fear that science and technology are encroaching on domains of life in a way that undermines human dignity, and they see this as a threat that needs to be resisted vigorously. They are right. There is a real crisis, and it needs our attention now, before irreparable damage is done to the fragile environment of mutually shared beliefs and attitudes on which a precious conception of human dignity does indeed depend for its existence. I will try to show both that the problem is real and that the most widely favored responses to the problem are deeply misguided and bound to fail. There is a solution that has a good chance of success, however, and it employs principles that we already understand and accept in less momentous roles. The solution is natural, reasonable, and robust instead of fragile, and it does not require us to try to put the genie of science back in the bottle—a good thing, since that is almost certainly impossible. Science and technology can flourish open-endedly while abiding by restrictive principles that are powerful enough to reassure the anxious and mild enough to secure the unqualified endorsement of all but the most reckless investigators. We can have dignity and science too, but only if we face the conflict with open minds and a sense of common cause.

## The Problem

Human life, tradition says, is infinitely valuable, and even sacred: not to be tampered with, not to be subjected to "unnatural" procedures, and of course not to be terminated deliberately, except (perhaps) in special cases such as capital punishment or in the waging of a just war: "Thou shalt not kill." Human life, science says, is a complex phenomenon admitting of countless degrees and variations, not markedly different from animal life or plant life or bacterial life in most regards, and amenable to countless varieties of extensions, redirections, divisions, and terminations. The questions of when (human) life begins and ends, and of which possible variants "count" as (sacred) human lives in the first place are, according to science, more like the question of the area of a mountain than of its altitude above sea level: it all depends on what can only be conventional definitions of the boundary conditions. Science promises—or threatens—to replace the traditional absolutes about the conditions of human life with a host of relativistic complications and the denial of any sharp boundaries on which to hang tradition.

Plato spoke of seeking the universals that "carve Nature at its joints,"* and science has given us wonderful taxonomies that do just that. It has identified electrons and protons (which have the mass of 1,836 electrons and a positive charge), distinguished the chemical elements from each other, and articulated and largely confirmed a Tree of Life that shows why "creature with a backbone" carves Nature better than "creature with wings." But the crisp, logical boundaries that science gives us don't include any joints where tradition demands them. In particular, there is no moment of *ensoulment* to be discovered in the breathtakingly complicated processes that ensue after sperm meets egg and they begin producing an embryo (or maybe twins or triplets—when do *they* get their individual souls?), and there is no moment at which the soul leaves the body and human life ends. Moreover, the more we understand, scientifically, about these complexities, the more practical it becomes, technologically, to exploit them in entirely novel ways for which tradition is utterly unprepared: *in vitro* fertilization and cloning, organ harvest and transplant, and,

---

* *Phaedrus* 265d-266a.

at the end of life, the artificial prolongation of life—of one sort or another—after most if not all the *sacred* aspects of life have ceased. When we start treating living bodies as motherboards on which to assemble cyborgs, or as spare parts collections to be sold to the highest bidder, where will it all end? It is not as if we could halt the slide by just prohibiting (some of) the technology. Technology may provide the *faits accomplis* that demonstrate beyond all controversy that the science is on the right track, but long before the technology is available, science provides the huge changes in conceptualization, the new vistas on possibility, that will flavor our imaginations henceforth whether or not the possibilities become practical. We are entering a new conceptual world, thanks to science, and it does not harmonize comfortably with our traditional conceptions of our lives and what they mean.*

In particular, those who fear this swiftly growing scientific vista think that it will destroy something precious and irreplaceable in our traditional scheme, subverting the last presumptions of human specialness which ground—they believe—our world of morality. Oddly enough, not much attention has been paid to the question of exactly how the rise of the scientific vista would subvert these cherished principles—in this regard, it is a close kin to the widespread belief that homosexual marriage would somehow subvert traditional "family values"—but in fact there is a good explanation for this gap in the analysis. The psychologist Philip Tetlock identifies values as *sacred* when they are so important to those who hold them that the very act of considering them is offensive.[1] The comedian Jack Benny was famously stingy—or so he presented himself on radio and television—and one of his best bits was the skit in which a mugger puts a gun in

---

* The philosopher Wilfrid Sellars, in his essay "Philosophy and the Scientific Image of Man" (in *Science, Perception, and Reality* [London: Routledge and Kegan Paul, 1963]), distinguished between the manifest image of everyday life, with its tables and chairs, trees and rainbows, people and dreams, and the scientific image of atoms and particles and waves of electromagnetic radiation, and noted that the task of putting these two images into registration is far from straightforward. The dimension of meaning, which resides solely—it seems—in the manifest image, is resistant both to reduction (the way chemistry, supposedly, reduces to physics) and to any less demanding sort of unification or coordination with the scientific image. The tension we are exploring here is a particularly vivid and troubling case of the tension between these two images.

his back and barks "Your money or your life!" Benny just stands there silently. "Your money or your life!" repeats the mugger, with mounting impatience. "I'm thinking, I'm thinking," Benny replies. This is funny because most of us think that nobody should even think about such a trade-off. Nobody should *have to* think about such a trade-off. It should be unthinkable, a "no-brainer." Life is sacred, and no amount of money would be a fair exchange for a life, *and if you don't already know that, what's wrong with you?* "To transgress this boundary, to attach a monetary value, to one's friendships, children, or loyalty to one's country, is to disqualify oneself from the accompanying social roles."[2] That is what makes life a sacred value.

Tetlock and his colleagues have conducted ingenious (and sometimes troubling) experiments in which subjects are obliged to consider "taboo trade-offs," such as whether or not to purchase live human body parts for some worthy end, or whether or not to pay somebody to have a baby that you then raise, or pay somebody to perform your military service. As their model predicts, many subjects exhibit a strong "mere contemplation effect": they feel guilty and sometimes get angry about being lured into even thinking about such dire choices, even when they make all the right choices. When given the opportunity by the experimenters to engage in "moral cleansing" (by volunteering for some relevant community service, for instance) subjects who have had to think about taboo trade-offs are significantly more likely than control subjects to volunteer—for real—for such good deeds. (Control subjects had been asked to think about purely non-sacred trade-offs, such as whether to hire a house-cleaner or buy food instead of something else.)[3]

So it is not surprising that relatively little attention has been paid to charting the paths by which science and technology might subvert the value of life. If you feel the force of the admonition, "Don't even think about it!", you will shun the topic by distracting your own attention from it, if at all possible. I know from experience that some readers of this essay will already be feeling some discomfort and even guilt for allowing themselves to broach these topics at all, so strong is the taboo against thinking the unthinkable, but I urge them to bear with me, since the policy that I will propose may have more going for it than their own.

The fact that the threat has not been well articulated does not mean it is not real and important. Let me try to make it plain by drawing some parallels. Like climate change, the threat is environmental and *global* (which means you can't just move to a different place where the environment hasn't yet been damaged), and time is running out. While global warming threatens to affect many aspects of the *physical* environment—the atmosphere, the flora and fauna, the ice caps and ocean levels—and hence alter our geography in catastrophic ways from which recovery may be difficult or impossible, the threat to human dignity affects many aspects of what we may call the *belief environment*, the manifold of ambient attitudes, presumptions, common expectations—the things that are "taken for granted" by just about everybody, and that just about everybody expects just about everybody to take for granted.

The belief environment plays just as potent a role in human welfare as the physical environment, and in some regards it is both more important and more fragile. Much of this has been well-known for centuries, particularly to economists, who have long appreciated the way a currency can become worthless almost overnight, for example, and the way public trust in financial institutions needs to be preserved as a condition for economic activity in general. Today we confront the appalling societal black holes known as failed states, where the breakdown of law and order makes the restoration of decent life all but impossible. (If you have to pay off the warlords and bribe the judges and tolerate the drug traffic…just to keep enough power and water and sanitation going to make life bearable, let alone permit agriculture and commerce to thrive, your chances of long-term success are minimal.) What matters in these terrible conditions is what people in general assume *whether they are right or wrong*. It might in fact be safe for them to venture out and go shopping, or to invest in a clothing factory, or plant their crops, but if they don't, in general, believe that, they cannot resume anything like normal life and rekindle a working society. This creates a belief environment in which there is a powerful incentive for the most virtuous and civic-minded to lie, vigorously, just to preserve what remains of the belief environment. Faced with a deteriorating situation, admitting the truth may only accelerate the decline, while a little creative myth-making might— *might*—save the day. Not a happy situation.

And this is what people fear might happen if we pursue our

current scientific and technological exploration of the boundaries of human life: we will soon find ourselves in a deteriorating situation where people—rightly or wrongly—start jumping to conclusions about the *non*-sanctity of life, the commodification of all aspects of life, and it will be too late to salvage the prevailing attitudes that protect us all from something rather like a failed state, a society in which the sheer security needed for normal interpersonal relations has dissolved, making trust, and respect, and even love, all but impossible. Faced with that dire prospect, it becomes tempting indeed to think of promulgating a holy lie, a myth that might carry us along for long enough to shore up our flagging confidence until we can restore "law and order."

That is where the doctrine of the soul comes in. People have immortal souls, according to tradition, and that is what makes them so special. Let me put the problem unequivocally: the traditional concept of the soul as an immaterial thinking thing, Descartes's *res cogitans*, the internal locus in each human body of all suffering, and meaning, and decisions, both moral and immoral, has been utterly discredited. Science has banished the soul as firmly as it has banished mermaids, unicorns, and perpetual motion machines. There are no such things. There is no more scientific justification for believing in an immaterial immortal soul than there is for believing that each of your kidneys has a tap-dancing poltergeist living in it. The latter idea is clearly preposterous. Why are we so reluctant to dismiss the former idea? It is obvious that there must be some *non*-scientific motivation for believing in it. It is seen as being needed to play a crucial role in preserving our self-image, our dignity. If we don't have souls, we are *just animals!* (And how could you love, or respect, or grant responsibility to something that was just an animal?)

Doesn't the very meaning of our lives depend on the reality of our immaterial souls? No. We don't need to be made of two fundamentally different kinds of substance, matter and mind-stuff, to have morally meaningful lives. On the face of it, the idea that all our striving and loving, our yearning and regretting, our hopes and fears, depend on some secret ingredient, some science-proof nugget of specialness that defies the laws of nature, is an almost childish ploy: "Let's gather up all the wonderfulness of human life and sweep it into the special hidey-hole where science can never get at it!" Although this fortress mentality has a certain medieval charm, looked at in the cold light of day, this idea is transparently desperate, implausible, and risky: putting all your eggs in one basket, and a remarkably vulnerable basket at that. It is vulnerable because it must declare science to be unable to shed any light on the various aspects of human consciousness and human morality at a time when exciting progress is being made on these very issues. One of Aristotle's few major mistakes was declaring "the heavens" to be made of a different kind of stuff, entirely unlike the matter here on Earth—a tactical error whose brittleness became obvious once Galileo and company began their still-expanding campaign to understand the physics of the cosmos. Clinging similarly to an immaterial concept of a soul at a time when every day brings more understanding of how the material basis of the mind has evolved (and goes on evolving within each brain) is a likely path to obsolescence and extinction.

The alternative is to look to the life sciences for an understanding of what does in fact make us different from other animals, in morally relevant ways. We are the only species with language, and art, and music, and religion, and humor, and the ability to imagine the time before our birth and after our death, and the ability to plan projects that take centuries to unfold, and the ability to create, defend, revise, and live by codes of conduct, and—sad to say—to wage war on a global scale. The ability of our brains to help us see into the future, thanks to the culture we impart to our young, so far surpasses that of any other species, that it gives us the powers that in turn give us the responsibilities of moral agents. *Noblesse oblige.* We are the only species that can know enough about the world to be reasonably held responsible for protecting its precious treasures. And who on earth could hold us responsible? Only ourselves. Some other species—the dolphins and the other great apes—exhibit fascinating signs of proto-morality, a capacity to cooperate and to care about others, but we persons are the only animals that can conceive of *the project of leading a good life*. This is *not* a mysterious talent; it can be explained.*

---

* My 2003 book, *Freedom Evolves*, is devoted to an explanation of how our capacity for moral agency evolved and continues to evolve. It begins with a quotation from a 1997 interview with Giulio Giorelli: "*Sì, abbiamo un'anima. Ma è fatta di tanti piccoli robot.*—Yes, we have a soul, but it's made of lots of tiny robots!" These "robots" are the mindless swarms of neurons and other cells that cooperate

Here I will not attempt to survey the many threads of that still unfolding explanation, but rather to construct and defend a perspective and a set of policies that could protect what needs to be protected as we scramble, with many false steps, towards an appreciation of the foundations of human dignity. Scientists make their mistakes in public, but mostly only other scientists notice them. This topic has such momentous consequences, however, that we can anticipate that public attention—and reaction—will be intense, and could engender runaway misconstruals that could do serious harm to the delicate belief environment in which we (almost) all would like to live.

I have mentioned the analogy with the ominous slide into a failed state; here is a less dire example of the importance of the belief environment, and the way small changes in society can engender unwanted changes in it. In many parts of rural America people feel comfortable leaving their cars and homes unlocked, day and night, but any country mouse who tries to live this way in the big city soon learns how foolish that amiably trusting policy is. City life is not intolerable, but it is certainly different. Wouldn't it be fine if we could somehow re-engineer the belief environment of cities so that people seldom felt the need to lock up! An all but impossible dream. At the same time, rural America is far from utopia and is sliding toward urbanity. The felicitous folkways of the countryside can absorb a modest amount of theft and trespass without collapse, but it wouldn't take much to extinguish them forever. Those of us who get to live in this blissfully secure world cherish it, for good reason, and would hate to abandon it, but we also must recognize that any day could be the last day of unlocked doors in our neighborhood, and once the change happened, it would be very hard to change back. That too is like global climate change; these changes are apt to be irreversible. And unlike global climate change, drawing attention to the prospect may actually hasten it, by kindling and spreading what Douglas Hofstadter once called "reverberant doubt."[4] The day that our local newspaper begins running a series about what percentage of local people lock their doors under what circumstances is the day that door-locking is apt to become the norm. So those who are in favor of diverting attention from too exhaustive an examination

---

to produce a thinking thing—just not an *immaterial* thinking thing, as Descartes imagined and tradition has tended to suppose.

of these delicate topics might have the right idea. This is the chief reason, I think, for the taboo against thinking about sacred values: it can sometimes jeopardize their protected status. But in this case, I think it is already too late to follow the tip-toe approach. There is already a tidal wave of interest in the ways in which the life sciences are illuminating the nature of "the soul," so we had better shift from distraction to concentration and see what we can make of the belief environment for human dignity and its vulnerabilities.

## The Solution

How are we to protect the ideal of human dignity from the various incursions of science and technology? The first step in the solution is to notice that the *grounds* for our practices regarding this are not going to be *local* features of particular human lives, but rather more *distributed* in space and time. There is already a clear precedent in our attitude toward human corpses. Even people who believe in immortal immaterial souls don't believe that human "remains" harbor a soul. They think that the soul has departed, and what is left behind is just a body, just unfeeling matter. A corpse can't feel pain, can't suffer, can't be aware of any indignities—and yet still we feel a powerful obligation to handle a corpse with respect, and even with ceremony, and even when nobody else is watching. Why? Because we appreciate, whether acutely or dimly, that how we handle *this* corpse *now* has repercussions for how other people, still alive, will be able to imagine their own demise and its aftermath. Our capacity to imagine the future is both the source of our moral power and a condition of our vulnerability. We cannot help but see all the events in our lives against the backdrop of what Hofstadter calls the *implicosphere* of readily imaginable alternatives—and the great amplifier of human suffering (and human joy) is our irresistible tendency to anticipate, with dread or delight, what is in store for us.[5]

We live not just in the moment, but in the past and the future as well. Consider the well-known advice given to golfers: *keep your head down* through the whole swing. "Wait a minute," comes the objection: "that's got to be voodoo superstition! Once the ball leaves the club head, the position of my head couldn't possibly affect the trajectory of the ball. This has to be scientifically unsound advice!" Not at all. Since we plan and execute all our actions in an anticipatory belief environment, and have only limited and indirect control over our time-pressured skeletal actions, it can well be the case that the only way to get the part of the golf swing that *does* affect the trajectory of the ball to have the desirable properties is to concentrate on making the later part of it, which indeed could not affect the trajectory, take on a certain shape. Far from being superstitious, the advice can be seen to follow quite logically from facts we can discover from a careful analysis of the way our nervous systems guide our muscles.

Our respect for corpses provides us with a clear case of a wise practice that does not at all depend on finding, locally, a special (even supernatural) ingredient that justifies or demands this treatment. There are other examples that have the same feature. Nobody has to endorse magical thinking about the gold in Fort Knox to recognize the effect of its (believed-in) presence there on the stability of currencies. Symbols play an important role in helping to maintain social equilibria, and we tamper with them at our peril. If we began to adopt the "efficient" policy of disposing of human corpses by putting them in large biodegradable plastic bags to be taken to the landfill along with the rest of the "garbage," this would flavor our imaginations in ways that would be hard to ignore, and hard to tolerate. No doubt we could get used to it, the same way city folk get used to locking their doors, but we have good reasons for avoiding that path. (Medical schools have learned to be diligent in their maintenance of respect and decorum in the handling of bodies in their teaching and research, for while those who decide to donate their bodies to medicine presumably have come to terms with the imagined prospect of students dissecting and discussing their innards, they have limits on what they find tolerable.)

The same policy and rationale apply to end-of-life decisions. We handle a corpse with decorum even though we *know* it cannot suffer, so we can appreciate the wisdom of extending the same practice to cases where we don't know. For instance, a person in a persistent vegetative state might be suffering, or might not, but in either case, we have plenty of grounds for adopting a policy that creates a comforting buffer zone that errs on the side of concern. And, once again, the long-range effect on community beliefs is just as important as, or even more important than, any locally measurable symptoms of suffering. (In a similar spirit, it is important that wolves and grizzly bears still survive in the wilder regions of our world even if we almost never see them. Just knowing that they are there is a source of wonder and delight and makes the world a better place. Given our invincible curiosity and penchant for skepticism, we have to keep checking up on their continued existence, of course, and could not countenance an official myth of their continued presence if they had in fact gone extinct. This too has its implications for our topic.)

What happens when we apply the same principle to the other boundary of human life, its inception? The scientific fact is that there is no good candidate, and there will almost certainly never be a good candidate, for a moment of *ensoulment*, when a mere bundle of living human tissue becomes a person with all the rights and privileges pertaining thereunto. This should not be seen as a sign of the weakness of scientific insight, but rather as a familiar implication of what science has already discovered. One of the fascinating facts about living things is the way they thrive on gradualism. Consider speciation: there are uncounted millions of different species, and each of them had its inception "at some point" in the nearly four billion year history of life on this planet, but there is literally no telling *exactly* when any species came into existence because what counts as speciation is something that only gradually and cumulatively emerges over very many generations. Speciation can emerge only *in the aftermath*. Consider dogs, the millions of members of hundreds of varieties of *Canis familiaris* that populate the world today. As different as these varieties are—think of St. Bernards and Pekinese—they all count as a single species, cross-fertile (with a little mechanical help from their human caretakers) and all readily identifiable as belonging to the same species, descended from wolves, by their highly similar DNA. Might one or more of these varieties or subspecies become a species of its own some day? Absolutely. In fact, every puppy born is a potential founder of a new species, but nothing about that puppy on the day of its birth (or for that matter on any day of its life) could be singled out as the special feature that marked it as the Adam or Eve of a new species. If it dies without issue, it definitely won't found a new species, but as long as it has offspring that have offspring…it might turn out, in the fullness of time, to be a good candidate for the first member of a new species.

Or consider our own species, *Homo sapiens*. Might it divide in two some day? Yes it might, and in fact, it might, in a certain sense, already have happened. Consider two human groups alive today that probably haven't had any common ancestors in the last thirty thousand years: the Inuit of Cornwallis Island in the Arctic, and the Andaman Islanders living in remarkable isolation in the Indian Ocean. Suppose some global plague sweeps the planet sometime in the next hundred years (far from an impossibility, sad to say), leaving behind only these two small populations. Suppose that over the next five hundred or a thousand years, say, they flourish and come to reinhabit the parts of the world vacated by us—and discover that they are not cross-fertile with the other group! Two species, remarkably similar in appearance, physiology and ancestry, but nevertheless as reproductively isolated as lions are from tigers. When, then, did the speciation occur? Before the dawn of agriculture about ten thousand years ago, or after the birth of the Internet? There would be no principled way of saying. We can presume that today, Inuits and Andaman Islanders are cross-fertile, but who knows? The difference between "in principle" reproductive isolation (because of the accumulation of genetic and behavioral differences that make offspring "impossible") and *de facto* reproductive isolation, which has already been the case for many thousands of years, is not itself a principled distinction.

A less striking instance of the same phenomenon of gradualism is *coming of age*, in the sense of being mature enough and well enough informed to be suitable for marriage, or—to take a particularly clear case—to drive a car. It will come as no surprise, I take it, that there is no special moment of *driver-edment,* when a teenager crisply crossed the boundary between being too immature to have the right to apply for a driver's license, and being adult enough to be allowed the freedom of the highway behind the wheel. Some youngsters are manifestly mature enough at fourteen to be reasonable candidates for a driver's license, and others are still so heedless and impulsive at eighteen that one trembles at the prospect of letting them on the road. We have settled (in most jurisdictions) on the policy that age sixteen is a suitable threshold, and what this means is that we simply refuse to consider special pleading on behalf of unusually mature younger people, and also refrain from imposing extra hurdles on those sixteen-year-olds who manage to pass their driving test fair and square in spite of our misgivings about the safety of letting them on the road. In short, we settle on a conventional threshold which we *know* does not mark any special internal mark (brain myelination, IQ, factual knowledge, onset of puberty) but strikes us as a good-enough compromise between freedom and public safety. *And once we settle on it, we stop treating the location of the threshold as a suitable subject for debate.* There are many important controversies to consider and explore, and this isn't one of them. Not as a general rule. Surprising new discoveries may in principle trigger a reconsideration at any time, but we foster a sort of inertia that puts boundary disputes out of bounds for the time being.

Why isn't there constant pressure from fifteen-year-olds to lower the legal driving age? It is not just that they tend not to be a particularly well-organized or articulate constituency. Even they can recognize that soon enough they will be sixteen, and there are better ways to spend their energy than trying to adjust a policy that is, all things considered, quite reasonable. Moreover, there are useful features of the social dynamics that make it systematically difficult for them to mount a campaign for changing the age. We adults have created a tacit scaffolding of presumption, *holding* teenagers responsible before many of them have actually achieved the requisite competence, thereby encouraging them to try to grow into the status we purport to grant them and discouraging any behavior—any action that could be interpreted as throwing a tantrum, for instance—that would undercut their claim to maturity. They are caught in a bind: the more vehemently they protest, the more they cast doubt on the wisdom of their cause. In the vast array of projects that confront them, this is not an appealing choice.

The minimum driving age is not quite a *sacred* value, then, but it shares with sacred values the interesting feature of being considered best left unexamined, by common consensus among a sizable portion of the community. And there is a readily accessible reason for this inertia. We human beings lead lives that cast long beams of anticipation into the foggy future, and we appreciate—implicitly or explicitly—almost any fixed points that can reduce our uncertainty. Sometimes this is so obvious as to be trivial. Why save money for your children's education if money may not be worth anything in the future? How could you justify going to all the trouble of building a house if you couldn't count on the presumption that you will be able to occupy it without challenge? Law and order are preconditions for the sorts of ambitious life-planning we want to engage in. But we want more than just a strong state apparatus that can be counted on not to be vacillating in its legislation, or whimsical in enforcement. We, as a society, do need to draw some lines—"bright" lines in legalistic jargon—and stick with them. That means not just promulgating them and voting on them, but putting an unequal burden on any second-guessing, so that people can organize their life projects with the reasonable expectation that these are fixed points that aren't going to shift constantly under the pressure of one faction or another. We want there to be an ambient attitude of *mutual* recognition of the stability of the moral—not legal—presumptions that can be taken for granted, something approximating a meta-consensus among those who achieve the initial consensus about the threshold: let's leave well enough alone now that we've fixed it. In a world where every candidate for a bright line of morality is constantly under siege from partisans who would like to change it, one's confidence is shaken that one's everyday conduct is going to be above reproach. Consider that nowadays, in many parts of the world, women simply cannot wear fur coats in public with the attitudes their mothers could adopt. Today, wearing a fur coat is making a political statement, and one cannot escape that by simply disavowing the intent. Driving a gas-guzzling SUV carries a similar burden. People may resent the activities of the partisans who have achieved these shifts in opinion even though they may share many of their attitudes about animal rights or energy policy; they have made investments—in all innocence, let us suppose—that now are being disvalued. Had they been able to anticipate this shift in public opinion, they could have spent their money better.

These observations are not contentious, I think. How, though, can we apply this familiar understanding to the vexing issues surrounding the inception—and manipulation and termination—of human life, and the special status it is supposed to enjoy? By recognizing, first, that we are going to have to walk away from the *traditional* means of securing these boundaries, which are not going to keep on working. They are just too brittle for the 21st century.

We know too much. Unlike traditional sacred values that depend on widespread acceptance of myths (which, even if true, are manifestly unjustifiable—that's why we call them myths rather than common knowledge), we need to foster values that can withstand scrutiny about their own creation. That is to say, we have to become self-conscious about our reliance on such policies, without in the process destroying our faith in them.

## Belief in Belief

We need to appreciate the importance in general of the phenomenon of *belief in belief*.[6] Consider a few cases that are potent today. Because many of us believe in democracy and recognize that the security of democracy in the future depends critically on *maintaining the belief* in democracy, we are eager to quote (and quote and quote) Winston Churchill's famous line: "Democracy is the worst form of government except for all the others that have been tried." As stewards of democracy, we are often conflicted, eager to point to flaws that ought to be repaired, while just as eager to reassure people that the flaws are not that bad, that democracy can police itself, so their faith in it is not misplaced.

The same point can be made about science. Since the belief in the integrity of scientific procedures is almost as important as the actual integrity, there is always a tension between a whistle-blower and the authorities, even when they know that they have mistakenly conferred scientific respectability on a fraudulently obtained result. Should they quietly reject the offending work and discreetly dismiss the perpetrator, or make a big stink?*

And certainly some of the intense public fascination with celebrity trials is to be explained by the fact that belief in the rule of law is

---

* As Richard Lewontin recently observed, "To survive, science must expose dishonesty, but every such public exposure produces cynicism about the purity and disinterestedness of the institution and provides fuel for ideological anti-rationalism. The revelation that the paradoxical Piltdown Man fossil skull was, in fact, a hoax was a great relief to perplexed paleontologists but a cause for great exultation in Texas tabernacles." See his "Dishonesty in Science," *New York Review of Books*, November 18, 2004, pp. 38-40.

considered to be a vital ingredient in our society, so if famous people are seen to be above the law, this jeopardizes the general trust in the rule of law. Hence we are not just interested in the trial, but in the public reactions to the trial, and the reactions to those reactions, creating a spiraling inflation of media coverage. We who live in democracies have become somewhat obsessed with gauging public opinion on all manner of topics, and for good reason: in a democracy it really matters what the people believe. If the public cannot be mobilized into extended periods of outrage by reports of corruption, or of the torturing of prisoners by our agents, for instance, our democratic checks and balances are in jeopardy. In his hopeful book, *Development as Freedom* and elsewhere,[7] the Nobel laureate economist Amartya Sen makes the important point that you don't have to win an election to achieve your political aims. Even in shaky democracies, what the leaders believe about the beliefs that prevail in their countries influences what they take their realistic options to be, so belief-maintenance is an important political goal in its own right.

Even more important than political beliefs, in the eyes of many, are what we might call metaphysical beliefs. Nihilism—the belief in nothing—has been seen by many to be a deeply dangerous virus, for obvious reasons. When Friedrich Nietzsche hit upon his idea of the Eternal Recurrence—he thought he had proved that we relive our lives infinitely many times—his first inclination (according to some stories) was that he should kill himself without revealing the proof, in order to spare others from this life-destroying belief.[8] Belief in the *belief that something matters* is understandably strong and widespread. Belief in free will is another vigorously protected vision, for the same reasons, and those whose investigations seem to others to jeopardize it are sometimes deliberately misrepresented in order to discredit what is seen as a dangerous trend.[9] The physicist Paul Davies has recently defended the view that belief in free will is so important that it may be "a fiction worth maintaining."[10] It is interesting that he doesn't seem to think that his own discovery of the awful truth (what he takes to be the awful truth) incapacitates him morally, but that others, more fragile than he, will need to be protected from it.

This illustrates the ever-present risk of paternalism when belief in belief encounters a threat: we must keep these facts from "the children," who cannot be expected to deal with them safely. And so people often become systematically disingenuous when defending a value. Being the unwitting or uncaring bearer of good news or bad news is one thing; being the self-appointed champion of an idea is something quite different. Once people start committing themselves (in public, or just in their "hearts") to particular ideas, a strange dynamic process is brought into being, in which the original commitment gets buried in pearly layers of defensive reaction and meta-reaction. "Personal rules are a *recursive* mechanism; they continually take their own pulse, and if they feel it falter, that very fact will cause further faltering," the psychiatrist George Ainslie observes in his remarkable book, *Breakdown of Will*.[11] He describes the dynamic of these processes in terms of competing strategic commitments that can contest for control in an organization—or an individual. Once you start living by a set of explicit rules, the stakes are raised: when you lapse, what should you do? Punish yourself? Forgive yourself? Pretend you didn't notice?

> After a lapse, the long-range interest is in the awkward position of a country that has threatened to go to war in a particular circumstance that has then occurred. The country wants to avoid war without destroying the credibility of its threat and may therefore look for ways to be seen as not having detected the circumstance. Your long-range interest will suffer if you catch yourself ignoring a lapse, but perhaps not if you can arrange to ignore it without catching yourself. This arrangement, too, must go undetected, which means that a successful process of ignoring must be among the many mental expedients that arise by trial and error—the ones you keep simply because they make you feel better without your realizing why.[12]

This idea that there are myths we live by, myths that must not be disturbed at any cost, is always in conflict with our ideal of truth-seeking and truth-telling, sometimes with lamentable results. For example, racism is at long last widely recognized as a great social evil, so many reflective people have come to endorse the second-order belief that *belief in the equality of all people regardless of their race* is to be vigorously fostered. How vigorously? Here people of good will differ sharply. Some believe that belief in racial differences is so pernicious that *even when it is true* it is to be squelched. This has led to some truly unfortunate excesses. For instance, there are clear clinical data about how people of different ethnicity are differently susceptible to disease, or respond differently to various drugs, but such data are considered off-limits by some researchers, and by some funders of research. This has the perverse effect that strongly indicated avenues of research are deliberately avoided, much to the detriment of the health of the ethnic groups involved.*

Ainslie uncovers strategic belief-maintenance in a wide variety of cherished human practices:

> Activities that are spoiled by counting them, or counting on them, have to be undertaken through indirection if they are to stay valuable. For instance, romance undertaken for sex or even "to be loved" is thought of as crass, as are some of the most lucrative professions if undertaken for money, or performance art if done for effect. Too great an awareness of the motivational contingencies for sex, affection, money, or applause spoils the effort, and not only because it undeceives the other people involved. Beliefs about the intrinsic worth of these activities are valued beyond whatever accuracy these beliefs might have, because they promote the needed indirection.[13]

So what sort of equilibrium can we reach? If we want to maintain the momentousness of all decisions about life and death, and take the steps that elevate the decision beyond the practicalities of the moment, we need to secure the appreciation of this very fact and enliven the imaginations of people so that they can recognize, and avoid wherever possible, and condemn, activities that would tend to erode the public trust in the presuppositions about what is—and

---

* There are significant differences in breast cancer, hypertension and diabetes, alcohol tolerance, and many other well-studied conditions. See Christopher Li, et al., "Differences in Breast Cancer Stage, Treatment, and Survival by Race and Ethnicity," *Archives of Internal Medicine* 163 (2003): 49-56; for an overview, see Health Sciences Policy Board (HSP) 2003, *Unequal Treatment: Confronting Racial and Ethnic Disparities in Health Care.*

should be—unthinkable. A striking instance of failure to appreciate this is the proposal by President Bush to reconsider and unilaterally refine the Geneva Convention's deliberately vague characterization of torture as "outrages on personal dignity." By declaring that the United States is eager to be a pioneer in the adjustment of what has heretofore been mutually agreed to be unthinkable, this policy is deeply subversive of international trust, and of national integrity. We as a nation can no longer be plausibly viewed as *above* thinking of arguable exceptions to the sacred value of not torturing people, and this diminishes us in ways that will be difficult if not impossible to repair.

What forces can we hope to direct in our desire to preserve respect for human dignity? Laws *prohibit*; traditions *encourage* and *discourage*, and in the long run, laws are powerless to hold the line unless they are supported by a tradition, by the mutual recognition of most of the people that they preserve conditions that deserve preservation. Global opinion, as we have just seen, cannot be counted on to discourage all acts of degradation of the belief environment, but it can be enhanced by more local traditions. Doctors, for instance, have their proprietary code of ethics, and most of them rightly covet the continuing respect of their colleagues, a motivation intensified by the system of legal liability and by the insurance that has become a prerequisite for practice. Then there are strict liability laws, which target particularly sensitive occupations such as pharmacist and doctor, preemptively removing the excuse of ignorance and thereby putting all who occupy these positions on notice that they will be held accountable whether or not they have what otherwise would be a reasonable claim of innocent ignorance. So forewarned, they adjust their standards and projects accordingly, erring on the side of extreme caution and keeping a healthy distance between themselves and legal consequences. Anyone who attempts to erect such a network of flexible and mutually supporting discouragements of further tampering with traditional ideas about human dignity will fail unless they attend to the carrot as well as the stick. How can we kindle and preserve a sincere *allegiance* to the ideals of human dignity? The same way we foster the love of a democratic and free society: by ensuring that the lives one can live in such a regime are so manifestly better than the available alternatives.

And what of those who are frankly impatient with tradition, and even with the values that tradition endorses? We must recognize that there are a vocal minority of people who profess unworried acceptance of an entirely practical and matter-of-fact approach to life, who scoff at romantic concerns with Frankensteinian visions. Given the presence and articulateness of these proponents, we do well to have a home base that can withstand scrutiny and that is prepared to defend, in terms other than nostalgia, the particular values that we are trying to protect. That is the germ of truth in multiculturalism. We need to articulate these values in open forum. When we attempt this, we need to resist the strong temptation to resort to the old myths, since they are increasingly incredible, and will only foster incredulity and cynicism in those we need to persuade. Tantrums in support of traditional myths will backfire, in other words. Our only chance of preserving a respectable remnant of the tradition is to ensure that the values we defend *deserve* the respect of all.*

---

* Thanks to Gary Wolf, Tori McGeer and Philip Pettit for asking questions that crystallized my thinking on these topics.

## Notes

[1] See Philip Tetlock, "Coping with Trade-offs: Psychological Constraints and Political Implications," in *Political Reasoning and Choice*, ed. Arthur Lupia, Matthew D. McCubbins and Samuel L. Popkin (Berkeley, California: University of California Press, 1999); "Thinking the unthinkable: sacred values and taboo cognitions," *Trends in Cognitive Science* 7 (2003): 320-324; and Philip Tetlock, A. Peter McGraw, and Orie V. Kristel, "Proscribed Forms of Social Cognition: Taboo Trade-Offs, Forbidden Base Rates, and Heretical Counterfactuals," in *Relational Models Theory: A Contemporary Overview*, ed. Nick Haslam (Mahway, New Jersey: Erlbaum, 2004), pp. 247-262, the latter also available online as Philip E. Tetlock, Orie V. Kristel, S. Beth Elson, Melanie C. Green, and Jennifer Lerner, "The Psychology of the Unthinkable: Taboo Trade-Offs, Forbidden Base Rates, and Heretical Counterfactuals," at http://faculty.haas.berkeley.edu/tetlock/docs/thepsy-1.doc.
[2] Tetlock, et al., op. cit., p. 6 of online version.
[3] Material in the previous two paragraphs is drawn from my *Breaking the Spell: Religion as a Natural Phenomenon* (New York: Viking Penguin, 2006), pp. 22-23.
[4] Douglas Hofstadter, "Dilemmas for Superrational Thinkers, Leading up to a Luring Lottery," *Scientific American*, June, 1983, reprinted with a discussion of reverberant doubt in *Metamagical Themas* (New York: Basic Books, 1985), pp. 752-755.
[5] Douglas Hofstadter, "Metafont, Metamathematics and Metaphysics," in *Visible Language*, August, 1982, reprinted with comments in Hofstadter, *Metamagical Themas*, pp. 290, 595.
[6] What follows is drawn, with revisions, from my *Breaking the Spell*, chapter 8.
[7] Amartya Sen, *Development as Freedom* (New York: Knopf, 1999); see also his "Democracy and Its Global Roots," *New Republic*, October 6, 2003, pp. 28-35.
[8] For a discussion of Nietzsche and his philosophical response to Darwin's theory of evolution by natural selection, see my *Darwin's Dangerous Idea: Evolution and the Meanings of Life* (New York: Simon & Schuster, 1995).
[9] Daniel C. Dennett, *Freedom Evolves* (New York: Viking Penguin, 2003).
[10] Paul Davies, "Undermining Free Will," *Foreign Policy*, September/October, 2004.
[11] George Ainslie, *Breakdown of Will* (Cambridge: Cambridge University Press, 2001), p. 88.
[12] Ibid., p. 150.
[13] George Ainslie, précis of *Breakdown of Will*, in *Behavioral and Brain Sciences* 28 (2005): 635-650, p. 649.

# 4

# Human Dignity and the Mystery of the Human Soul

## Robert P. Kraynak

Biotechnology and the life sciences have astonished the world in recent years, but they have also disoriented people by raising a whole new set of ethical issues. In response, a new branch of moral philosophy has emerged—bioethics—whose task is to grapple with the ethical challenges of cloning, stem cell research, genetic engineering, *in vitro* fertilization, drug therapy, new techniques for arresting the aging process, and aspirations to conquer death itself. While the policy debates about these issues are complex, they usually revolve around a few moral principles that might be summed up in three terms—utility, the advancement of knowledge, and human dignity.

The first term, utility, is broadly understood to mean promoting the greatest happiness of mankind by relieving human suffering and improving the human condition. This is often the first principle people cite when they argue that advances in biotechnology are needed in order to cure genetic diseases or to help infertile couples have children. The second principle, the advancement of knowledge, is usually combined with the first under the rubric of "progress": the biotechnical revolution is part of the inevitable development of modern science which not only has practical benefits but also intrinsic value in advancing our understanding of the universe and man

While these two principles are cited to expand research, a third principle is often raised to slow down or prohibit scientific experimentation on the grounds that it "violates human dignity." This expression refers to the powerful moral intuition that certain practices are wrong because they treat people as sub-humans or even as non-humans, for example, when human beings are treated like "guinea pigs" for experimentation without proper consent, or when human beings are used as disposable objects for research and destruction.

While all three moral principles are important for bioethics, this paper will focus on human dignity—the definition and grounding of human dignity as well as the practical question of whether it provides a workable guideline for decisions about biotechnology. The position I will take is that human dignity is a viable moral concept for bioethics, but one that needs clarification. To clarify the concept, I will compare three models of man—the model of scientific materialism, according to which man is a complex machine; the model of classical philosophy which views man as a rational soul united to a body; and the Biblical view of man as a creature made in the image of God. My argument is that human dignity implies a special moral status for human beings and that this special status ultimately requires a belief in the human soul. Scientific materialism denies the soul and thereby undermines human dignity, but most materialists find they cannot do without the soul and restore it by various strategies. Classical philosophy is more sensible in claiming that human beings have rational souls united to physical bodies, but the theoretical underpinnings of this doctrine are highly speculative. Surprisingly, the Bible and Christian theology may make the strongest case for human dignity because they recognize that human dignity is a mystery: the special status of man cannot be reduced to any set of essential attributes but rests on the mysterious "election" of man as the only creature in the universe made in the image of God. I will conclude by showing why human dignity, grounded in the mystery of the soul, should make scientists think twice about experiments aimed primarily at advancing earthly happiness and scientific knowledge.

## Scientific Materialism: Man as Complex Machine and as Master of the Machine

When we speak about "human dignity" or "the dignity of man," we usually mean the special moral status of human beings in the natural universe as well as the respect due to individual humans because of their essential humanity.[1] The central point of human dignity is that membership in the human species is somehow special and therefore a matter of moral significance that includes duties and rights which most cultures recognize and which reason can justify as objectively good. Interestingly, the most common objection to respecting human dignity is not moral relativism but the alleged "truth" of scientific materialism that man is a complex machine without soul or special moral status and we should simply "get over it" for our own good. The argument I will make is that most scientific materialists ultimately find this view untenable and restore the soul in some fashion to account for morality and their own scientific activities.

This pattern can be seen in the philosophy of Thomas Hobbes, one of the original spokesmen for scientific materialism.[2] Hobbes argued that the universe is nothing more than "bodies in motion" and that everything happens by one body touching another body without action-at-a-distance by immaterial causes, such as the spirits and ghosts of popular religion or the intangible substances of medieval Scholasticism or the forms and essences of Aristotle. Following the logic of materialism, Hobbes sought to explain all of man's behavior by a stimulus-response model of "appetites and aversions" in which the senses receive motions from external bodies, the signals are passed to the heart and brain, an image is formed that triggers a response, and the body moves accordingly. In this view, the mind is just a processor of sense images, and complex human emotions are reduced to selfish passions—especially the irrational desire for power and the rational fear of death. Hobbes denied that human beings have souls and said the will is not free to choose but is merely "the last appetite in deliberation." He even used the metaphor of an "engine" driven by springs and wheels to describe man at the beginning of *Leviathan* in order to emphasize his mechanical conception of human behavior.

In addition, Hobbes explicitly rejected Descartes's view that the universe is made of two distinct substances, material bodies immaterial minds. Hobbes was a strict materialist in asserting that thinking or consciousness is simply a motion in the brain and that language is a motion of the tongue (he denied, in other words, that mental states of inner awareness existed in addition to brain waves). He opposed the dualism of matter and mind as both unnecessary and as politically dangerous insofar as it led to beliefs in souls and spirits that could be exploited by religious leaders for rebellion against political authority. Hobbes also denied the essential difference of humans and animals and therefore rejected any notion of human dignity based on a hierarchy of beings in the universe as a dangerous illusion that led to vainglorious claims of superiority and wars of religion. He asserted that all human beings are equal in their vulnerability to being killed and that mankind would be better off if everyone accepted their status as mortal machines without inherent dignity. For Hobbes, this was the whole truth about man—the low but solid ground on which to build an enlightened, secular civilization that could avoid the anarchy of the state of nature and establish lasting civil peace.

Despite his determined effort to be a thorough-going materialist, Hobbes seemed to admit that the human mind could not simply fit the model of a machine. He recognized that the activity of science itself, especially political science, stood outside the determinism of nature because the mind could construct an artificial world of speech based on free choices of the will in defining words—the very words needed for the social contracts of politics and the method of exact science. As Hobbes claimed, "we know only what we make," by which he meant that the mind could construct systems of knowledge outside the world of mechanical causality, and that these logical constructs were the only certain knowledge. Hobbes therefore contradicted himself by assuming something like an immaterial mind or soul which distinguished human beings from animals and enabled them to overcome nature. In the last analysis, then, Hobbes acknowledged that the whole truth about man included body and soul.

It would be an oversimplification to say that all scientific materialists have been Hobbesians, but Hobbes provided the model of mechanical man for later materialists to refine and develop. His daring conception became a prototype for behavioral psychology and its offshoots—for the physical-chemical model of mental and emotional states as well as for robotics and artificial intelligence. Indeed, if we jump ahead a few centuries, we can see that B. F. Skinner's "behaviorism" is a development of Hobbes's scientific materialism and suffers from many of the same problems.

Like Hobbes, Skinner is critical of those who bemoan the loss of man's lofty place in the universe and worry about the human soul. In *Beyond Freedom and Dignity* (1972), he responds to C. S. Lewis's fears about "the abolition of man" by saying that the only thing "being abolished is autonomous man—the inner man...defended by the literatures of freedom and dignity; his abolition is long overdue."[3] Commenting as well on fears that he lowers humans to the level of animals, Skinner says: "'animal' is a pejorative term only because 'man' has been made spuriously honorific...whereas the traditional view supports Hamlet's exclamation, 'How like a god!' Pavlov, the behavioral scientist, emphasized, 'How like a dog!' But that was a step forward."[4] Of course, Skinner adds, "man is much more than a dog, but like a dog he is within range of scientific analysis." In his campaign to deflate human dignity, Skinner cites as progress the impact of Copernicus, Darwin, and Freud in diminishing the special status of humanity. But why is this progress?

Like Hobbes, Skinner favors scientific materialism because it gives a realistic, naturalistic view of man and is more conducive to the survival and material welfare of the human species than earlier conceptions. Skinner develops Hobbes, however, by adding the theory of "behavior modification" through the reinforcement of values in a controlled environment like his notorious "Skinner box"—an invention influenced by Rousseau's ideas about highly controlled social environments and Darwin's ideas about evolutionary change in response to natural environments.* While recognizing the role of genetic inheritance, behavioral scientists like Skinner believe human nature is more malleable than Hobbes thought, and they consciously seek to modify man in new ways for the benefit of the human species.

The difficulty for Skinner is that the use of science to get outside of nature leads to a major contradiction in his scientific materialism:

---

* The Skinner box is an idea that Skinner may have developed from Rousseau's *Emile* (1762), a work that features the role of a tutor as the invisible manipulator of the child's environment; see Skinner, *Beyond Freedom and Dignity*, pp. 89, 124.

man is not only a complex machine but also the master of "the machine" who is free to modify "the machine" according to a new vision of man. The implication is that Skinner has his own version of freedom and dignity which presupposes an essential difference between humans and animals and which even exaggerates man's dignity by loosening all limits: man is now seen as the sovereign master of nature—the being who creates himself and invents his own moral law. While Skinner understands the term "good" as the survival of the species as well as pleasure and non-aggression, he also suggests that "good" and "bad" are malleable according to the conditioning of behavioral engineers. Thus, human dignity still resides in something unique to man, but that unique capacity is not the "inner agent" of the rational soul obeying a higher moral law. Rather, it lies in man's freedom to experiment on man for whatever purposes might be posited by the "conditioners" and "reinforcers."[5] It is remarkable to read in Skinner's work the wild oscillation between the exaggerated debasement of man (how like a dog!) which implies robotic behavior and the exaggerated glorification of man (how like the master of the universe!) which implies a "super-soul" capable of autonomous self-creation.

A similar pattern can be found in Daniel Dennett, who is famous for promoting modern science over religion by using the popular metaphor of "cranes" and "skyhooks": cranes are explanations that use scientific materialism, while skyhooks resort to miracles or non-material causes to explain things. In *Darwin's Dangerous Idea*, Dennett claims that the greatest "crane" of all is Darwinian evolution, which can be used to explain everything—the origins of the universe, the origins of life from non-life, the evolution of living species from prior species, and the evolution of man, including man's genetic makeup and cultural life (the "genes and memes" of humanity). Darwin's central idea, according to Dennett, is that the well-designed universe we inhabit actually arose from the opposite of design—from the mindless, purposeless, directionless forces of evolution, which provides "a scheme for creating Design out of Chaos without the aide of Mind."[6]

Darwin's scheme, of course, is natural selection, which Dennett explains in mathematical terms as an "algorithm"—a system for sorting out options using a simple mechanical rule repeated an indefinite number of times until a single option is left. Unlike other algorithms which sort by logic or merit, natural selection creates winners by allowing random variations to survive, a process which adds up to a pattern or design over a long period of time. Dennett's ambition is to apply the Darwinian algorithm to everything—e.g., our universe and its laws arose from a myriad of accidental tries with other combinations that did not survive.[7] This enables him to argue that the universe and man are accidental products of evolutionary forces, but they still have meaning and purpose once they are "frozen" in place. Thus, scientific materialism can be vindicated while avoiding moral relativism and affirming a culture based on modern liberalism, democracy, and respect for the dignity of persons.

If we look at Dennett's argument with critical distance, however, we can see that it follows the typical contradictory pattern of scientific materialism: it combines dogmatic materialism in describing a universe that is indifferent to man (it's all just "frozen accidents") with idealistic moral principles that presuppose the unique status of man and an ultimate purpose to human existence. Dennett is so insistent on man's special dignity that he even criticizes the sociobiologist E. O. Wilson and the behavioralist B. F. Skinner for mistakenly reducing human goals to those of other animals (survival, procreation, and pleasure/pain). Dennett repeatedly asserts that "we are not like other animals; our minds set us off from them";[8] and "what makes us special is that we, alone among species, can rise above the imperatives of our genes."[9] Dennett sees man aiming at higher purposes than passing on genes and dismisses the idea of "survival of the fittest" as an "odious misapplication of Darwinian thinking" by the Social Darwinist Herbert Spencer.[10] In contrast to Spencer, Dennett strongly condemns oppression, slavery, and child abuse as "beyond the pale of civilized life."[11] Yet, all of this is supposedly consistent with the accidental nature of the universe: "the world is sacred," even though "it just happened to happen" and human reason is just "a by-product of mindless purposeless forces."[12]

In response to Dennett, I would say that he has contradicted himself by reintroducing "skyhooks" in his understanding of man. He claims the universe has no purpose, but man still has a moral purpose—to be decent, humane, and just, and to pursue scientific knowledge. He assumes, in other words, that a ground exists for a higher moral law in the nature and dignity of man, even though there is nothing wrong, from a Darwinian perspective, with the strong dominating the weak or the "survival of the fittest." What is missing in Dennett is the humility to acknowledge that he assumes an essential difference between humans and animals based on something like a rational soul, even though he reduces man to accidental evolutionary forces. When the materialist conception makes morality impossible, he turns to notions of dignity that are unsupported by his cosmology and says, "there is a huge difference between our minds and the minds of other species, enough even to make a moral difference."[13] Thus, he implicitly embraces a dualism of substances (matter vs. mind or nature vs. freedom) that divides humanity into two orders of causality which cannot interact except by external mastery. This actually exaggerates human dignity by making man the master of the universe, possessing a "super-soul" with creative will and infinite worth. The narrowness of materialism and the incoherence of dualism should lead us to rethink the problem with greater intellectual humility.

## Classical Greek Philosophy: Man as an Embodied Rational Soul

Scientific materialism is untenable, I have argued, because it tries to banish the soul as a basis for human dignity but smuggles it back in by various strategies. Materialists also deny a hierarchy of being in the universe, but they finally admit that man is "higher" than other animals because of human reason and embrace a higher moral law directed to an objective human good. These contradictions should awaken an interest in classical Greek philosophy and its view that man is a living being with a rational soul united to a body who finds dignity in perfecting his reason—elevating man to the top of a natural hierarchy but not quite equal to the highest substance in the universe.

To understand this perspective, we might begin with the observation that much of classical philosophy is a kind of "glorified" common sense. Common sense tells us that human beings are neither a single substance like matter, nor two separate substances, but a combination of body and soul, which are not entirely distinct from each other because they interact on a regular basis. The body clearly exists as a substance because it differentiates one individual human being from another. But the body's shape is more than the sum of its parts because it moves together on its own power as an integral whole, requiring a form united with matter. This is the first meaning of "soul": the self-moving power of a body with form that functions as a unified whole.

In this sense, all animals are a union of body and soul because they move on their own power as integral wholes; and this is precisely Aristotle's point in his classic work, *On the Soul*.[14] His thesis is that "the soul is the first principle of animal life"—meaning, the soul is the cause of life in living beings. For Aristotle, life is a kind of mystery because living beings have bodies that move on their own and this implies the intangible power of "soul" (*anima* in Latin; *psyche* in Greek). The puzzle is that the soul is not the same as the body, yet it is also not separate from the body: "the soul does not exist without a body and yet is not itself a kind of body." Aristotle uses a variety of expressions to capture this relation: "the soul is the actuality of the body" and "the soul exists in a body" and "the product of the two is an ensouled thing." Aristotle's expressions are attempts to describe the unity of matter and form in a being whose body seems lifeless without an immaterial cause that gives it motion and function. In this view, the soul actualizes the potential of the body to do its proper work.

What surprises the reader of Aristotle is the claim that all living beings have "souls"—there are plant souls, animal souls, and human souls. While shocking at first, Aristotle's idea follows common sense in distinguishing living beings by three different capacities: (1) self-motion, (2) sense perception, and (3) thinking. All living things are distinguished from non-living things by the power of self-motion—either by growing (including feeding and reproducing) or by moving from place to place (local motion). Plants are self-moving in the sense of feeding, growing, and reproducing; hence, they have "plant souls." Animals have self-motion and sense perception, and even some capacity for desiring and wishing that seems to involve "imagination," if not intellectual activity. Hence, they have "animal souls." Human beings have "human souls" because their souls include all three powers—self-motion, sense perception, and thinking. Aristotle, of course, spends a lot of time trying to explain how the human soul thinks or uses the intellect. And he comes up with his puzzling lines that in sense perception "the soul receives the form [of the object] without the matter," like an imprint in wax; but in thinking, "the intellect becomes each thing"—that is, the mind somehow fuses with the object of knowledge. Hence, "the soul in a way is all existing things."

We do not have to clarify the meaning of these difficult lines in order to understand what Aristotle is saying about man and his dignity in the natural universe. It is a sophisticated version of common sense: the natural universe is divided into species or kinds that display an ordered hierarchy of being—with non-living beings at the bottom, followed in ascending order by living beings with souls, such as plants (beings with self-motion), animals (beings with self-motion and sense perception), and humans (beings with self-motion, sense perception, and abstract thinking). Man is therefore a rational animal at the top of a hierarchy of living beings, who possesses a lofty dignity but not the infinite worth of an absolutely unique being. As a living being, man shares characteristics with other animals while also being essentially different; he is neither a beast nor a god but an "embodied rational soul." Accordingly, Aristotle says in the *Nicomachean Ethics*, "Man is not the best thing in the universe," because the heavenly bodies are more perfect; they move in eternal circular motion which man can contemplate and admire but cannot emulate. In this reckoning, human dignity is comparative rather than absolute—man is a living reflection of the divine intelligence that orders the cosmos, but man is not the highest substance in the universe.

Overall, I would argue that Aristotle's view of man as an embodied rational soul makes more sense than either materialism or dualism. It puts man back together, so to speak, into a unified whole of body and soul, and it recognizes man's proper place in the natural hierarchy as a rational animal above the beasts but below the "gods" (understood loosely as the heavenly bodies and the eternal laws of the rational universe). The problem with classical philosophy is that, even though it is supported by common sense, it rests on theoretical premises that are highly speculative. To really establish it, two points must be demonstrated: (1) that the mind is more than the brain yet is somehow still in the brain, like a rational soul in a body; and (2) that the order of the universe is not an accident but a necessary rational order with intelligent beings at the top. I believe these two points can be plausibly defended using the insights of modern philosophers such as John Searle and Paul Davies, but they remain speculative and are at best probable truths.

John Searle supports Aristotle by showing that the mind's relation to the brain is like an embodied rational soul. In his recent book, *Mind*, he argues that the debates about mind and body have reached an impasse because "neither dualism nor materialism is acceptable, yet they are presented as the only possibilities." Materialism is inadequate because it dishonestly denies the real existence of conscious states by trying to reduce them to motions of the brain. Yet, consciousness is just as real as the physical particles of a table because all it claims to be is a mental state of inner awareness that is capable of causing bodily actions (e.g., when I tell my arm to go up, it goes up). Searle also rejects dualism because the mind is not a different substance from the brain and can be explained by neurological processes, a view he endorses under the label "biological naturalism."[15]

Searle's primary argument is that mental states arise from the neurons and synapses of the brain but operate on a different level. This is a distinction of "levels" not of substances, like the different states of molecules in a table which are in motion at the micro level while being "solid" at the macro level in their lattice structures. By analogy, the brain cells that fire across synapses at the physical-chemical level are the same cells that produce conscious states at the mental level—which means that conscious states are "features" of the brain (like the table's solidity) that are more than just motions of the brain. Despite this clever analogy, Searle has to admit that the precise causal relation of consciousness to neurological processes is "largely unknown"[16] and "we really do not know how free will exists in the brain."[17] If he were a bit more humble, Searle might also admit that calling the mind a "feature" of the brain is really what Aristotle meant by a rational soul united to a human body or an embodied rational soul.

We may still ask, however, why the rational soul confers a special moral status on man and is worthy of dignity and respect. It would deserve respect only if the natural universe exists as a rational order with intelligent beings at the top for some necessary reason—a view that can be derived from a remarkable essay by Paul Davies entitled,

"The Intelligibility of Nature."[18] Davies's thesis is that we live in a universe that is highly intelligible—indeed, it is written in a "cosmic code" with mathematical precision—and that such a universe could not have emerged by accident. Accidents are random processes, and they are not sufficient to explain the universe's evolution from its original simplicity to the highly organized and complex structures of today, including life and consciousness. Random processes are structurally arbitrary (why should a boundary be here or there?) and statistical odds weigh heavily against the chance creation of order in a finite amount of time: it assumes "an unreasonable ability for matter and energy to achieve complex organizational states." A more plausible inference is that the universe's features emerged by a different type of causality—"self-organizing complexity," meaning formal causes of some kind that organize matter and energy into ordered wholes, like galaxies, living cells, and human minds.

While "self-organizing complexity" hearkens back to Aristotle's formal causality, Davies finds it not in an eternal order of the universe but in the expanding and evolving universe of modern cosmology: "The universe began in an essentially featureless state, consisting of a uniform gas of elementary particles, or possibly even just expanding empty space; and the rich variety of physical forms and systems that we see in the universe today has emerged since the big bang as a result of a long and complicated sequence of self-organizing physical processes.... Consciousness should be viewed as an emergent product in a sequence of self-organizing processes that form part of a general advance of complexity occurring throughout the universe." Davies's bold conclusion is that "the emergence of mind is in some sense inevitable" and that it is unscientific to regard intelligent life as "either a miracle or a stupendously improbable accident"; for "the laws of nature encourage…the emergence of intelligent organisms with the ability to understand nature at the theoretical level." In other words, nature is directed toward intelligent life and even seems to aim at conscious understanding of itself as its natural end.

Davies is cautious enough to say that this does not necessarily imply the guiding hand of an intelligent God, but he does say "we may legitimately talk about 'cosmic purpose.'" He hedges a bit by referring to his view as "teleology without teleology" because the laws of nature, once given, operate with both determinism and openness—implying that "re-running the cosmic movie" would produce intelligent, rational beings in an intelligible universe but not necessarily the human species as we know it. Nevertheless, a universe evolving toward a hierarchy of being with rational beings at the top is a necessary and inevitable development of nature's self-organizing complexity. It even leads to the prediction "that life and consciousness should be widespread in the universe, and not restricted to Earth." Indeed, Davies argues in *Are We Alone?* that intelligent life should exist in other realms of the universe and its discovery would vindicate "the dignity of man" as a rational creature.[19] It would refute the false model of an indifferent universe driven by blind mechanical causes by showing how favorable the universe really is to intelligent beings.

## The Bible and Christian Faith: Man as a Rational Creature Made in the Image of God

While the classical theory of human dignity is more plausible than materialism or dualism, it is not entirely satisfying either. It accords with common sense in viewing humans as rational animals that are higher than plants and other animals, but it rests on theoretical premises that are speculative (such as the causal relation of the mind to the brain and self-organizing complexity). One could reply that reason cannot do any better than use elements of classical philosophy and modern science to give a plausible account of man's dignity as an embodied rational soul at the top of a natural hierarchy. Yet reason could do better if it acknowledged that most of these things are genuine mysteries—questions that will never be fully answered by reason or science, such as how and why the universe began (creation), why reason is such an integral feature of the universe (rational order), how the mind or rational soul can be united to a physical body (the unity of soul and body), whether the soul can be separated from the body after death (the immortality of the soul), and what ultimate purpose reason is meant to serve (the final end). When such mysteries are acknowledged, reason's limits are exposed; and the mind may be opened to faith in revealed truths, such as those of the Bible and Christian faith.

The principal claim of the Bible and Christian faith is that the universe was created by a miracle of an all-powerful God whose will is mysterious but benevolent. Although the beginning of the universe is shrouded in mystery, the Bible indicates that God gave the universe a certain rational order: it is divided into heavens and earth, and the earth is filled with plants and animals that reproduce "after their kinds" like biological species, and the creation is an ordered hierarchy with a special status for human beings as the only creatures made in the image and likeness of God. The claim that humans are made in the image of God—the *Imago Dei*—is the Biblical and Christian charter of human dignity which gives them an exalted rank above the plants and animals but a little lower than the angels or God. One of the challenges of the Bible is to figure out what constitutes the divine image in man: is it reason, language, free will, a physical trait (such as upright posture), immortality, capacities for love, holiness, and justice? For Christian theologians like St. Augustine, who was influenced by Plato and classical philosophy, it seemed obvious that the divine image in man referred to reason. Hence, Augustine wrote in his commentaries on *Genesis* that "it is especially by reason of the mind that we are to understand that man was made in the image and likeness of God"; even the erect form of the body testifies to this view, since it enables man to look up and contemplate the heavens.[20]

Yet, if one actually examines the Bible, one is struck by how difficult it is to make such inferences. There are only a few references to the *Imago Dei* in both the Old and New Testaments, and they are ambiguous about what precisely constitutes the divine image in man, from which I draw the conclusion that the Bible avoids equating human dignity with any particular traits in order to teach people that it is not a set of attributes that confers human dignity. Rather, human dignity and the duties implied by it (such as the command to "love one another") are ultimately grounded in God's mysterious love for man above all the creatures of the universe, giving every human being an inherent dignity independent of their physical and mental traits. In short, the Bible grounds human dignity in God's "mysterious election" rather than in essential attributes. This broadens the meaning of humanity and extends the concept of the soul beyond rational consciousness to include the mysterious divine image, while still acknowledging reason as a secondary feature of humanity that permits natural and social hierarchies according to the perfections of reason in certain areas of life.

To clarify this point, I will examine briefly some passages referring to the *Imago Dei*, starting with the most famous passage in *Genesis*: "Then God said, 'Let us make man in our image, after our likeness; and let them have dominion over the fish of the sea, and over the birds of the air, and over the cattle, and over all the earth....' So God created man in his own image, in the image of God he created him, male and female he created them" (*Genesis* 1:26-27). A second passage draws a parallel between God and Adam: "When God created man, he made him in the likeness of God. Male and female he created them, and he blessed them and named them man (*adam*).... When Adam had lived a hundred and thirty years, he became the father of a son in his own likeness, after his image, and named him Seth" (*Genesis* 5:1-3). A third passage occurs in the story of the Flood when God blesses Noah's family: "Be fruitful and multiply, and fill the earth. The fear and the dread of you shall be upon every beast of the earth.... For your lifeblood I will surely require a reckoning.... Whoever sheds the blood of man, by man shall his blood be shed; for God made man in his own image" (*Genesis* 9:5-7).

These are the only references in *Genesis* (and in the entire Hebrew Bible) to the *Imago Dei*. They show that God created the natural world as a hierarchy with the human species at the top, possessing a special right of dominion over the lower species. In the first grant of dominion, man is commanded to subdue the birds, fish, and cattle, but his food is restricted to plants (*Genesis* 1:29-30). When Adam and Eve are created in the Garden, they are further restricted by the prohibition not to eat of the tree of the knowledge of good and evil, lest they shall die. After they disobey, whatever dignity they previously possessed is henceforth combined with depravity and mortality; but their dignity is not entirely lost. In fact, in the story of Noah, the grant of dominion is renewed and the image of God reaffirmed. According to the second grant, the primitive vegetarianism is expanded to include animal flesh as food; but the blood must be drained (*Genesis* 9:4). In addition, man is elevated by the respect that must be shown to human life. This almost resembles a right to life, except that it includes the death penalty for taking a life, which seems to imply, as the scholar Umberto Cassuto notes, that a "murderer has...erased the divine likeness from himself by his act of murder."[21]

We may thus infer that the divine image is a sign of special favor from God—a comparative rank entitling man to limited dominion over creatures that is a mirror of God's total dominion over all creation. Yet, the divine image can be partially lost, either by the whole human species, as in the Fall, or by individuals, as a result of committing murder. In addition to stressing dominion, the passages from *Genesis* emphasize procreation, as if procreation were an image of God's power of creation—which would explain the reference to male-female sexual differentiation as part of the divine image and the command to "be fruitful and multiply." Although procreation enables people to make children in their image—just as God made Adam in God's image, so Adam makes Seth in his image—one cannot be sure if this is the basis of human dignity. For the lower animals also procreate "according to their kinds" and are commanded to "be fruitful and multiply" (*Genesis* 1:22). Perhaps the Bible is saying that procreation with the conscious intention of passing on personal identity and subduing the earth is the divine image in man.

The challenge of *Genesis* is that it offers a glimpse into human dignity by referring to the divine image without precisely defining it. Dignity includes man's superior rank in the created hierarchy; and it confers special worth to human life and procreation, although the lifeblood and procreation of other animals also receive certain blessings (as if they too shared in the divine image to some extent). If this is true, however, what remains of the special dignity of man? The only answer that makes sense to me is that the lifeblood and procreation which man shares with other animals have a deeper meaning for the human species: they are pale reflections of something man alone possessed before the Fall, namely, immortal life. The implication is that *immortality* is the lost image of God in man—a suggestion supported by the account of the Fall, which is primarily about the loss of immortality, as well as by the longevity of Adam and the early patriarchs, who lived up to 900 years, as a kind of afterglow of immortality that God finally ended by setting a limit to human life at 120 years (*Genesis* 6:3). As compensation for the limited life span of mortals, the surrogate immortality that Adam gained through his son Seth continues through the procreation of families and tribes that endure for generations. Man's dignity, in the sense of original immortality or surrogate immortality (through children and long life) is therefore a comparative notion since it is the highest degree of perfection in the created hierarchy.

After these passages in *Genesis*, the only other books in the Old Testament that directly address human dignity are *Psalms*, *Wisdom*, and *Ecclesiasticus*. Psalm 8 does not include the phrase "image of God," but it uses the unmistakable language of *Genesis* to describe man's lofty place in the universe. The psalmist expresses his wonder that God created the vast heavens and yet cares above all for the human creature: "What is man that thou art mindful of him?.... Yet thou hast made him a little less than God [or a little less than the angels or divine beings] and dost crown him with glory and honor. Thou hast given him dominion over the works of thy hands". (*Psalms* 8:4-8) These lines are a classic example of Biblical minimalism: Man's dignity and glory are expressed with loving wonder, and man's dominion over the lower animals is asserted. But no reason is given for God's favor. The selection of the human species for special care is comparable in its mystery to the special election of Israel from among the myriad tribes and nations, a reflection of the inscrutable will of YHWH Who Is What He Is without giving reasons.

By contrast, the books of *Wisdom* and *Ecclesiasticus* (included in most Christian Bibles but not in the Hebrew Bible) supply reasons for man's dignity, possibly reflecting Greek philosophical influences. *Wisdom* 2:23-24 says, "For God created man for incorruption, and made him in the image of his own eternity, but through the devil's envy, death entered the world." This is the most explicit identification of the image of God in man with the attribute of immortality or divine eternity. The passage in *Ecclesiasticus* 17:1-12 also follows the pattern of defining the image of God in terms of attributes: "The Lord created man out of earth, and turned him back to it again. He gave to men few days…but granted them authority over things upon the earth. He endowed them with strength like his own, and made them in his own image. He placed the fear of them in all living beings and granted them dominion over beasts…. He gave them ears and a mind for thinking. He filled them with knowledge and understanding and showed them good and evil…. [He] allotted to them the law of life…[and an] eternal covenant." In this passage, the echoes of *Genesis* are evident in the references to human dominion; but the emphasis on attributes such as God-like strength (a puzzling notion) and reason or understanding through the senses and language gives a more precise meaning to the *Imago Dei*.

Yet, it is unclear if any of these attributes is as important as the simple fact of God's election of man for special care and the election of Israel for an eternal covenant. In this sense, the *Imago Dei*—as God's mysterious election of certain beings for divine favor—is the premise of the entire Old Testament, which may explain why it appears prominently in *Genesis* up to the first covenant (with Noah) and then drops out of sight.

It is not until the New Testament that the original language of *Genesis* about the *Imago Dei* reappears in the Bible. Here, we find a dozen references to the image, likeness, and figure of God as well as other references to the children of God and to partakers of the divine nature. Some of these terms are reserved for Jesus Christ, who is called "the image (*eikon*) of the invisible God" (*Colossians* 1:15). These descriptions seem to connect the *Imago Dei* of *Genesis* with the central article of the Christian faith, the Incarnation, in which the invisible God becomes a visible man in Jesus Christ. As Paul says, "though he was in the form of God, he did not count equality with God a thing to be grasped, but emptied himself, taking the form of a servant, being born in the likeness of men" (*Philippians* 2:5-7). The point of using the language of image and likeness from *Genesis* to explain the birth of Christ may be inferred from Paul's theology: while God originally created man in the divine image, that image has been partially lost and needs to be restored by Christ, who is the real image of God. Unlike the foolish pagans, who "exchange the glory of the immortal God for images of mortal men or animals" (*Romans* 1:20-23), Christians see the real image of God in the immortal man, Jesus Christ. Christ combines in his person the image of God (immortality) and the likeness of fallen men (mortality) and therefore is able to restore the lost image of God to man (to restore lost immortality).

The lesson of the Bible seems to be that the *Imago Dei* includes the rational soul or intellect of man but does not equate human dignity with it. The Bible even uses the image of God to avoid designating a set of qualities as the essential attributes of man, thereby precluding a Christian theory of human nature in the strict sense. Instead of focusing on attributes, the Bible presents man in terms of his relations to God: originally man was close to the image of God, then he fell away, and eventually the lost image of God was restored through the redemptive sacrifice of Christ. The Bible, in other words, is more interested in the theory of salvation (soteriology) than in the theory of man (anthropology), even though it permits speculation about the essential attributes of man in certain books. In sum, human dignity based on the *Imago Dei* refers primarily to mysterious election while still mentioning reason and lost immortality, which gives man a special moral status because he is a rational but fallen creature made in the image of the eternal God.

## Guidelines for Bioethics: Utility, Knowledge, and Dignity

Bioethics can benefit from these meditations because it needs more than utility and the advancement of knowledge as guiding principles; it needs a principle like respect for human dignity based on the special moral status of human beings as creatures with rational souls mysteriously tied to bodies but even more mysteriously elected by God as creatures with immortal souls that are an image of eternity. Perhaps this is what people mean when they say that man is body, soul, and spirit—physical body, rational mind, and immortal spirit. Perhaps it is the "human person" whose unique and irreplaceable personality is partly known to reason but fully known only to God, who gives everyone on earth a personal calling or mysterious personal destiny. In other words, science tells us about the body and especially the physical-chemical reactions of the brain; philosophy tells us about the rational soul united to the body; but religion takes us into the mysterious realm of the divine image of eternal destiny in each human being. If this is the whole truth about man, what are the implications for biotechnology?

While analyzing specific policies is highly technical (and beyond the scope of this essay), I would like to conclude by sketching some of the implications of human dignity for limiting utility and the quest for theoretical knowledge. Let me state briefly five lessons:

(1) First and foremost, the mystery of the human soul as the basis of human dignity implies a certain reverence and awe before the unknown and unknowable causes of human existence in the partly rational but mysterious universe. This suggests caution about scientific experimentation on human beings for the sake of relieving suffering

or advancing knowledge. The pride of science should be tempered by the recognition that science and reason will never be able to understand fully the most important things about the universe and man—for example, why we get old and die or why our body cells wear out or why cell replacement diminishes; these are biological questions in one sense and in other sense spiritual questions about why our bodies are mortal and finite. Because science can deal only with one dimension of this issue, we should moderate the ambitions of science and accept the fact that it will not be able to produce the "miracle" of unending life or the knowledge of aging and death that it promises.

(2) Second, genetic engineering in particular will not be able to succeed in changing or perfecting human nature. Genetic engineering is part of the utopian dream of the modern scientific and political project to remake man according to blueprints of perfect rationality and perfect justice. This project assumes the dualism of man as a machine for mastery and as master of the machine; but this is a false dualism. Scientists may learn how to connect certain genes with certain traits like diseases or abnormal aggression. But they will never develop an exact science that connects genes with all the traits that make up a human being. The basis of the personality is the human soul, and the soul cannot be reduced to the body or the brain because the soul will always be mysterious. We may find links between genes and aspects of traits like depression, aggression, sexual identity, and self-esteem. But what about talents like musical ability, higher intellectual pursuits, artistic creativity, spiritual awareness of mortality and immortality? The notion that these are explicable in terms of genes and traits is a false pretense of scientific materialism. The mysteries of the human soul will never be reducible to the 30,000 genes or the 3 billion nucleotides of the human genome.

(3) Third, since human dignity is based on the mystery of the human soul, we do not have to fear human cloning as much as some critics suggest,[22] even though it is a bad idea, because it will probably produce nothing more than unnecessary suffering in its defective human products. Even if we could clone Charles De Gaulle and put him in a general's uniform, he still would not be Charles De Gaulle—whose personality and character are partly a product of his genes but are also a product of his rational and divine soul, not to mention his historical times and national culture. The cloned version

of Charles De Gaulle created in the year 2007 and put in a general's uniform may look like De Gaulle, but he will not have De Gaulle's soul and may just as well be content flipping hamburgers in uniform rather than acting as the heroic savior of France.

(4) Fourth, cloning is still a violation of human dignity because it violates the God-given natural methods of procreation through male-female reproduction, which is part of the teaching of *Genesis* about human beings made in the image and likeness of God. Sexual reproduction is partly a natural biological process, but it is also a divine mystery because the human species could have been made to reproduce by asexual reproduction or by way of three sexes rather than male-female procreation. Biotechnology threatens the natural order of things because it seems to imply that everything can be reinvented by science and the human will—by man as master of the machine. But the uncertainty of tampering with God's creation should be reinforced by a cautionary sense of awe before the mystery of life and procreation.

(5) Fifth, the techniques of the biotechnical revolution that are the most justifiable are those that most modestly follow the course of nature and respect the mysterious unity of man as body and soul. Thus, the procedures of *in vitro* fertilization that essentially replicate the natural processes in couples who cannot conceive on their own are the most defensible in terms of respecting human dignity. Specifically, fertilizing the egg and sperm of married couples outside the womb and then replacing the embryo in the mother's womb are corrections of defects in accordance with nature's ways, not a willful effort to conquer and remake nature. Likewise, drug therapies that respect the limitations of knowledge regarding the physiology of moods and behavior are justifiable if they do not willfully assume, for example, that depression or aggression are merely physical and chemical rather than possibly spiritual maladies. Healing the body and mind by healing the soul has always been practiced, more or less successfully, and it can offer limited hopes in relieving a certain amount of human suffering without expecting science to master the human mind. In sum, we can accept certain features of the biotechnical revolution that acknowledge the partial truths of modern science, but they must be tempered by the awareness of the whole truth about man as the mysterious unity of body, rational soul, and an image of the divine eternity.

# Notes

[1] See Francis Fukuyama, *Our Posthuman Future: Consequences of the Biotechnology Revolution* (New York: Farrar, Straus & Giroux, 2002), p. 160.
[2] Thomas Hobbes, *Leviathan,* ed. Edwin Curley (Indianapolis, Indiana: Hackett, 1994 [1651]).
[3] B. F. Skinner, *Beyond Freedom and Dignity* (New York: Knopf, 1972), p. 200.
[4] Ibid., p. 201.
[5] Ibid., pp. 104-107.
[6] Daniel C. Dennett, *Darwin's Dangerous Idea: Evolution and the Meanings of Life* (New York: Simon & Schuster, 1995), p. 50.
[7] Ibid., p. 185.
[8] Ibid., p. 370.
[9] Ibid., p. 365.
[10] Ibid., pp. 389-393.
[11] Ibid., pp. 516-517.
[12] Ibid., p. 520.
[13] Ibid., p. 371.
[14] Aristotle, *On the Soul,* in *A New Aristotle Reader,* ed. J. L. Ackrill (Princeton, New Jersey: Princeton University Press, 1987).
[15] John R. Searle, *Mind: A Brief Introduction* (Oxford: Oxford University Press, 2004), p. 113.
[16] Ibid., p. 133.
[17] Ibid., p. 234.
[18] Paul Davies, "The Intelligibility of Nature," in *Quantum Cosmology and The Laws of Nature: Scientific Perspectives on Divine Action,* ed. Robert J. Russell, Nancy Murphy, and Christopher J. Isham (Vatican City: Vatican Observatory, and Berkeley, California: Center for Theology and Natural Sciences, 1993), pp. 145-161.
[19] Paul Davies, *Are We Alone? Philosophical Implications of the Discovery of Extraterrestrial Life* (New York: Basic Books, 1995), p. 129.
[20] St. Augustine, *On the Literal Interpretation of Genesis,* in *The Fathers of the Church,* vol. 84, trans. Roland J. Teske, S. J. (Washington, D.C.: Catholic University of America Press, 1991).
[21] Umberto Cassuto, *Commentary on the Book of Genesis,* 2 vols., trans. Israel Abrahams (Jerusalem: Magnes Press, 1984).
[22] The President's Council on Bioethics, *Human Cloning and Human Dignity: An Ethical Inquiry* (Washington, D.C.: Government Printing Office, 2002).

# Commentary on Kraynak
## Daniel C. Dennett

In my primary essay in this volume, I proposed a naturalistic defense of the values of human dignity against the encroachments of science and technology, arguing that it was more robust than the traditional defenses, which I described as brittle and vulnerable. "We need to articulate these values in open forum. When we attempt this, we need to resist the strong temptation to resort to the old myths, since they are increasingly incredible, and will only foster incredulity and cynicism in those we need to persuade."[1] I concentrated on the strengths of my proposal rather than the shortcomings of the traditional alternatives, in part because I didn't want to be suspected of choosing weak examples to quote and criticize. (Finding mediocre opponents to ridicule is usually easy and seldom instructive.) Now that Robert Kraynak's essay has been delivered into my hands, I have a good example of just what I meant by a traditional defense, giving me a golden opportunity to illustrate the problems inherent in such an approach.

Kraynak sets out to defend what he conceives of as a middle ground between dualism and materialism, inspired by Aristotle's tripartite division of plant (or vegetative) souls, animal souls, and rational, human souls. "As a living being, man shares characteristics with other animals while also being essentially different; he is neither a beast nor a god but an 'embodied rational soul.'"[2] I agree with this, so far as it goes. It is Kraynak's unfortunate supplement, drawn from Christianity, to the effect that this embodied rational soul is immortal, immaterial, and "mysterious," that causes all the problems. How can I, an unflinching materialist, agree with Kraynak that what sets human beings aside from all other creatures is an embodied rational soul (as contrasted with a mere animal soul)? No problem. As Kraynak himself observes, I am not the kind of materialist Hobbes or Skinner were, denying the existence of freedom and dignity:

> Dennett's ambition is to apply the Darwinian algorithm to everything—e.g., our universe and its laws arose from a myriad of accidental tries with other combinations that did not survive.* This enables him to argue that the universe and man are accidental products of evolutionary forces, but they still have meaning and purpose once they are "frozen" in place. Thus, scientific materialism can be vindicated while avoiding moral relativism and affirming a culture based on modern liberalism, democracy, and respect for the dignity of persons.[3]

Just so. As Giulio Giorello once said, as the headline to an interview with me in *Corriere della Sera,* Milano, in 1997: *Sì, abbiamo un'anima. Ma è fatta di tanti piccoli robot.* "Yes, we have a soul, but it's made of lots of tiny robots!" This has been my motto for almost a decade, and its import stands in stark contrast to Kraynak's vision. The "tiny robots'" in question are cells (such as neurons) and even tinier robots (such as motor proteins and neurotransmitter molecules) that have evolved to form amazingly ingenious armies of operatives, uniting to form an organization—as Aristotle said—that sustains not just life, like the vegetative soul, and not just locomotion and perception, like the animal soul, but imaginative, rational, conscious thought. Kraynak accepts that Aristotle's first two souls can be material organizations, as Aristotle himself maintained, but he thinks the rational soul must be composed according to altogether different principles. And in support of this he even quotes the passage from Aristotle that I

---

* Kraynak cites my *Darwin's Dangerous Idea,* p. 185; this is not quite accurate, but let it pass.

had alluded to in my essay. Kraynak observes that Aristotle held that "'Man is not the best thing in the universe' because the heavenly bodies are more perfect; they move in eternal circular motion which man can contemplate and admire but cannot emulate."[4] But the great philosopher was wrong about this, as I pointed out:

> One of Aristotle's few major mistakes was declaring "the heavens" to be made of a different kind of stuff, entirely unlike the matter here on Earth—a tactical error whose brittleness became obvious once Galileo and company began their still-expanding campaign to understand the physics of the cosmos. Clinging similarly to an immaterial concept of a soul at a time when every day brings more understanding of how the material basis of the mind has evolved (and goes on evolving within each brain) is a likely path to obsolescence and extinction.[5]

Kraynak thinks that the soul has to stand outside the purview of the natural sciences—has to be "mysterious." This is transparently wishful thinking. The soul is not going to stay mysterious, and it's a good thing it isn't, since as we come to understand how it works, we will also be able to *explain* why and how human minds are morally competent in a way animal minds are not. We don't have to declare that this is a "mysterious election"—one of the least satisfying dodges I have ever seen. Courage, Professor Kraynak! We can explain these matters, just as we have explained reproduction and self-repair and metabolism, for instance.

Kraynak thinks I am contradicting myself, "reintroducing 'skyhooks'" in my understanding of man:

> What is missing in Dennett is the humility to acknowledge that he assumes an essential difference between humans and animals based on something like a rational soul, even though he reduces man to accidental evolutionary forces.... Thus, he implicitly embraces a dualism of substances (matter vs. mind or nature vs. freedom) that divides humanity into two orders of causality which cannot interact except by external mastery.[6]

Nonsense. This is a curious passage, since as examples of a "dualism of substances" Kraynak offers two candidates, only one of which, matter vs. mind, could be considered a dualism of substances. The opposition of "nature vs. freedom" is a telling category mistake. Neither nature nor freedom is a substance, and they are not suited for opposition—unless you are presupposing, as Kraynak apparently does, that freedom (free will) *cannot* be natural, *must* be a sort of magical abridgment of the laws of nature. This idea has a long tradition, but so have its rebuttals, unremarked by Kraynak. There is no problem of "two orders of causality"; all causality is physical. The space of reasons fits comfortably within the material world of living, evolved things.

More debilitating than his assumption—he offers no argument—about the impossibility of a natural account of freedom is his presumptuous rhetoric:

"When Adam had lived a hundred and thirty years, he became the father of a son in his own likeness, after his image, and named him Seth" (*Genesis* 5:1-3). A third passage occurs in the story of the Flood when God blesses Noah's family: "Be fruitful and multiply, and fill the earth. The fear and the dread of you shall be upon every beast of the earth.... For your lifeblood I will surely require a reckoning.... Whoever sheds the blood of man, by man shall his blood be shed; for God made man in his own image" (*Genesis* 9:5-7).

These are the only references in *Genesis* (and in the entire Hebrew Bible) to the *Imago Dei*. They show that God created the natural world as a hierarchy with the human species at the top, possessing a special right of dominion over the lower species. In the first grant of dominion, man is commanded to subdue the birds, fish, and cattle, but his food is restricted to plants (*Genesis* 1:29-30). When Adam and Eve are created in the Garden, they are further restricted by the prohibition not to eat of the tree of the knowledge of good and evil, lest they shall die. After they disobey, whatever dignity they previously possessed is henceforth combined with depravity and mortality; but their dignity is not entirely lost.[7]

What does he think he is doing here? These passages from scripture don't "show" anything. Surely he knows that most of the people in the world—the people he should be attempting to reason with in this open forum on human dignity—don't believe any of this! My friend Sally, who is always right, has informed me that human dignity is a gift from space aliens who visited the planet about six million years ago. Take my word for it—there's nothing to discuss. Sally never makes a mistake! I take it that everyone can see that this claim of mine is simply an unacceptable move in the game. Kraynak's flat assertion of the truth of these passages from the Bible is no more acceptable. I don't object to his using scripture to try to make points, and it doesn't matter whether the passages are true or not. (I think they are obviously false—the Garden of Eden never existed, and nobody fathered a child at age 130.) But even if those of us who do not believe in the literal truth of the Bible are wrong, Kraynak has no right to assume this. He must argue for the truth of these passages, explain their truth, give reasons for believing them. Anything else is simply rude. We have to begin tuning our ears to these speech acts, and recognize them for what they are: personal fouls. Kraynak several times chides me and Searle for lack of "humility," when it is his arrogant, in-your-face assertion of Christian dogma that would be truly offensive if it weren't so comically ineffective.

Once we set aside such inappropriate contributions to the conversation, we have plenty to talk about. Human dignity is well worth protecting, and we can do it without first converting everybody to fundamentalist Christianity. Isn't my appeal to science equally presumptuous? No, on two counts. First, there is no sectarian science—no Muslim geology or Christian mathematics or Hindu biology. Every religion in the world can be reasonably assumed to accept the scientific method—after all, they rely on it when collecting their alms and building their temples—so this is one of the few areas of truly common understanding around the world. (Music is arguably another, but it isn't so much a method of understanding as a means of focusing and enhancing experience—you can't solve a problem or explain a puzzle with a piece of music.) Second, at every point my appeal to the claims and presuppositions of science may be challenged. It is for this reason that my faith in science is not any sort of religious faith. It is based entirely on the proven record of scientific success, and makes no appeal to authority beyond the reasoning ability of each individual in the conversation. It has been fashionable in some academic groves in recent years to downplay the power of such methods, insisting that all conversations—however biased or illogical—are on a par, but fortunately that fad is going extinct, and people are resuming their appreciation of the truly thrilling power of open-ended rational questioning. If you "don't get it" all you have to do is ask, persistently and politely, for an explanation of the baffling points. This may sometimes be met with impatience and rudeness, but everyone knows that, officially, it is the responsibility of the scientific researcher to *explain* and *defend* every last claim. That contrasts sharply with the celebration of faith and mystery found in most religions, and this is what simply disqualifies them from playing the leading role in the peaceful, mutually respectful explorations we are now engaging in. The sacred texts of the world's religions may be used as rich sources of ideas, but brandishing them as above criticism and then celebrating the "faith" with which one excuses oneself from defending them is an abuse of religious freedom.

## Notes

[1] From my essay in this volume, p. 58.
[2] From Kraynak's essay in this volume, p. 70.
[3] From Kraynak's essay, p. 67.
[4] From Kraynak's essay, p. 70.
[5] From my essay, p. 45.
[6] From Kraynak's essay, p. 68.
[7] From Kraynak's essay, p. 75.

# Commentary on Dennett

## Robert P. Kraynak

Daniel Dennett is a leading spokesman in our times for Darwinian natural science and, more broadly, for scientific materialism. Known for his long white beard and sense of humor, he is often compared to Santa Claus. But this comparison is very misleading. Dennett's intellectual mission, one might say, is to tell the world that there is no Santa Claus—no "comforting myths" about God, creation, intelligent design, the human soul, or ultimate purpose and meaning in the cosmos.

Dennett likes to shock audiences by saying that such beliefs are like appeals to mythical "skyhooks"—to miracles from heaven that have been discredited by modern science, which has shown all educated and intelligent people (the "brights," as he likes to call his superior group) that the universe is just an accident, the laws of nature are accidents, the emergence of life, human beings, and society are simply the incremental accidents of Darwinian evolution. "Get over it!" Dennett implores us: there are only material causes in a material world that is indifferent to man and that has order (if not purpose) only because the incremental accidents that shaped the world have been "frozen" in place over time. We live in a universe of "frozen accidents," and that is where we must make our home.

Dennett also likes to argue against philosophers of mind who still believe that human consciousness arises from an immaterial substance like a rational soul or in an irreducible free will which gives human beings the power to choose independently of material causation. Nonsense, says Dennett, we are complex machines, and the mind is just the motion of brain cells and neurological processes that will one day be replicated by the fancy robots of Artificial Intelligence. We may still speak of human "souls," Dennett argues mischievously, as long as we understand them to be made up of tiny robots. And we may still speak of "free will" as long as we mean the way our genetically programmed selves react to the environment rather than the rational choice of ultimate ends.

None of this would be very surprising if Dennett followed his Darwinian materialism to its logical conclusions in ethics and politics. After all, scientific materialists have been around for a long time, attacking religion, miracles, immaterial causes, and essential natures. Think of Lucretius and his poem about the natural world consisting of atoms in the void, or Hobbes's mechanistic universe of "bodies in motion," or B. F. Skinner's "behaviorism," Ayn Rand's "objectivism," E. O. Wilson's "sociobiology," Darwin's Darwinism, and even Nietzsche's "will to power." But all of these materialist debunkers of higher purposes and soul-doctrines drew conclusions about morality that were harsh and pessimistic, if not cynical and amoral. Lucretius saw that a universe made up of atoms in the void was indifferent to man, and he counseled withdrawal from the world for the sake of philosophical "peace of mind"—letting the suffering and injustices of the world go by, like a detached bystander on the seashore watching a sinking ship, and treating the spectacle of people dying with equanimity as impersonal bundles of atoms in the void. Hobbes, Skinner, Rand, and Nietzsche saw humans as essentially selfish creatures of pleasure, power, and domination who in some cases can be induced by fear and greed to lay off killing each other. Darwin never spelled out the moral implications of his doctrine, but presumably he could not have objected to the strong dominating the weak or to nature's plagues and disasters as ways of strengthening the species. Herbert Spencer's Social Darwinism—the survival of the fittest in a competitive world—is a logical conclusion of Darwinian natural science.

But such conclusions are alien to Daniel Dennett. He is a Darwinian materialist in his cosmology and metaphysics while also strongly affirming human dignity as well as a progressive brand of liberalism in his ethics and politics. Herein lies the massive contradiction of his system of thought. He boldly proclaims that we live in an accidental universe without divine and natural support for the special dignity of man as a species or as individuals; yet he retains a sentimental attachment to liberal-democratic values that lead him to affirm a humane society that respects the rights of persons and protects the weak from exploitation by the strong and from other injustices. He also objects to B. F. Skinner and the sociobiologists for reducing man to the desires for pleasure, power, and procreation. And he condemns Social Darwinism as "an odious misapplication of Darwin's thinking" and expresses outrage at child abuse, the exploitation of women, and President Bush's attempt to rewrite the Geneva Convention's definition of torture as violations of personal dignity. In short, he is a conventional political liberal of the Cambridge, Massachusetts, type whose moral doctrine is a version of neo-Kantian liberalism that assumes the inherent worth and dignity of every human being. But none of this follows logically from his Darwinian materialism and it even contradicts it, which means Dennett's humane liberalism is a blind leap of faith that is just as dogmatic as the religious faith he deplores.

In my essay, "Human Dignity and the Mystery of the Human Soul," I sought to expose some of these contradictions in Dennett's book, *Darwin's Dangerous Idea* (1995). How could he say that the universe is an accident—"it just happened to happen"—while claiming that "the world is sacred" and that life is basically good? How can he say that the human mind is a result of mindless and purposeless evolutionary forces and that animal species are not essentially different from each other, while also maintaining that "there is a huge difference between the human mind and the minds of other species, enough even to make a moral difference"? How can he destroy the foundations of human dignity in cosmology and metaphysics, while continuing to affirm human dignity and human rights in ethics and politics? Thomas Jefferson was more consistent when he proclaimed that our natural and human rights are "endowments of our Creator" and derived from "the Laws of Nature and of Nature's God" that give human beings a special moral status as rational beings in a universe possessing the moral order of a benevolent Creator. The moral philosopher Kant was also more thoughtful when he argued that human dignity could be sustained only by the dualism of nature and freedom.

Perhaps, then, Dennett really is Santa Claus, because he gives us free gifts like the goodness of life, the dignity of human beings, and democratic human rights without any logical or theoretical support for them, and indeed with a materialist doctrine that subverts them at every point. Perhaps Dennett's materialist humanism is even a residue of Christian humanism with its emphasis on the special status of human beings as rational creatures in the cosmos (a trenchant point made by John Gray in his review of Dennett's book on free will).*

In Dennett's essay for this volume we can detect signs of uncertainty about whether his earlier position can be sustained. The title, "How to Protect Human Dignity from Science," acknowledges that there is a real problem here—a potential conflict between modern science and technology, on the one hand, and the grounds for defending human dignity, on the other. He realizes that the underlying assumption of human dignity is the special moral status of man in the universe and that this status was upheld traditionally by the doctrine of the human soul. Dennett even admits that science cannot easily provide an alternative grounding for human dignity and that biotechnology might lead to treating humans as commodities for sale and as objects for manipulation and destruction. Dennett is also uncharacteristically silent about Darwinian materialism, even though his main point is that the doctrine of the human soul is discredited in the 21st century and that natural science will have to produce a substitute that will be more "workable" in defending human dignity: "We can have dignity and science too," he says nervously.

Dennett's argument is strange because it often sounds like a plea for a new kind of mythology for human dignity. He talks about the "belief environment" surrounding cherished moral ideas, such as the sacredness of life and the dignity of persons, and he praises the value of "belief in belief"—of upholding the necessary assumptions of moral

---

* John Gray, "Review of *Freedom Evolves* by Daniel C. Dennett," *The Independent*, Feb. 8, 2003: "The ringing tone of Dennett's declaration of human uniqueness provokes a certain suspicion regarding the scientific character of his argument. After all, the notion that humans are free in a way other animals are not does not come from science. Its origins are in religion—above all, in Christianity."

order, such as freedom of the will and the special status of human beings, even if they are unprovable or illusory. Dennett even speaks sympathetically of Paul Davies's view that freedom of the will may be a necessary fiction for morality (like a combination of Plato's noble lie and Kant's postulates of practical reason). Yet, Dennett insists that belief in an immaterial and immortal human soul cannot serve as the basis for human dignity any longer, as it did in the Western tradition under the influence of Christianity and Platonism. Belief in the soul is "discredited," so we have to find something else to defend the human dignity that even Dennett seeks to preserve.

In reflecting on Dennett's provocative analysis, I would raise two critical questions: Why is he so sure that belief in the human soul is discredited? And what alternative does Dennett offer?

The first question is obviously a momentous one that I will answer with a few brief points. The doctrine of the human soul will never be "discredited" as long as the relation of mind to matter or of conscious reasoning to the brain remains mysterious; and it remains an awesome mystery. Most neuroscientists and philosophers honestly admit that they have few clues about how mental activities such as consciousness, free will, language, and even much of common sense arise from the firing of brain cells across synapses. Therefore, some kind of immaterial substance—call it "the rational soul"—must be at work here; and since the soul is mysteriously connected to the body, the best definition of man's essence is "an embodied rational soul." This view of man is just as workable today as it was centuries ago in Greek philosophy; and, in fact, modern science heightens the case for the mysterious existence of man as an embodied rational soul rather than dispelling it. Science properly done teaches us to "live with mystery" rather than to embrace one-dimensional materialism dogmatically.

Likewise in cosmology, the more we learn from science, the more we see how mysterious the universe really is and how purely naturalistic causal explanations are inadequate. Nature is not a self-contained whole because the laws of nature themselves are contingent and had to be "selected" by some mysterious power outside of nature; this is one way that science points toward God as the intelligent selector of the laws of nature. In addition, Big Bang Cosmology takes us back to a beginning point or "singularity" that preceded everything—including the laws of nature, the formation of space and time, and the formation of matter and energy. Cosmologists admit that what happened "in the beginning" is in principle a mystery because it is beyond science to comprehend; what they resist is calling it the miracle of a mysterious power because this too implies God as the Creator. Furthermore, the appearance of rational beings such as man at the top of a hierarchy of living beings, capable of rationally analyzing the process, appears to be the result of self-organizing complexity rather than a mindless accident, as Paul Davies argues. Yet rationality as a primary feature of matter and of the universe is itself mysteriously selected. Because the Bible presents the creation of the world and the creation of man at the top of a hierarchy as the mysterious acts of a still more mysterious power, and because science properly done points toward these mysteries, it is both scientific and reasonable to place faith and trust in the Bible's teaching about man's dignity as an embodied rational soul made in the image of God. Belief in the *Imago Dei* is thus more reasonable than Daniel Dennett's completely unjustified leap of faith.

The second question about Dennett's analysis is easier to answer than the first: Dennett offers nothing to replace the traditional doctrine of the human soul as the distinguishing feature of human beings and the foundation of our essential humanity. He claims that natural science can find a substitute for the soul-doctrine but offers no new grounding. At most, Dennett appeals to the social conventions of a liberal democratic society or a pragmatic test, like the late Richard Rorty's appeal to historical contingency: we in modern liberal democratic societies act in such a way as to respect human dignity by not desecrating human corpses, for example, so pragmatically it works for us. In other words, respecting human dignity is a social convention of our times in the modern Western world. But this is patently inadequate because it simply means living off the moral capital accumulated by the Judeo-Christian tradition. I conclude therefore that Daniel Dennett's leap of faith from materialism to ethical idealism is not only rationally unjustified, it also points toward genuine religious faith as the logical path to the beliefs that he and others so ardently cherish.

# Commentary on Dennett

## Alfonso Gómez-Lobo

In this note I would like to address a single issue in Professor Dennett's paper. I decided to do it not because I consider his views on this particular question in any way offensive or subversive, but because I find them rather perplexing on his own assumptions. First, I should say in truly Socratic fashion where I think there is sufficient agreement for the conversation to take place. I have a positive appreciation of science and I do not see scientific truth as in any way a threat to anything I hold dear. I wholeheartedly admit *bona fide* scientific evidence as a valid move in the dialogue. On the other hand, I hesitate to accept the extrapolation of scientific results beyond the self-imposed limits of science itself, as well as arguments based on the mere existence of a technological practice.

The issue I want to examine is whether the following claims by Professor Dennett are true or false:

> The questions of when (human) life begins and ends…are, according to science, more like the question of the area of a mountain than its altitude above sea level: it all depends on what can only be conventional definitions of the boundary conditions. Science promises—or threatens—to replace the traditional absolutes about the conditions of human life

with a host of relativistic complications and the denial of any sharp boundaries on which to hang tradition.[1]

The above claims are important to the contents of this volume because, if true, they leave us in the position of Plato's bad butcher: we would have "to splinter a limb (or part, *meros*) into pieces" since there would be no "natural joints (*arthra*)" at which to effect the proper cut.[2] In other words, there would be no way of deciding objectively whether very young (and very old) human beings have inherent dignity and therefore should be respected. This would be a purely "conventional" matter, i.e., something to be decided...by whom? By the majority (which often means by the most powerful and influential within that group)? By right-wing politicians? By left-wing ideologues? This, of course, makes it extremely difficult, in my view, "to ensure that the values we defend *deserve* the respect of all," as Professor Dennett rightly demands.

How does Professor Dennett argue for his claims? He first gives us a picture of the "wonderful taxonomies" science has given us. He even uses Plato's imagery and terminology: "[Science has]...articulated [from *arthra*] and largely confirmed a Tree of Life that shows why 'creature with a backbone' carves Nature better than 'creature with wings.'" And then he adds: "But the crisp, logical boundaries that science gives us don't include any joints where tradition demands them. In particular, there is no moment of ensoulment to be discovered in the breathtakingly complicated processes that ensue after sperm meets egg and they begin producing an embryo...."

The last statement is puzzling. Surely Professor Dennett does not speak of ensoulment in his own voice. In other parts of his text he rejects Cartesian dualism and also seems to reject dualism altogether. But the notion of ensoulment requires dualistic assumptions: only if there is one substance, a body, and a different substance, a (Cartesian) soul, does it make sense to claim that a soul comes into a body that previously was not human and now makes it human.

If someone rejects dualism (and I think this can only be done by means of metaphysical arguments and not by merely scientific ones) then the natural position to adopt is a form of monism, the view namely that we are a single integrated substance that is alive and that, at a certain stage of maturity, will exhibit certain mental activities that we associate with freedom and reason. On this approach the soul can be understood not as a separate entity that comes to occupy the body, but as the genetic information contained in the DNA that provides the dynamism for the development of a human organism.

The view just presented is not only consistent with present-day science, it also allows us to see that talk about "a mere bundle of living human tissue becoming a person" is a remnant of the rejected dualistic metaphysics. This discredited picture requires one substance, "a mere bundle of living human tissue," what biology textbooks would more accurately call "an embryo" or "a fetus," and a second item that was not previously there, not even in latent form, that provokes a drastic change, a change that *ex hypothesi* does not preserve the substance's identity. Since the previously existing organism continues to exist after the arrival of the new item, the resulting "person" would be a new entity, a composite of the body and something arriving at a later point in time.

It makes much better sense to accept the scientific evidence, under the assumption that each one of us is essentially an integrated human organism. On this view, the gradual changes that take us to adulthood seem to preserve identity (we say that it is the same organism that is growing and maturing), and those changes may be interpreted as a successive activation of functions that were already latent "in the genes." None of this is old myth, and all of it is consistent with present common knowledge.

Let us press on and ask whether contemporary science shows gradualism or a clear articulation at the inception of a human life. Since I am not a scientist, I am here relying on biology and embryology textbooks in use at American universities.[3] The picture that emerges, in summary, is this: through meiosis human organisms produce gametes, that is, cells that have half the standard number of human chromosomes. Each gamete (either sperm or egg) is a specialized cell that lies at the end of a line of development and is thus unipotent. By itself it cannot go any further. Neither an egg nor a sperm is an organism, and each of them is destined to die within a short period of time. If, however, a sperm manages to penetrate the *zona pellucida* of the egg and the two fuse, then a radical change takes place: a new cell emerges that stands at the beginning of a line of development. It has the full complement of human chromosomes and is strictly totipotent. There is no gradualism here of the sort found in the emergence of a new species nor a process analogous to the "coming of age." The empirical evidence shows that the gametes cease to exist and a zygote, the first stage in a new organism, begins to exist within a short period of time.

There is much more in the embryology literature that could be quoted, but this suffices to make Plato's good butcher happy: here we have uncovered an *arthron*, an "articulation" or "joint," that allows him to make an elegant cut.

What this entails for the defense of values that deserve the respect of all is this: no scientific progress is sufficient to make us abandon the rational moral conviction that it would be wrong intentionally to kill an innocent adult human being. If we reject dualism as part of the old myths and accept the basic, commonsense conviction that we are unified human animals, then we should accept that as long as we are alive we are the same being,[4] and if an adult is endowed with dignity then it follows that he or she also was endowed with dignity in earlier phases of his or her life, back to the beginning. I submit that this conception of the acknowledgement of dignity deserves the respect of all because in principle no human being is excluded.

## Notes

[1] From Dennett's essay in this volume, p. 40.
[2] *Phaedrus* 265e.
[3] Cf. Neil A. Campbell and Jane B. Reece, *Biology*, 6th ed. (San Francisco, California: Benjamin Cummings, 2002); William J. Larsen, *Essentials of Human Embryology* (New York: Churchill Livingstone, 1998); Keith L. Moore and Trivedi V. N. Persaud, *Before We Were Born: Essentials of Embryology and Birth Defects*, 6th ed. (Philadelphia: Saunders, 2003).
[4] Some people reject the trans-temporal identity of an adult and the zygote he or she once was on the basis of the possibility of twinning. A critique of this view is offered in Gregor Damschen, Alfonso Gómez-Lobo, and Dieter Schoenecker, "Sixteen days? A reply to B. Smith and B. Brogaard on the beginning of human individuals," *Journal of Medicine and Philosophy* 31 (2006): 165-175.

# 5
# Human Dignity from a Neurophilosophical Perspective

Patricia S. Churchland

This essay on human dignity and bioethics will have six parts. In the first, I argue that dignity is an important concept whose meaning is inherently ambiguous and cannot be settled by appeals to religious authority, conceptual analysis, or philosophical argument; instead, the meaning of human dignity—and its specific consequences for today's biomedical controversies—must be worked out pragmatically, in a spirit of compromise. In the second part, I suggest that we can gain some clarity about human dignity by examining where morality comes from, and in particular the biological and social origins of human moral behavior. In the third part, I argue that moral progress is possible, but that misplaced moral certitude can do more harm to human dignity than good. In part four, I describe historical cases in which medical progress was impeded by moral and theological opposition, and I predict that those who today are morally opposed to embryonic stem cell research will fall silent once the clear medical benefits begin to emerge. Part five considers a deeper question concerning human dignity: whether modern biology has exposed human dignity itself as something that doesn't really exist. Part six addresses the related question of whether, in the light of modern neuroscience, holding people morally responsible makes any sense.

## I. How Do We Figure Out What Adherence to the Idea of Human Dignity Requires of Us?

Consider a few obvious facts. First, "human dignity" is not a precise concept, in the way that "electron" or "hemoglobin" are precise. Nor is it merely conventional, in the way that "meter" or "gallon" are conventional. It is not a matter of etiquette, as thank-you notes are. It does not connote a matter of fact, as "the Earth revolves around the Sun" does. Regarding our fellow humans as worthy of dignity, and being considered worthy of dignified treatment ourselves, are important to us. But what that entails is not precisely defined. The idea varies—across cultures, within cultures, across history, and within a single person's lifetime. More exactly, it varies even among those persons of goodwill who are themselves exemplars of moral rectitude. For example, some of the morally wise consider contraception a moral abomination, while others view it as a moral obligation. Both may claim moral certitude; both claim religious blessing.[*]

In our recent history, some people viewed smallpox vaccination as morally heinous on the grounds that it usurped the power of God, while others considered it a moral duty to vaccinate all children against this disease. Some sacred books command us to kill anyone who is deemed a witch;[†] other wise texts state that burning of heretics and blasphemers is morally indecent.[‡] In some cases, the very same sacred book is inconsistent on the question of the morality of slavery.[§]

The variation in moral practice, which is often correlated with variation in religious preference, implies that we cannot settle what "human dignity" means by appealing to universally shared ideology.

---
[*] See Adam Schulman's introductory essay in this volume.
[†] The Old Testament—see *Exodus* 22:18: "Thou shalt not suffer a witch to live."
[‡] Among the earliest, Friedrich von Spee's work of 1631, *Cautio Criminalis, or a Book on Witch Trial*, trans. Marcus Hellyer (Charlottesville, Virginia: University of Virginia Press, 2003).
[§] See, for example, *Exodus* 21:2-6: "If thou buy a Hebrew servant...." and *Exodus* 22:2-3: "If a thief...have nothing, then he shall be sold for his theft." On the other hand, see also *Exodus* 21:16, where "stealing a man" is grounds for execution, and *Deuteronomy* 23:15-16, where it is forbidden to hand over an escaped slave to his master. As Bernard Shaw wryly noted, no one believes the Bible means what it says; everyone believes it means what *he* says.

Can philosophers deploy a tool known as "conceptual analysis" to reveal the requirements? No more than they can use conceptual analysis to discover whether fire is rapid oxidation or whether mortgage rates will rise next month. There is no final and indisputable source of truth about what "human dignity" entails, to which philosophers, even word-wise, reflective philosophers, have privileged access. There is no "essence" that is somehow fixed in some realm, if only we had access, or by deploying pure reason, if only we were smart enough.

What is conceptual analysis? If "conceptual analysis" merely taps into how the concept is currently used by ordinary people, then all the variation, ambiguity, vagueness, and open-endedness inherent in ordinary usage of "human dignity" is immediately laid bare. On this construal, conceptual analysis is essentially an anthropological enterprise. On the other hand, if conceptual analysis is deployed in hopes of dissipating all that ambiguity and vagueness and settling whether, for example, human dignity must be attributed to the fertilized egg, then the hopes are vain. There is no purely analytical technique that gets you from here to there. Some philosophers do covertly import into their "analysis" a favored moral conviction, but this over-reaches strictly analyzing the concept as it lives and breathes, and goes on to endorse a particular moral view. In which case, one might as well avoid the whole charade of conceptual analysis and just endorse the moral view forthrightly.

Is there any source of special knowledge to which philosophers uniquely can appeal? There is none. Plato famously believed that important concepts, complete with all their entailments, did exist in the realm of the intellect, later waggishly dubbed Plato's heaven. Alas, Plato's heaven is merely a fantasy, as Aristotle well knew. Concepts are part of living languages and are imbued with beliefs, associations, and analogies. They change over time, they sometimes vanish or come into existence; they are the categories brains use for making sense of the world. They are not fixed and frozen Platonic essences that are reachable via some semi-magical procedure such as Platonic intellection.

How then do we resolve moral disagreements about a certain practice? Can we embrace a principle of universal human dignity and still use contraception and support stem cell research? Like all social activities, resolution of these issues is a complex sociological dance. To a first approximation, it involves people of goodwill trying to come to a workable solution. That may sound mundane, but it embodies the wisdom of humans as diverse as Aristotle, John Locke, Benjamin Franklin, John Dewey, Nelson Mandela, and Confucius. It involves recognition that no single person, no single profession, no single religious sect, no single sacred text, can be counted on to deliver the correct answer to moral questions.

As I am fond of telling my students, there is no Wise Guru sitting atop a mountain holding all moral truths in his pocket. How could there be? Such a guru would need to know about all social conditions and all possible scientific advancements. No human being falls into that privileged category. Nor is there a specific recipe for how people of goodwill work together to find a solution. But we do have history to learn from. In addition to examples of what to avoid, we do have examples where no bloody crusade was launched, no heretic burned, no infidel beheaded, no city sacked, and no idol smashed. Instead, fair-minded compromises were worked out. From these examples, we can hope to learn the morally decent ways of resolving disagreements about the uses of new medical technologies.

## II. The Biological and Cultural Sources of Morality

We may be able to find common ground on the meaning and implications of human dignity by examining the origins of human moral behavior. Put simply, where does morality come from?

The answer has two parts. First, the evolution of the brain of social animals provides the neurobiological platform for social dispositions such as cooperation, reciprocity, group defense and prevention of disorder.[1] This is the neuro-genetic component. Second, conditions of life, accidents of history, and the capacity for cultural accretion stimulate the emergence of various superstructures on this biological platform. The first is biology, while the second is politics, in the broadest sense. Let me explain a bit further.

Humans are social animals, and as individuals our flourishing very much depends on the behavior of others in our group. Sociability confers a wide range of benefits on the individual. Living within a pack, a wolf can help hunt large animals such as deer and elk, rather than scrounge for mice. Benefits multiply: group defense against predators, shared resources for care of the young, warmth in the group huddle during winter storms, grooming to remove parasites from the hide, a division of labor whereby those who know where to find water or where the caribou cross the river can guide the rest of the pack. The life span of a loner chimpanzee is much shorter than that of his conspecifics who live in a troop.

The brains of social animals are wired to feel pleasure in the exercise of social dispositions such as grooming and cooperation, and to feel pain when shunned, scolded, or excluded. Neurochemicals such as vasopressin and oxytocin mediate pair-bonding, parent-offspring bonding, and probably also bonding to kith and kin. Other neurotransmitters, such as serotonin and dopamine, play a role in the astonishing complexity that is social life, as do hormones such as testosterone.[2]

Typically, young social mammals learn the prevailing practices and settle into a fairly stable pattern of social life. Humans, like other social animals, including chimpanzees, bonobos, baboons, monkeys, wolves, and ravens, have social instincts. These basic social instincts, enabled by the genes and tuned to local practices by the reward system, are the platform for cooperation and maintenance of the social order, and they provide the neurobiological foundation for ethics in its broader sense. More particularly, they provide the basis for love of mates and offspring, for the affection of kin, and for the default respect accorded to other group members. A plausible hypothesis is that the desire to extend to all humans the respect and dignity once more or less limited to small groups probably originates here.

In human society, the benefits of group membership are even more far-reaching and extensive than in baboons and chimpanzees, mainly because humans have a drive to share and accumulate knowledge. To a greater extent than other mammals, humans are consummate imitators.[3] The capacity to imitate a skill learned by an elder puts the young human at a singular advantage: he or she does not have to learn everything by trial and error. Jointly, the drive to learn by imitation and to upgrade that knowledge with new ideas is what yields the gradual accumulation of clever ways of doing things that can be passed on from one generation to the next. That is, it yields culture. A child can learn from the elders how to make fire and keep it going, how to prepare for winter, how to set a broken bone.

These benefits acknowledged, the costs of social life are mainly the costs associated with sharing resources, inhibiting the impulses to exploit the weakness of others, assisting in group defense, and maintaining the social order by, among other things, punishing those who violate group norms or threaten the group as a whole. Of course these may not be recognized as costs by the animal making its way in social life, but they are costs in the straightforward biological sense that risking loss of life and limb in defense of the group can get the animal injured or killed.

The greater reach of altruism in humans than in other primates has long been a puzzle, because the costs of helping strangers seem to outweigh the benefits to gene spread. A recent model by Samuel Bowles[4] suggests a solution: If our ancestral groups engaged in lethal intergroup competition, where the group successful in battle takes the resources of the vanquished, and if this was accompanied by practices of "reproductive leveling" such as monogamy and food sharing beyond the family, then genes disposing individuals to altruistic behavior would tend to spread through the population.

Social dispositions are only part of our motivational package, of course. Our brains are also wired to see to the welfare of ourselves and our offspring at the expense of those unrelated to us. If we are lucky, these impulses will not conflict with social impulses, but of course they often do. Even the rules of thumb conflict: charity begins at home; love your neighbor as yourself. Suppose one can enhance one's welfare at the expense of another? Depending on conditions, social and otherwise, this can lead to great complexity in behavior, including all the familiar ways of flouting the social norms: cheating, deceiving, hoarding, refusing to reciprocate, etc. Historically, it has also led to branding some humans as "not fully human," and hence not deserving of dignity. Taking as slaves members of alien groups, where the slaves are considered "not of our kind," has had a long, if sorry, history, and if Bowles's theory is correct, in-group altruism and out-group aggression naturally co-occur. Because humans are very smart, these inclinations to violate social norms while seeming not to can be manifested in subtle as well as not so subtle ways. Hence we see complicated forms of deception, hypocrisy, extended forms of slavery, cabals, factions, power struggles masked as moral struggles, and all the other forms of human tragedy explored by Shakespeare. As with other social animals, humans augment the basic social dispositions with rewards for socially acceptable behavior and punishments for its opposite.

The point of much of cultural structure is to deter behavior that runs counter to the accepted practices. Stories about the glory of courage and the humiliation of cowardice instill the values of out-group aggression and in-group defense; songs about kindness rewarded and sharing blessed, about truthfulness praised and deceit despised, solidify social values. Rituals involving praise for warriors and punishment for cheaters reinforce the cultural lines of demarcation. The local religion may depict both the basic social dispositions and their detailed local expression as gifts from spirits or gods and as deserving otherworldly goods after death. Sacrifices, of animals and humans, are often employed with the effect of dramatizing the power of the other-worldly source.

Once trained, the child has an automatic negative response to the very idea of stealing, as well as to cowardice. And history and anthropology both teach us that, with adolescence, a bloodlust for outgroup massacres often manifests itself.[5] The youth's desires change. He is apt to acquire narrow-minded convictions about what is right and what is wrong, about who is truly a group member, and who is not. The salient thing about this cultural activity is that a group's ethical standards may tend to be internalized as absolute; absolutely true, infallible, correct, applicable for all time under all conditions, and beyond explanation. Moral certitude is not inevitable, but it is common, more so in the young than in the broadly experienced, less so in certain kinds of temperaments (e.g., Aristotle, Gandhi, Lincoln, the Dalai Lama, Nelson Mandela) than in others.

To sum up: Both biology and "politics"—understood broadly to include cultural anthropology, sociology, and group psychology—help us to understand how and why moral standards of behavior developed among humans, as well as how and why we are tempted to violate those standards. The next question is whether, given such a realistic account of the origins and function of morality, it makes sense to speak of "moral progress," i.e., of one society being better than another at preserving "human dignity."

## III. Can There Be Moral Progress?

Aristotle viewed moral understanding as a kind of skill—a skill in navigating the social world. He realized that, through one's experience of life, one could achieve an increasingly deep understanding of what is conducive to the flourishing of human societies and what undermines that flourishing. Skills may improve over time, but they may also degenerate, and that is true of social skills as well. It is, I think, fair to say that some moral progress has been achieved in some societies. For example, trial by one's peers, though an imperfect institution, is, all things considered, a more stable and efficacious system than trial by ordeal. The rule of monarchs by divine right has the defect that the monarch may have a diseased brain or a feeble brain; the education of females tends to reduce collective poverty; bribing government officials leads to a loss of faith in the system as a whole; and so on. Plainly, there are better and worse ways of organizing society.[6]

Not infrequently, it may be difficult to discern whether a proposed law will aid or impede human flourishing in the long run. As many moral thinkers, including Aristotle and John Dewey, have realized, sometimes the consequences are very hard to predict, and cautious legislation may be viewed as a kind of social experiment. For example, in the early part of the 19th century, many people predicted utter catastrophe if women were allowed to vote in elections to Federal and state office. Yet these predictions have turned out to be wholly false. Prohibition of the sale and consumption of alcohol in the 1920s in the United States was acclaimed by temperance groups as a monumental moral achievement, but eventually it became evident that the legislation had addressed a bad problem and made it worse. This is probably also true of the current prohibition of other addictive drugs, such as marijuana, cocaine, and heroin.

As John Stuart Mill realized, legislating private morality (i.e., not what I do to others but what I do to myself) generally causes more trouble than it cures.[7] If you make my private life your business, the door is open to no end of busybody intrusion, no end of ugly harassment in the name of morality, and no end of enforcement costs. Moral certitude about the right way to lead one's private life tends, in the enthusiastic, to generate the impulse to force others to fall into line. Much moral courage and breadth of experience are needed to face the fact that such an impulse can lead to immense and unnecessary wretchedness.

Some well-intentioned advice, even from exemplary moral thinkers, can turn out to be poor advice. At one point, Jesus advised that we should live as the lilies in the field, without care for the long term. As historical research makes clear, he advised thus because he believed the end of the world was nigh. Since the world did not end, it was very bad advice indeed, and Sunday school teachers now hastily contrive an excuse for not taking it seriously. St. Paul also believed the end of the world was nigh and, in the midst of some rather moving ruminations about kindness, also rendered exceptionally poor advice, especially on the topic of sexuality. These lapses are not surprising.

Even thoughtful, experienced, balanced people may be ignorant of certain facts or may themselves be blinded by certain hopes and passions. Everyone sees the world from some perspective or other, influenced by one's own idiosyncratic experience, framed by one's own idiosyncratic brain, with its particular balance of emotions, fears, beliefs, and temperament. This means that we are all limited, in some respect or other. We do the best we can, but there is no guarantee that it is The Best Absolutely. To be sure, there are plenty of people who advertise their preeminent wisdom, including, sometimes, allegedly infallible guides to life. Self-styled wise men will always attract followers, since there are plenty of desperate people vulnerable to their promises.

To sum up: It does make sense to speak of moral progress; some societies are unquestionably better than others at treating people decently, i.e., with due respect to their dignity; and societies can learn from their mistakes and improve their performance in this regard. But it is an unfortunate fact that morally self-righteous attempts to improve human society—sometimes undertaken in the name of preserving human dignity—have sometimes led to the mistreatment of human beings and to much human suffering. Good intentions based on moral certitude are no guarantee that human beings will actually benefit.

## IV. Vaccines, Anesthesia, and Stem Cells

Now let us consider some of the burning issues of contemporary bioethics, and in particular the advent of new medical technologies that some observers believe pose a threat to human dignity.

What about stem cell research? More exactly, what about the research use of human embryos for therapeutic (not reproductive) purposes? Let us accept for this discussion the prevailing criterion that the embryos at issue have not yet advanced to the stage of cell differentiation (so there are no brain cells at all). Is a blastocyst (a ball of about 200 undifferentiated cells) something that commands the dignity, rights, and privileges accorded a full-term human infant? And what about assisted suicide for the terminally ill patient, suffering in agonizing pain, who pleads for it? If her religion allows it, but yours does not, why should yours prevail? On what basis can you assume that you know better? As I argued in Section I, attention and reflection to the everyday use of the concept "human dignity" cannot give us the answers. Life is harder than that.

What I can do is tell you how I am inclined to approach these questions, as I draw upon historical examples, and as I try to apply the ideas of diverse thinkers—e.g., Aristotle, Confucius, Aquinas, Dewey, Mill, and the Dalai Lama. I shall avoid putting my eggs in one basket. I shall do the best I can, but I do not wish to claim it is Absolutely The Best, and I do not wish to claim special moral authority, though I do not think I should be taken less seriously than the Pope or Pat Robertson. I only wish to suggest that we reason together.

Past moral and theological opposition to novel medical technologies sheds some light on contemporary bioethical controversies. Smallpox is a highly contagious, painful and disfiguring viral disease. Mortality of those infected is about 20–40%. In the mid-18th century in Europe, on average one in thirteen children died of smallpox, and many more were left blind owing to corneal ulcerations. As early as 1000 BC, physicians in India used a form of inoculation to prevent the spread of infection. They rubbed the pus of an infected person into a small cut of a healthy person, who then contracted a mild form of smallpox and was immune thereafter. The Chinese variant was to powder a smallpox scab and inhale the powder into the nasal cavity. Eventually the British and Americans learned of the inoculation practices and began to try them, though some patients did still die in spite of inoculation, and some died as a result of the inoculation itself. Overall, however, it produced a transformative reduction in the rate of infection. In 1757 Jenner became famous for having safely vaccinated a boy with cowpox, after noticing that milkmaids were immune to smallpox. Cowpox vaccination produced very mild and local symptoms but provided immunity against smallpox.

Arch-conservative theologians and medical men, both Catholic and Protestant, bitterly opposed inoculation as well as vaccination with cowpox. The struggle went on for some thirty years.[8] The theological opposition turned on the conviction that smallpox is a judgment of God on the sins of the people, and that to avoid the disease was to risk further punishment. Inoculation was described as a tool of Satan that would distance man from God. For example, Rev. Edward Massey in England preached an impassioned sermon in 1772 entitled *The Dangerous and Sinful Practice of Inoculation*. Personal threats were leveled at medical practitioners, and primitive bombs were thrown into homes. Not all theologians were opposed, and some, especially among the Puritans, took an active role in promoting vaccination. One theologian, attempting to defend the science, argued that Job's boils were actually smallpox pustules caused by the devil. So, he concluded, if Job's agony was devilish in origin, then avoiding the agony is consistent with God's law.

By the middle of the 19th century, pro-vaccination forces had succeeded in getting large numbers of people vaccinated, and the number of deaths plummeted. The death rate of children in Europe due to smallpox fell from one in thirteen to one in sixteen hundred. In London, in 1890, only one person died of smallpox, while a hundred years earlier smallpox had taken thousands.

That vaccination against a horrible viral disease was once fought as a violation of God's law is rarely remembered today. That vaccination was opposed at all scarcely seems possible, and the opposition seems anything but moral. But the opposition was entirely real; it was also powerful, impassioned, widespread, and—but for the courage of a few—could have been successful. The opponents never did take the pulpit to admit they were wrong.

The opposition was defeated not by argument, but by the obvious benefits of vaccination. Quite simply, it became more and more difficult to convince people that the misery of smallpox was morally superior to the benefits of immunization. The bishops and priests and reverends who once thundered about the sin of inoculation drummed up other topics on which to thunder.

Incidentally, it may be worth noting that today, arch-conservative Christian groups, such as the Family Research Council, appear to continue this tradition of favoring misery and death over vaccination against a virus. They oppose routine vaccination of young girls against cervical cancer. The vaccination against human papilloma virus (HPV) is highly effective and can prevent some 10,000 new cases (and 3,500 hundred deaths) in the United States per year. Worldwide, 300,000 women die of cervical cancer each year. Cervical cancer is in fact the second leading cause of cancer deaths in women. "Abstinence is the best way to prevent HPV," says Bridget Maher of the Family Research Council. "Giving the HPV vaccine to young women could be potentially harmful, because they may see it as a license to engage in premarital sex," Maher claims.[9] The Christian Coalition of Florida also opposes routine vaccination, on much the same grounds: "We're concerned about the age of the kids and the message we're sending," said Bill Stephens, the coalition's executive director. Stephens said the coalition might be more apt to support the legislation if it included education about abstinence.[10] According to *Fortune* magazine, Dr. Hal Wallis, head of the Christian conservative group, Physicians Consortium, said, "If you don't want to suffer these diseases, you need to abstain, and when you find a partner, stick with that partner." The founder of the National Abstinence Clearinghouse also opposed the vaccine. This organization was formed "to promote the appreciation for and practice of sexual abstinence (purity) until marriage." Leslee Unruh, the organization's founder, was quoted as stating, "I personally object to vaccinating children against a disease that is 100 percent preventable with proper sexual behavior."[11] Phil Gingrey, a Republican representative from Georgia, has claimed, "States should require vaccinations for communicable diseases, like measles and the mumps. But you can't catch HPV if an infected schoolmate coughs on you or shares your juice box at lunch. Whether or not girls get vaccinated against HPV is a decision for parents and physicians, not state governments."[12] If the deeper motivation for opposition to the vaccine is that cervical cancer is a deserved result of failure to adhere to sexual abstinence outside of marriage, as AIDS has been claimed to be God's punishment for homosexual activity, one would have to question the morality of such a position. In any case, even if abstinence may be the surefire way to prevent sexually transmitted diseases, as a social policy it cannot be said to have had a successful history.

\*

The history of opposition to anesthesia as a method of relieving pain during surgery and childbirth is equally dismaying, and also surprising. What could be morally objectionable about relieving pain? Quite a lot, apparently. Arch-conservative theologians and physicians regarded pain as God's punishment for sin, as part of God's divine plan, as making the person closer to God as he begs for mercy. To interfere with that plan was to play into the hands of the devil. It was to usurp God's power and take it unto oneself or—as one might say now—to "play God."

Ether and chloroform, the best of the early anesthetics, were particularly potent and if used carefully, were also reasonably safe. William Morton, a dentist in Boston, demonstrated the use of ether at Massachusetts General Hospital in 1846, and chloroform was introduced by James Young Simpson in Scotland in 1847. In Scotland, Simpson's use of chloroform was widely denounced in the pulpit. One clergyman asserted that "chloroform is a decoy of Satan. It may appear to be a blessing, but it will harden society and rob God of the deep earnest cries for help." Use of anesthesia in childbirth, even in Caesarian sections, was strenuously opposed even by some who thought its use in amputation and tooth extraction was just barely acceptable. Their justification was that the procedure tried to circumvent God's curse upon Eve as she and Adam left the Garden of Eden: "I will greatly multiply your pain in childbearing. In pain shall ye bring forth children" (*Genesis* 3:16).

As with vaccination, the benefits were so profound and so immediately appreciated that religious opposition eventually fell silent. No one today would consider it a moral necessity to avoid anesthesia during a breach delivery. But the opposition in the 19th century was sincere, backed by Biblical text, devoutly embraced, and supported by unwavering moral certitude. Again, there is no evidence of clerics coming to the pulpit to announce a change of mind, the clear benefits notwithstanding. Rather, this embarrassing bit of theological history was left in the back of the closet.

There are plenty of other examples of religious condemnations of scientific technologies that have greatly benefited mankind, including contraceptive techniques, *in vitro* fertilization (which allegedly violates human dignity[13]), division (dissection) of the dead body (Boniface VIII in 1300[14]) and organ donation by living donors (Pope Pius XII, 1956), as well as religious blessings of such practices as female subjugation*, slavery, forced conversions, and genital mutilation of females.

Part of the point of these historical interludes is that claims to know what God wants are no guarantee against moral failure. Humility, whatever one's religious inclinations or moral convictions, is surely appropriate. The main point, however, is that moral attitudes can change when the benefits of a technology are clear and demonstrable. As the benefits of a technology become plain, it becomes more and more difficult to convince large numbers of people that enduring the misery of disease is morally superior to enjoying the benefits of health. Ideology, however laced it may be with moral certainty, generally has a tendency to quietly fold its tents once the benefits of a technology are manifest and reasonable regulations have been worked out. Moral certitude itself can be a moral menace when it stymies the compromises and negotiations of fair-minded, sensible people.

If past experience is a guide, I predict that the opposition to stem cell research will likely weaken once the benefits of that research begin to emerge. Even now, parents whose infants have diabetes do not find it credible that a microscopic fertilized egg is a person. Someone who has macular degeneration and is blind at twenty or who is a quadriplegic at fifteen does not find it reasonable that a ball of undifferentiated cells—not a neuron in sight—is really his equal in rights and obligations. As I write this, new research is showing that when newly born retinal cells from mice pups are injected into the eyes of retina-damaged mice, they link up to existing retinal cells and restore

---

* According to 1 *Timothy* 2:8-11, women are required to learn in silence and to submit to men in silence.

a functional retina, providing the best evidence so far for cell replacement therapy in the central nervous system.[15] Once the therapeutic benefits become undeniable, the Biblical texts will be reinterpreted to show that God approves of scientific advances that ameliorate suffering, just as they were in the cases of anesthesia and vaccination. It will be seen as obvious that, just as a fertilized apple seed is not an apple tree and a fertilized chicken egg is not a chicken, so a fertilized egg is not a person. It will be acknowledged that just as fertilization is an important step in reproduction, so is the development of a nervous system. Neural development will turn out to be vastly more important in reaching agreement on when a person has come into being.\* Religious leaders who have supported well-regulated stem cell research will gather adherents. Common sense will prevail.

Why do I believe this is likely? Because when ideology conflicts with obvious benefits for human health and flourishing, common sense typically, if slowly, triumphs.

So, as a practical matter, I believe that mankind will by and large prove successful in meeting the challenges of modern biomedical technology, reaping its great fruits while pragmatically avoiding the threats it might pose to human dignity. But there remains, in the minds of some, a theoretical problem concerning human dignity and modern science: to the extent that evolutionary theory, neurobiology, and genetics can give an account of our moral behavior and how it arose, some are afraid that human dignity itself will be explained away. I turn to this question next.

## V. If Ethics Is Rooted in Social Instincts Supplied by Our Genes, Doesn't That Mean Human Dignity Is Not Real?

Occasionally someone may suggest that, if our thoughts and ideas are merely the product of the brain and its activities, then they cannot be

---

\* As Robert Pasnau observes, Aquinas believed that God would not put "the rational soul" into a body that was not prepared, and the body of the developing human fetus was not prepared for the rational soul until about three months of gestation. He selected that date because by then the fetus begins to move. See Robert Pasnau, *Thomas Aquinas on Human Nature: A Philosophical Study of* Summa theologiae *1a 75-89* (Cambridge: Cambridge University Press, 2002).

real—not genuinely real. Consequently, it will be concluded, neuroscientists must believe that human dignity is not something real. But this worry rests on a misunderstanding, the nature of which can be readily explained.

When we remember the mad scene in *King Lear*, when we shoot a basketball, run to catch the ferry, hum "Greensleeves," or recognize a flower as goldenrod, networks of neurons in the brain are responsible for the result. In no case is the achievement the result of a single neuron. In no case is the achievement owed to a nonphysical soul.[16]

Representations more generally—in perception, thought, emotion, motor planning—are distributed over many neurons, typically millions of neurons in the case of mammals. Even the rhythmic behavior of walking, chewing, breathing, and so forth, is not the product of a single "rhythmic generator," but is an emergent property that arises from the interactions of many neurons. By emergent property, I do not mean anything spooky or metaphysical. I merely mean that the property is a function of both the intrinsic properties of neurons in the network and the dynamics of their interactions. I mean it is a network property.[17] The network provides the neural mechanism whereby the phenomenon is produced.

Discovering the mechanisms whereby networks yield their effects is horrendously complex. Nevertheless, neuroscience is beginning to piece together the story of how neurons collectively work together to represent colors, locations in space, decisions to move, odors, sounds, and temporal durations. Quite a lot is known about how populations of neurons represent in these ways, though much of the story is still ahead of us.

So the first point is simple: representations are network properties. The second point, to which I now turn, is that representations of the social world are also network properties, and they too are real and they too mediate behavior. Of course, if there is no social world for the animal (e.g., if it is completely isolated from others) then it will not have a social world to represent.

Chimpanzees have been shown to represent the goals of others; an individual chimpanzee can represent what another chimpanzee can and cannot see from its point of view.[18] Chimpanzees represent the niceties of social structure, and they know who is the offspring of whom. Young males can represent a weakness on the part of the alpha male and will orchestrate a challenge for dominance of the troop. With normal serotonin levels, participants in a donnybrook represent when it is prudent to back off the fight. These cognitive activities are the function of the orchestrated activity of neurons in neural networks. The representation of another animal's intention to ask for grooming is as real as the representation of a location of a food cache or the representation of movement. It as every bit as real as the activity of a single neuron; it just happens to be the activity of large numbers of neurons organized into a coherent network. Detailed understanding of exactly how all this works still eludes us, but every year brings new advances that make the problems more tractable.[19]

When social animals such as humans represent another as deserving dignified treatment, that cognitive/emotional state is achieved by networks of neurons. Representations of highly abstract ideas (e.g., infinity) and complex thoughts (e.g., mortgages) probably depend on the use of language, but linguistic representations nevertheless are still the business of neural networks. Social representations—of goals, intentions, sympathy, respect, fairness, kindness, exploitation, slavery—are as real as any other representation.

Notice, moreover, that many representations are not exact or precise, but typically have fuzzy boundaries. Depending on what is learned, in the myriad ways in which things can be learned, one's representation of the nature of the tides or of toilet training or of social justice may be modified—revised, augmented, deepened. A three-year-old's understanding of "fairness" is much less rich and elaborated than that of Abraham Lincoln.[20] In any event, it is simply a misunderstanding of neuroscience to conclude that, because there is a biological substratum underlying our representations of justice, morality, dignity and the like, those representations have no reality.

Even if it is accepted that such moral representations are real, some observers worry that the causal account of mental activity promised (and increasingly delivered) by neuroscience undermines our belief in free will and moral responsibility. But this too, I argue, is based on a misunderstanding.

## VI. If My Decisions and Choices Are the Outcome of Brain Activity, and if the Brain Is a Causal Machine, Am I Responsible for Anything?

Let me begin by simplifying. The fundamental point about holding an individual responsible ultimately rests on the need for safety of individuals in the group. We understand reasonably well the conditions permitting social traits to spread through a population, and they include the capacity to detect and remember who are the socially dangerous individuals and the willingness to punish them—as well as to punish those who will not share the burden of exacting punishment.[21]

Darwin had the basic story right when he remarked in *The Descent of Man*, "A tribe including many members who, from possessing in high degree the spirit of patriotism, obedience, courage and sympathy, were always ready to aid one another and to sacrifice themselves for the common good would be victorious over most other tribes; and this would be natural selection."[22]

Monogamous pair bonding is typical in certain species, such as marmosets, Canada geese and prairie voles. The behavior exists not because Divine Law or Pure Reason decrees its universal propriety, but owing to the utility of monogamy for their way of making a living. The species have evolved so that most individuals have high concentrations of receptors for the peptides oxytocin and vasopressin in limbic structures of the brain.[23] The limbic pathways connect to the dopamine-mediated reward system (mainly the ventral tegmental area and the nucleus accumbens). Thus, when a pair of voles copulates each comes to associate great pleasure with that particular mate. In social animals (including human beings), bonding with kith and kin probably involves these same biochemical pathways.

Fundamentally, punishment of cheaters (in the broadest sense) is justified because social traits such as cooperation and sharing cannot spread through a population unless cheaters are punished. Dispositions to punish are likely also to be regulated by neural modulators such as dopamine in the reward system, serotonin in frontal structures, and oxytocin in limbic structures. The precise nature of the punishment—shunning, beating, biting or whatever—may, in some species such as humans, be a matter for negotiation and cultural standards.

In varying degrees, human groups also recognize that under special circumstances the form of punishment calls for a closer look. Special circumstances may include being involuntarily intoxicated, being very young, sleep-walking, having an epileptic seizure, or being severely brain damaged. Insanity has always been a complicated issue for judicial systems, and it remains so now, though agreement on the necessity for public safety is pretty much universal.[24]

There are many forms of mental abnormality, some that render the individual merely eccentric, others that distort the representation of reality to such a degree that custodial care is essential. There are no easy answers regarding how to diagnose those forms of insanity, or exactly when responsibility is diminished. Nor is it at all obvious, in many cases, what justice requires. In his book *The Ethical Brain,* Michael Gazzaniga has suggested that issues involving insanity and criminal justice will not be made easier even when we can identify differences in the brains of those who are classified as insane and those who are not.[25] I suspect he is right, mainly because asylums for the criminally insane will have to be as secure as regular prisons, and because many people believe that—insanity notwithstanding—the possibility of punishment acts as a strong deterrent.

In any event, far from being undermined by neuroscience's insights into human behavior and its causes, moral responsibility is actually put on a firmer and more realistic basis, the more we understand about the neurological substratum of our moral life.

## Conclusion

Treating all members of our species with dignity is, certainly, a worthy aim. What must remain sobering to all thoughtful people, however, is that—as a matter of historical fact—those who espoused such a principle have often been willing to take coercive action, sometimes brutally coercive, to achieve their version of human dignity. Such coercion may be exercised even in matters of private morality, where the welfare of others is entirely irrelevant. In the name of religion, so-called heretics have been burned, blasphemers hunted down, private lives invaded and made miserable, cities sacked, and the peace overturned. For your own good, and in the name of your own dignity, it may be argued, you must suffer terrible pain and submit to smallpox or Parkinson's disease or spinal paralysis.

We have much more to fear from the moral dogmatist who brandishes his unshakable certainty about what God supposedly wants and intends concerning human dignity than from the calmly tolerant person who will listen to others, and who will work toward a peaceful compromise that is conducive to human flourishing. If someone professes certainty regarding a fact, we can always test his claim against the evidence. By contrast, if someone expresses certitude regarding what God intends, it is much harder to test his claim. In any case, it would be inconsistent with human decency to assume that feeling certain is itself conclusive evidence of possessing the truth.

## Notes

[1] See Edward O. Wilson, *On Human Nature* (Cambridge, Massachusetts: Harvard University Press, 1988); Matt Ridley, *The Origins of Virtue: Human Instincts and the Evolution of Cooperation* (New York: Viking, 1996); Frans de Waal, *Good Natured: The Origin of Right and Wrong in Humans and Other Animals* (Cambridge, Massachusetts: Harvard University Press, 1996).

[2] For a comprehensive review, see Thomas R. Insel and Russell D. Fernald, "How the brain processes social information: Searching for the social brain," *Annual Review of Neuroscience* 27 (2004): 697-722. See also Frances P. Champagne and James P. Curley, "How social experiences influence the brain," *Current Opinion in Neurobiology* 15 (2005): 704-709.

[3] Michael Tomasello, Malinda Carpenter, Josep Call, Tanya Behne, and Henrike Moll, "Understanding and sharing intentions: The origins of cultural cognition," in *Behavioral and Brain Sciences* 28 (2005): 675-691; Michael Tomasello, *The Cultural Origins of Human Cognition* (Cambridge, Massachusetts: Harvard University Press, 1999).

[4] Samuel Bowles, "Group Competition, Reproductive Leveling and the Evolution of Human Altruism," *Science* 314 (2006): 1569-1572.

[5] Richard W. Wrangham and Dale Peterson, *Demonic Males: Apes and the Origin of Human Violence* (New York: Mariner Books, 1996); Patricia S. Churchland, "Of gangs and genocide: Chimp behavior provides clues to the neural basis for aggression in humans," *Science and Theology News*, August 11, 2006.

[6] See William D. Casebeer, *Natural Ethical Facts: Evolution, Connectionism, and Moral Cognition* (Cambridge, Massachusetts: MIT Press, 2001).

[7] John Stuart Mill, *On Liberty*, ed. Gertrude Himmelfarb (London: Penguin, 1974 [1859]).

[8] Andrew Dickson White, *A History of the Warfare of Science with Theology in Christendom* (Gloucester, Massachusetts: Peter Smith, 1978 [1896]), chapter XIII, section 5.

[9] Deborah MacKenzie, "Will Cancer Vaccine Get to All Women?," *The New Scientist*, April 18, 2005.

[10] Shannon Colavecchio-van Sickler, "Vaccine bill finds tough opposition," *St. Petersburg Times*, February 26, 2007.

[11] Janet Guyon, "The Coming Storm Over a Cancer Vaccine," *Fortune*, October 31, 2005, p. 123.

[12] Fran Eaton, "HPV Vaccine Effort Encounters Strong Opposition," *Health Care News*, June 1, 2007, available online at www.heartland.org/Article.cfm?artId=21151.

[13] In 1968, Pope Paul VI issued the encyclical *Humanae vitae* (i.e., "Of human life"), all contraceptive devices, including condoms, intrauterine devices, the pill and patches, as well as sterilization techniques (vasectomy and tubal ligation), forbidding because of the "the inseparable connection, established by God, which man on his own initiative may not break, between the unitive significance and

the procreative significance which are both inherent to the marriage act" (*Humanae vitae* II.12). He used the same argument in forbidding *in vitro* fertilization. (The official English translation of *Humanae vitae*, quoted here, may be found online at www.vatican.va/holy_father/paul_vi/encyclicals/documents/hf_p-vi_enc_25071968_humanae-vitae_en.html.)

*Catholic Insight* explains that IVF is "in opposition to the dignity of procreation and the conjugal union." See John B. Shea, MD, "What the Church teaches about human reproduction," *Catholic Insight*, September, 2006, available online at www.catholicinsight.com/online/church/humanae/article_684.shtml. According to Australian physician John Billings, "this moral attitude [separation of sex and possible procreation] has produced in our own time an anti-child society." See John Billings, MD, *Gift of Life and Love* (Apostolate of Catholic Truth, Sixth Printing, 1997), quoted in Fr. Joseph Hattie, "The prophecies of Paul VI," *Catholic Insight*, July/August 2003, available online at www.catholicinsight.com/online/church/humanae/article_131.shtml).

In the 1968 encyclical, Paul VI goes on to say: "Consequently, unless we are willing that the responsibility of procreating life should be left to the arbitrary decision of men, we must accept that there are certain limits, beyond which it is wrong to go, to the power of man over his own body and its natural functions—limits, let it be said, which no one, whether as a private individual or as a public authority, can lawfully exceed" (*Humanae vitae*, II.17). Having witnessed for myself, as a child growing up in rural Canada, the unspeakable misery caused in many families by inability to control family size, I cannot but find these claims morally dubious. Common sense generally prevails here too, as many educated Catholics ignore the injunction against contraception.

[14] Boniface's bull, *Detestande feritatis* (i.e., "Of Abhorred Wounds") of 1300, forbade the division of the body, and did so in the strongest terms, with excommunication and denial of an ecclesiastical burial as automatic penalties for violation. Some historians have argued that Boniface's intent was only to prohibit the friends of dead crusaders from extracting the bones, boiling them, and returning them home for burial. See, for example, Daniel Boorstin, *The Discoverers* (New York: Random House, 1983). More recent and thorough historical analysis reveals a much more complicated story that has little to do with the crusaders and was intended to apply quite broadly.

Among other things, the evidence suggests that Boniface, a sickly man, had a strong concern with his own body and a deep personal abhorrence of the fairly common practice of bodily division before burial, perhaps fearful that he might be carved up before fully dead. He may also have worried about what division might imply for the doctrine of saintly "refreshment," perhaps envisaging his own canonization. His reasons for the decree remain obscure, however, since he published the decree without providing any arguments. In any case, his decree was broadly ignored, though not actually nullified by later Popes. For example, Boniface's successor, Clement V gave Philip the Fair permission to have his corpse divided so as to maximize the number of churches in which his remains could be buried. See

Katherine Park, "The Criminal and the Saintly Body: Autopsy and Dissection in Renaissance Italy," *Renaissance Quarterly* 47:1 (Spring, 1994), pp. 1-33, and Elizabeth A. R. Brown, "Authority, the Family, and the Dead in late Medieval France," *French Historical Studies* 16:4 (Autumn, 1990), pp. 803-832. Many thanks to Michael Stack for translating from Latin into English Boniface's bull, and for thorough reading and criticism of my manuscript.

[15] See Robert E. MacLaren, et al., "Retinal repair by transplantation of photoreceptor precursors," *Nature* 444 (2006): 203-207. Millions of otherwise normal people are affected by macular degeneration or retinitis pigmentosa and become blind.

[16] See Paul M. Churchland, *The Engine of Reason, the Seat of the Soul* (Cambridge, Massachusetts: MIT Press, 1996), and Patricia S. Churchland, *Brain-Wise: Studies in Neurophilosophy* (Cambridge, Massachusetts: MIT Press, 2002).

[17] For the best account of this see Carl F. Craver, "Beyond reductionism: Mechanism, multifield integration and the unity of science," in *Studies in the History and Philosophy of Biological and Biomedical Sciences* 36 (2005): 373-396.

[18] Michael Tomasello, Josep Call, and Brian Hare, "Chimpanzees understand psychological states: The question is which ones and to what extent," *Trends in Cognitive Science* 7 (2003): 153-156.

[19] Carl F. Craver and William Bechtel, "Mechanisms and mechanistic explanation," in *The Philosophy of Science: An Encyclopedia*, ed. Sahotra Sarkar and Jessica Pfeiffer (New York: Routledge, 2005).

[20] Tanya Behne, Malinda Carpenter, and Michael Tomasello, "One-year-olds comprehend the communicative intentions behind gestures in a hiding game," *Developmental Science* 8 (2005): 492-499.

[21] See Matt Ridley, *The Origins of Virtue: Human Instinct and the Evolution of Cooperation* (New York: Viking, 1996).

[22] Charles Darwin, *The Descent of Man, and Selection in Relation to Sex*, 2nd edition (New York: Appleton, 1909 [1877]), chapter V, p. 135.

[23] Larry J. Young, Brenden Gingrich, Miranda M. Lim, and Thomas R. Insel, "Cellular mechanisms of social attachment," *Hormonal Behavior* 40 (2001): 133-138.

[24] See Owen D. Jones and Timothy H. Goldsmith, "Law and Behavioral Biology," *Columbia Law Review* 105 (2005): 405-502.

[25] Michael Gazzaniga, *The Ethical Brain* (Chicago: University of Chicago Press [distributed for Dana Press], 2005).

# Commentary on Churchland

## Gilbert Meilaender

"Human Dignity from a Neurophilosophical Perspective" is about many things, but the concept of "human dignity" does not seem to be one of them. No reader of this essay could possibly come away from it with a clearer notion of what we might mean by dignity. It is, of course, true, as Churchland notes, that dignity is not a precise concept and that it is sometimes a matter of dispute. But that is no excuse for failing to help us think better about it. This is the paper's fundamental flaw, but there are a few others worth noting here.

The paper breathes a spirit of condescension entirely at odds with its rhetoric. Seldom will one find attitudes of "unwavering moral certitude" rejected with such certitude, or "humility" endorsed in language so permeated by its opposite. Indeed, the paper is a reminder that the "calmly tolerant person," while certain of his or her own rectitude and good will, can be extraordinarily intolerant. The bad effect of this on moral argument is that such a "calmly tolerant person" tends to confuse assertion with argument. Those of us who are not fully persuaded by Churchland's paper may at least take some comfort in the fact (stated in her concluding sentence) that "feeling certain is itself inconclusive evidence for truth."

Churchland's account of the origins of morality relies upon the importance of social cooperation, which each of us requires if we are to survive. (In passing, lest we confuse causes with reasons, we should note that this is less an account of the origins of morality than an explanation of its point.) And surely this is part of the point of morality. Yet, one of the oldest puzzles about morality is that what my group needs to survive and flourish may be my own willingness to suffer or die. "Men need virtues as bees need stings," Peter Geach once wrote. "An individual bee may perish by stinging, all the same bees need stings: an individual man may perish by being brave or just, all the same men need courage and justice."[1] The best Churchland can do to make place for this truth is to note that altruistic behavior in the past might (via a complicated scenario that is purely speculative) have spread throughout the population.

However we account for such sacrificial behavior, Churchland's depiction of a neurobiological foundation for morality cannot explain our experience of intentional action. A person is not simply a place where certain psychological states occur. A person is present in his actions without disappearing entirely into them—present in but also distanced from them. Activities of the brain do surely provide, as Churchland puts it, "a biological substratum" for the mind's thoughts and intentions, but those mental activities in turn interact with and shape the brain. Our thoughts are both located in the brain and distanced from it—which is why we are capable of what Thomas Nagel has called "the view from nowhere."

If we think of morality in Churchland's way, moral education—"stories about the glory of courage and the humiliation of cowardice…; songs about kindness rewarded and sharing blessed"—is not initiating the young into a set of obligations that unfold the meaning of human flourishing. It is, instead, simply training them in behaviors that "solidify social values." There is all the difference in the world between indoctrinating the young in a set of norms we find useful and initiating the young into a set of norms that bind us also, even when we wish they did not. "We castrate and bid the geldings be fruitful," was C. S. Lewis's description of what moral education becomes on a view such as she espouses.[2]

Churchland's discussion of embryonic stem cell research is so lacking in nuance as to be embarrassing. She takes the distinction between therapeutic and reproductive embryo research to be obvious and in no need of clarification or argument. She evidently thinks (though she puts forward this view only while donning the robes of the prophet peering into a distant future) that bettering the human condition—and, more particularly, our own condition or that of others dear to us—is the only consideration that really matters in moral evaluation. She seems to think the analogy of fertilized apple seed to embryo as apple tree is to person an illuminating one, even though her discussion does not tell us how or when one becomes a person—without which information we could scarcely know what even to think about the analogy.

But when these and other flaws are set to the side, we are still left with the fact that this paper sheds no light on what we mean by human dignity—and, hence, no light on how it might be endangered or protected. Churchland speaks of "threats" to human dignity, but she eschews the first task of an author: to help her readers understand why people have cared about her subject.

They have cared in some considerable measure because they have thought that there might be ways of failing to recognize or demeaning the dignity of persons that did not necessarily involve harming them and that might even, in certain respects, benefit them. Nothing she says helps us think better about whether human dignity is in any way undermined when (say) parents attempt to determine the sex of their child, when those without diagnosed illness medicate themselves in order to feel "better than well," when we attempt to enhance performance (of various sorts) by means of drugs, when someone is tortured. These are all instances in which we may have recourse to the language of dignity in order to express moral concern or condemnation; yet, nothing Churchland says helps us in any way to understand or evaluate such language.

It is hardly surprising, therefore, that she is utterly tone deaf to the sorts of reasons Roman Catholics might have for rejecting contraception, or the reasons Catholics and others might have for thinking *in vitro* fertilization a violation of human dignity, or for worrying about cutting up dead bodies in order to seek knowledge or living bodies in order to get organs for transplant. I see no evidence that she could even begin to explain why, from their perspective, these people view such practices as violations of human dignity. And unless and until one is capable of that, the most dignified thing to do would be to remain silent.

## Notes

[1] Peter T. Geach, *The Virtues: The Stanton Lectures, 1973-74* (London: Cambridge University Press, 1977), p. 17.
[2] C. S. Lewis, *The Abolition of Man* (Oxford: Oxford University Press, 1943), chapter 1: "Men Without Chests."

# Part II.
# Human Nature and the Future of Man

# 6

# Human Uniqueness and Human Dignity: Persons in Nature and the Nature of Persons

## Holmes Rolston III

"Humanity itself is a dignity." Immanuel Kant sought a universal human dignity with his respect for persons.[1] His highprincipled claim continues, endorsed by the nations of the Earth, in the Preamble to the United Nations' *Universal Declaration of Human Rights*: "[R]ecognition of the inherent dignity...of all members of the human family is the foundation of freedom, justice, and peace in the world."[2]

Such dignity is a core concept getting at what is distinctively human, commanding special moral attention. Our dignity figures in our personal identity, first at basic levels, where dignity is inalienable and common to us all, and further at developmental levels, where dignity can be achieved or lost, recognized or withheld. A person who has "lost his dignity" behaviorally is not thereby a person whom we can treat as without dignity in the native entitlement sense. A person's dignity resides in his or her biologically and socially constructed psychosomatic self with an idiographic proper-named identity.

At both levels, we should think of a *gestalt*, more than some quantitative scalar quality. Dignity is an umbrella concept (something like freedom, love, justice, integrity), which makes it at once inclusive and comprehensive, and yet raises issues of scope and precision.[3] The plan here is to see whether we can make some progress toward recognizing distinctive human worth by articulating the ways in which humans differ from nonhuman animals. We will spiral around a constellation of interrelated capacities, as often consulting what scientists are discovering as we are listening to the humanists. Awareness of the gulf separating humans from all other species can sensitize us to our potential for dignity.

This could be important in an age when it is philosophically and scientifically fashionable to "naturalize" all phenomena, human behavior included. The skeptic will say that we here are resisting accepting human continuity with animal nature, exaggerating the dichotomy between humans and their nonhuman ancestors. Our reply is that just this human capacity to present arguments such as those we are here producing establishes this discontinuity and the dignity for which we are arguing. Paradoxically, the more we discover that we are products of an evolutionary process, descended from the apes, the more we find that the capacity we humans have to demonstrate this— requiring paleontology, genomics, cladistics, anthropology, cognitive science, neuroscience, philosophy, and ethics—distinguishes us from the rest and disrupts the continuity demonstrated. Our concern here is not primarily medical, but this search might highlight understanding of what in humans we especially seek to protect, both in medicine and elsewhere in human affairs.

## Nature and Culture

Human dignity results from both (1) the *nature* of and in human nature and (2) the *culture* in which humans comprise their character. Humans live embodied lives. This embodiment, not itself undignified, is necessary but not sufficient. Our human biology opens up vast new possibility spaces in which our dignity can be (indeed must be) further nurtured in culture. In this respect, mixing our biological finitude with cultural refinements, we radically differ from animals. This search for such dignity, it now seems, is an all and only human assignment.

This search is anti-reductionist; we resist the claim that a human is "nothing but" an animal. Peter Richerson and Robert Boyd find "that the existence of human culture is a deep evolutionary mystery on a par with the origins of life itself.... Human societies are a spectacular anomaly in the animal world."[4] The human transition into culture is exponential, non-linear, reaching extraordinary epistemic powers. To borrow a term from the geologists, humans have crossed an unconformity. To borrow from classical philosophers, we are looking for the unique *differentia* of our *genus*.

Animals do not form cultures, at least not cumulative transmissible cultures. Information in wild nature travels intergenerationally largely on genes; information in culture travels neurally as persons are educated into transmissible cultures. Animals inherit some skills by copying the behavior of others, but genetics remains the dominant mode of intergenerational information transfer. The determinants of animal and plant behavior are never anthropological, political, economic, technological, scientific, philosophical, ethical, or religious. The intellectual and social heritage of past generations, lived out in the present, re-formed and transmitted to the next generation, is regularly decisive in culture.

The term "culture" is now commonly used of some animals, which is done partly by discovering behavior of which we were previously unaware, but also by revising the scope of the term "culture" to include behavior transmitted by imitation. In this sense culture is present not only among primates, but among birds, when they learn songs or migration routes from conspecifics. If so, we need another term, super-culture, for the human cultural capacities, or at least more precision in distinguishing kinds of culture.

Opening an anthology on *Chimpanzee Culture,* the authors doubt, interestingly, whether there is much of such a thing: "Cultural transmission among chimpanzees is, at best, inefficient, and possibly absent." There is scant and in some cases negative evidence for active teaching of the likeliest features to be transmitted, such as tool-using techniques. Chimpanzees clearly influence each other's behavior, and seem to intend to do that; they copy the behavior of others. But there is no clear evidence that they attribute mental states to others. They seem, conclude these authors, "restricted to private conceptual worlds."[5]

One way to gauge this is to inquire about intentional teaching, which involves the effort to transfer ideas from mind to mind. There is little critical evidence for such teaching in nonhuman animals; the best such evidence is still equivocal. One can trim down the meaning of "teaching," somewhat similarly to reducing the definition of "culture," and find noncognitive accounts of teaching. Interestingly, a recent study suggests a form of teaching not in the primates, where it is usually looked for, but in wild meerkats. Adults differentially cripple prey for their young to hunt, depending on how naive the juvenile hunter is.[6] Many predators release crippled prey before their young, encouraging their developing hunting skills.[7]

But if teaching is found wherever individuals have learned to modify their behavior so that the naive learn more quickly, then teaching is found in chickens in the barnyard, when the mother hen scratches and clucks to call her chicks to newfound food, with the chicks soon imitating her. The meerkat researchers conclude that they exhibit only simple differential behavior, responding to the handling skills of the pups, without the presence of ideas passing from mind to mind. There need not even be recognition (cognition) of pupil's ignorance; there is only modulated behavior in response to the success or lack thereof of the naive, with the result that the naive learn more efficiently than otherwise. There is no intention to bring about learning, and such behavior falls far short of customary concepts of teaching, undoubtedly present in ourselves.

Indeed, teaching in this differential behavior sense is found even in ants, when leaders lead followers to food.[8] If we are going to interpret such animal activities as (behavioral) teaching, then we need a modified account of (ideational) teaching, where teacher deliberately instructs disciple. In this sense of teaching, Bennett G. Galef concludes, "As far as is known, no nonhuman animal teaches."[9] Richard Byrne finds that chimpanzees may have glimmerings of other minds, but he sees little evidence of intentional teaching.[10]

Although chimpanzees collaborate to hunt or get food, Michael Tomasello and his colleagues conclude "with confidence" that "chimpanzees do not engage in collaborative learning.... They do not conceive of others as reflective agents—they do not mentally simulate the perspective of another person or chimpanzee simulating their perspective.... There is no known evidence that chimpanzees, whatever their background and training, are capable of thinking of other interactants reflectively."[11] "Nonhuman primates in their natural habitats…do not intentionally teach other individuals new behaviors."[12] Daniel Povinelli and his colleagues conclude of chimps: "There is considerable reason to suppose that they do not harbor representations of mental states in general…. Although humans, chimpanzees, and most other species may be said to possess mental states, humans alone may have evolved a cognitive specialization for reasoning about such states."[13] Without some concept of interactive teaching, of ideas moving from mind to mind, from parent to child, from teacher to pupil, a cumulative transmissible culture is impossible.

Humans, then, can participate intensively in the knowledge and skills that each other has acquired. Such capacity to encounter ideas in others who serve as role models gives rise to estimates of the worth of these others and, reciprocally, of their estimate of one's own worth. This will at first include estimates by the disciple of how expert is the teacher, and by the teacher of how well the disciple is doing. These are already value judgments; they will begin simply but, once launched, will grow more complex, involving deeper senses of achievement and worth among the interactants. For example, we are here engaged in such "collaborative learning" about human dignity, in conversation with both scientists and humanists. But this involves respect for the wisdom and perspective of others, and efforts both to recognize and to improve upon them, and that brings us to the threshold of human dignity.

This collaborative learning is what has produced human cultures. Human dignity includes the capacity for growing into and assimilating a cumulative transmissible culture. So part of one person's dignity may be that he is Scots, raised not only on that landscape but into that culture. She is a southern lady, declining now in her latter years, and altered in her original views on racial segregation (the result of collaborative learning), but still firm in her classic embodiment of the culture of the Old South and what it meant to be a woman of dignity. Animals, failing such cultural heritages, fail in such possibilities of dignity.

# Human Dignity and Animal Integrity

This "separatist" approach we are using here, distinguishing humans from animals, could have undesirable results if it led us to devalue (nonhuman) animal life. Research over recent decades has increasingly shown sophistication in animal minds.[14] One ought to respect life, both animal and human. Nevertheless, human life carries a dignity that merits an especially high level of respect. Recognition of the intrinsic values in nature needs careful analysis, ongoing in environmental ethics. This will include a welcome appreciation of animal integrity. But we should also be discriminating about human uniqueness, and that obligation is encapsulated in the idea of "human dignity."

We would not, for instance, attribute "dignity" to rocks or trees, nor even to the Grand Canyon or a giant sequoia, though we might find them majestic or sublime.*

We would puzzle over whether a bear or an eagle has "dignity," while never denying their charismatic excellence. We say that the Thomson's gazelles run with grace, without thinking that their flight from the approaching cheetah is dignified. There are parallel problems with "virtue," going back to the Greek *areté*. "Virtue" has the root idea of some effective "strength"; *areté* was at times applied to "excellence" in animals, found in diverse forms in diverse kinds. Nevertheless, "virtue" and *areté*, like "dignity," have come principally to refer to the highest human potentials and achievements. Can we be discriminating about our human dignity without losing discernment of the worth of animal excellences?

Critics will ask whether it might be a mistake to look to other beings less complex than we are to understand what we are (the genetic

---

* Etymology is not much help here. The Latin *dignitas* refers to worth, merit, desert, and honor, but also to rankings of all kinds. In Middle English, the modern uses are present, such as worth, honor, nobleness, as well as rankings applied to nonhumans. The *Oxford English Dictionary* (2nd ed., Oxford: Oxford University Press, 1989) cites from 1594: "Stones, though in dignitie of nature inferior to plants"; and from 1657: "the dignity and value of Fruit-trees." Even planets have more dignity in some positions of the Zodiac than others. From 1751: "There is no kind of subject, having its foundation in nature, that is below the dignity of a philosophical inquiry." The word "human" is derived from *humus*, Latin for "earth" or "soil," but that is of little help in understanding its present meaning.

fallacy). If there has been any evolutionary emergence in humans, the whole idea of an emergent quality is that it cannot be predicted or understood by looking at (or reducing things to) the simpler precedents. True, we do not learn what it means to be human by studying chimpanzees. Nevertheless, with animals as a foil, if we can gain some account of the thresholds we have crossed, we might get a more focused picture of the human uniqueness and of our resulting dignity.

Terrence W. Deacon puts this pointedly: "Hundreds of millions of years of evolution have produced hundreds of thousands of species with brains, and tens of thousands with complex behavioral, perceptual, and learning abilities. Only one of these has ever wondered about its place in the world, because only one evolved the ability to do so."[15] Oriented by such a worldview, a person can choose his or her goals, thoughts, and career in ways that animals cannot; this capacity to give self-direction to one's own life, with whatever realization of it has been accomplished, is worthy of intrinsic respect. These traits are both threshold and aristocratic.

Biologically, there is a distinctiveness to being human not found in other animals. This dignity is *ipso facto* democratically present in human beings, a legacy of our phylogeny, unfolding and actualized in the ontology of each person. Simultaneously, this suite of traits opens up the space of possibilities such that, psychologically, there can be comparative success and failure in this actualization. One can more or less realize these ideational, idiographic, existential, and ethical opportunities common in basic senses to us all, but in which some are more and less gifted, fortunate, encouraged, resolute, and successful than others. Dignity matures with the continued perseverance of a meaningful life project.

A chimp cannot ask, with Socrates, whether the unexamined life is worth living, much less be shamed for not having done so, or troubled by failure to live up to its goals. "Man is the only animal that blushes. Or needs to." Mark Twain takes from *Pudd'nhead Wilson's New Calendar* this folk wisdom about embarrassed dignity, impossible for animals.[16] "They knew that they were naked" (*Genesis* 3:7). If, in the course of medical treatment, one covers up the patient's nakedness, there is decency, dignity. With animals, there is nothing to cover. If we should discover that animals can blush or know that they are naked, we might have to revise our beliefs about their dignity. Until then, let this separate human dignity from animal integrity.

## Ideational Uniqueness

> But, if a universe were to crush him, man would still be more noble than that which killed him, because he knows that he dies and the advantage which the universe has over him; the universe knows nothing of this. All our dignity consists, then, in thought.[17]

Pascal's insights have been reinforced in contemporary biology and animal behavior studies. As philosophers from ancient Greece onward have claimed, humans are "the rational animals." Scientific research continues to confirm this ideational uniqueness. Humans are remarkable among all other species in their capacities to process thoughts, ideas, symbolic abstractions figured into interpretive gestalts with which the world is understood and life is oriented. Evidence of that comes from studies in the nature of language and in neuroscience. This is a constitutive dimension of our worth, our dignity.

Stephen R. Anderson, a linguist, concludes:

> When examined scientifically, human language is quite different in fundamental ways from the communication systems of other animals.... Using our native language, we can produce and understand sentences we have never encountered before, in ways that are appropriate to entirely novel circumstances.... Human languages have the property of including such a discrete infinity of distinct sentences because they are *hierarchical* and *recursive*. That is, the words of a sentence are not just strung out one after another, but are organized into phrases, which themselves can be constituents of larger phrases of the same type, and so on without any boundary.[18]

The result is "massive differences in expressive capacities between human language and the communicative systems of other animals":[19]

No other primate functions communicatively in nature even at the level of protolanguage, and the vast gulf of discrete, recursive combinability must still be crossed to get from there to the language capacity inherent in every normal human. We seem to be alone on our side of that gulf, whatever the evolutionary path we may have taken to get there.[20]

This ideational uniqueness involves complex use of symbols. Ian Tattersall concludes:

We human beings are indeed mysterious animals. We are linked to the living world, but we are sharply distinguished by our cognitive powers, and much of our behavior is conditioned by abstract and symbolic concerns.[21]

Similarly, Richard Potts concludes:

In discussing the evolution of human critical capacities, the overarching influence of symbolic activity (the means by which humans create meaning) is inescapable. Human cultural behavior involves not only the transmission of nongenetic information but also the coding of thoughts, sensations, and things, times, and places that are not visible. All the odd elaborations of human life, socially and individually, including the heights of imagination, the depths of depravity, moral abstraction, and a sense of God, depend on this *symbolic coding of the nonvisible*.[22]

This means of course that humans can form a symbolic sense of self, with its dignity.

The nature and origins of language is proving, according to some experts in the field, to be "the hardest problem in science."[23] Kuniyoshi L. Sakai finds: "The human left-frontal cortex is thus uniquely specialized in the syntactic processes of sentence comprehension, without any counterparts in other animals."[24] The result is our mental incandescence.

We now neuroimage blood brain flow to find that such thoughts can reshape the brains in which they arise. Genes make the kind of human brains possible that facilitate an open mind. But when that happens, these processes can also work the other way around. Minds employ and reshape their brains to facilitate their chosen ideologies and lifestyles. Our ideas and our deliberated practices configure and reconfigure our own sponsoring brain structures.

Joaquín M. Fuster, a neuroscientist, finds that in human brains there is an "emergent property" that is "most difficult to define":

> As networks fan outward and upward in associative neocortex, they become capable of generating novel representations that are not reducible to their inputs or to their individual neuronal components. Those representations are the product of complex, nonlinear, and near-chaotic interactions between innumerable elements of high-level networks far removed from sensory receptors or motor effectors. Then, top-down network building predominates. Imagination, creativity, and intuition are some of the cognitive attributes of those emergent high-level representations.[25]

This is what philosophers call "top down" causation (an emergent phenomenon reshaping and controlling its precedents), as contrasted with "bottom up" causation (simpler precedent causes fully determinative of more complex outcomes). Quantitative genetic differences add up to qualitative differences in capacity, an emerging cognitive possibility and practical performance that exceeds anything known in previous evolutionary achievements. This native endowment and potential, more and less actualized across a person's career, comes to constitute his or her dignity. Some trans-genetic threshold seems to have been crossed.

Geneticists decoded the human genome, confirming how little humans differ in their protein molecules from chimpanzees,* only to

---

* Humans may differ in protein molecules from chimpanzees by only some 3 percent. But they do have nearly 400 percent more cerebral cortex. Also, the microscopic fine structures of synaptic connections are much more open and complex; see Michael Balter, "Brain Evolution Studies Go Micro," *Science* 315(2007): 1208-1211. The human postsynaptic membrane contains over a thousand different proteins in the signal-receiving surface. "The most molecularly complex structure known [in the human body] is the postsynaptic side of the synapse," according to Seth Grant, a neuroscientist (quoted in Elizabeth Pennisi, "Brain

realize that the startling successes of humans doing just this sequencing of their own genome as readily proves human distinctiveness. Humans have made an exodus from determination by genetics and natural selection and passed into a mental and social realm with new freedoms.

J. Craig Venter and over 200 geneticist co-authors, completing the Celera Genomics sequencing of the human genome, caution:

> In organisms with complex nervous systems, neither gene number, neuron number, nor number of cell types correlates in any meaningful manner with even simplistic measures of structural or behavioral complexity.... Between humans and chimpanzees, the gene number, gene structures and functions, chromosomal and genomic organizations, and cell types and neuroanatomies are almost indistinguishable, yet the developmental modifications that predisposed human lineages to cortical expansion and development of the larynx, giving rise to language, culminated in a massive singularity that by even the simplest of criteria made humans more complex in a behavioral sense.... The real challenge of human biology, beyond the task of finding out how genes orchestrate the construction and maintenance of the miraculous mechanism of our bodies, will lie ahead as we seek to explain how our minds have come to organize thoughts sufficiently well to investigate our own existence.[26]

This "massive singularity" of our ideational uniqueness introduces massive dignity.

## Idiographic Uniqueness

*"Man, in a word, has no nature; what he has is...history."* José Ortega y Gasset pinpoints, with emphasis, the human idiographic uniqueness. He continues: "Expressed differently: what nature is to things, history, *res gestae,* is to man."[27] More carefully put, nature too has a

---

Evolution on the Far Side," *Science* 314 (2006): 244-245.

history—natural history, but humans superimpose on their nature a remarkable capacity to experience and to individuate their narrative careers. Humans have a capacity for enacted individuality that is not otherwise known in the animal world. This makes possible biography, transcending the biology on which it is superimposed.

Again, we must use some care. All nature is natural *history*, generating distinct individuals as well as historical times and geographical places, and one sometimes needs to make that point. Each bat is particular. A mother bat, who has been out all night catching insects, can return to Bracken Cave in Texas and find and feed her own pup in total darkness, among millions of other bat pups. Such animal skills result from the biological requirement that mothers and their young recognize each other, if the best-adapted are to survive. Humans and many animals have immunologically unique bodies. Such particularity is welcome in the natural world.

Meanwhile, humans remain unique in their escalated degrees of freedom, their voluntary intentional actions, guided by these new powers of cognitive and symbolic thought, analytic reason, and conscious aspiration. While most creatures respond to somatic biological and ecological circumstances, humans are drawn into a future by constructed visions of their fullest flourishing, by their ideologies. We enact ourselves as interpreted story; each person enjoys constructing his or her idiographic storied residence on Earth.

In the vocabulary of neuroscience, we map brains to discover that we have "mutable maps." Michael Merzenich, a neuroscientist, reports his increasing appreciation of "what is the most remarkable property of our brain: its capacity to develop and to specialize its own processing machinery, to shape its own abilities, and to enable, through hard brainwork, its own achievements."[28] For example, with the decision to play a violin well, and with resolute practice, string musicians alter the structural configuration of their brains, to facilitate the differential use of left and right arms, fingering the strings with one and drawing the bow with the other.[29] Likewise, musicians enhance their hearing sensitivity to tones, enlarging the relevant auditory cortex by 25% compared with non-musicians.[30]

With the decision to become a taxi driver in London, and with long experience driving about the city, drivers likewise alter their brain structures, devoting more space to navigation-related skills than do non-taxi drivers. "There is a capacity for local plastic change in the structure of the healthy adult human brain in response to environmental demands."[31] Similarly, researchers have found that "the structure of the human brain is altered by the experience of acquiring a second language."[32] Or by learning to juggle.[33]

So our minds shape our brains. The authors of a leading neuroscience text use the violin players as an icon for us all and conclude: "It is likely that this is an exaggerated version of a continuous mapping process that goes on in everyone's brain as their life experiences vary."[34] This brain is as open as it is wired up; the self we become is registered by its synaptic configurations, which is to say that the information from personal experience, both explicit and implicit, goes to pattern the brain. The informing of the mind, our psychological experiences reconfigure brain process, and there are no known limits to this global flexibility and interactivity. "Plasticity is an intrinsic property of the human brain."[35]

Nature endows human persons with the capacity for distinctively particular, self-reflective biographies. Embodied we humans are, and limited by flesh and blood, but there are no such limits to what humans can think or to the imagination of our minds. The possibility space is endlessly open. In a study of infinity, John D. Barrow considers what is in effect a mental infinity (though technically a massively large number):

> By counting the number of neural configurations that the human brain can accommodate, it has been estimated that it can represent about $10^{70,000,000,000,000}$ possible "thoughts"—for comparison there are only about $10^{80}$ atoms in the entire visible Universe. The brain is rather small, it contains only about $10^{27}$ atoms, but the feeling of limitless thinking that we possess derives not from this number alone but from the vastness of the number of possible connections that can exist between groups of atoms. This is what we mean by complexity, and it is the complexity of our minds that gives rise to that feeling that we are at the centre of unbounded immensities. We should not be surprised. Were our mind significantly simpler, then we would be too simple to know it.[36]

Animal minds are too simple to know such things. That we humans have such potential to forge endless thoughts and imaginations, and to incorporate these into our unique biographies, is evidence of our dignity.

Despite the contributions of science in confirming such uniqueness, this search for the dignity latent in idiographic uniqueness will not be straightforward science. Science has little interest in particulars for their particularity after they have been included as instances of a universal type. It has little interest, for instance, in proper names as essential to its content. An ethical account, however, will retain an interest in particulars both for their constitutive power in enriching the universal model and as loci of value. It admires proper names no less than theoretical models.

The human mind creates for itself a unique person, a human being placed in a community of other humans, with its own embodied self-consciousness in the midst of others equally idiographic. Humans are reared over decades in families, from which they acquire their identities, characters, habits, neighborhoods, networks of support, commitments, worldviews. Animals too can be social, but an animal's surroundings do not constitute for it this self-reflective ideational, narrative, biographical identity. The person can follow a biography, cradle to grave, as no animal can.

The person knows the name of his or her father, mother, sisters, brothers, hometown, the favored or disliked math teacher, the day of his or her marriage, a career (or hopes thereof). With chimpanzees, if a brother departs and disperses to another troop for a year and then returns, brother does not remember and recognize (re-cognize) brother. Chimps take their family and troop cues from whoever is nearby and do not have the concept of "brother." But humans cognize such family relationships; this family identity enters into their personal identity—a narrated story line. A human life makes sense from a distinctly individual point of view, in ways that differ from animal life.

Michael Tomasello continues:

> Any serious inquiry into human cognition, therefore, must include some account of these historical and ontogenetic processes, which are enabled but not in any way determined

by human beings' biological adaptation for a special form of cognition.... My central argument...is that it is these processes, not any specialized biological adaptations directly, that have done the actual work in creating many, if not all, of the most distinctive and cognitive products and processes of the species *Homo sapiens*.[37]

Other mammals are also constituted by their relationships, but they do not display these kinds of self-reflective cognitive understandings. We can form ideas of other minds, and of our own mind in encounter with other minds, and this, already by virtue of that capacity alone, accentuates human talents. But in the exercise of this skill, we form estimates of the embodied mental states in ourselves and in others whom we encounter. In such activity the possibility of dignity gained or lost arises.

Such powers and performance will variously be limited by disease, juvenile condition or aging, economic and cultural circumstances, failure of will, past successes and defeats, sometimes by coercion from others, but dignity can remain in the potential for development, for regeneration, or in the courage and resolution with which one faces such threats, struggling to retain a dignified quality of life.

## Existential Uniqueness

Only humans are "persons," enjoying "existential uniqueness." "Human being" is perhaps a biological term, but "person" refers to the further existential dignity associated with an experiencing subjectivity with personal identity, a phenomenological "I" conserved with ongoing agency and responsibility. We can wonder whether neuroscience has (or ever will have) access to how the multiple streams of perception, images, and ideas are melded into such an experiencing "I." Mark F. Bear and his colleagues, somewhat revealingly, call this problem "the Holy Grail of neuroscience."[38] The difficulty is in understanding how thoughts in the conscious mind form, re-form, or, more accurately, *in-form* events in this brain space to construct an inhabited first-person with direct self-awareness.

The term "personality" is sometimes used of animals, usually to mark individual variations of temperament, arousal, sociability, curiosity, and similar traits. Jennifer A. Mather and Roland C. Anderson give an account of the "personalities of octopuses."[39] They hardly intend that these are persons; rather they borrow that term to describe their differentiated individuality. This is more accentuated in higher animals. But such "personality" is a behavioral, not an existential claim, more metaphorical than literal.

With humans we need, somewhat provocatively, the term "spirit" to get past the consciousness that is present in animals and capture this self-reflective inwardness. We need what the Germans call *Geist* or what existentialist philosophers call *Existenz*. Each person has a lone ecstasy, an *ek-stasis,* a "standing out," an *existence,* where the I is differentiated from the not-I. Only in humans is there such *genius* (recalling the Latin connotations).

Animals do not feel ashamed or proud; they do not have angst. They do not get excited about a job well done, pass the buck for failures, have identity crises, or deceive themselves to avoid self-censure. They do not resolve to dissent before an immoral social practice and pay the price of civil disobedience in the hope of reforming their society. They do not say grace at meals. They do not act in love, faith, or freedom, nor are they driven by guilt or to seek forgiveness. They do not make confessions of faith. They do not conclude that the world is absurd and go into depression. They do not get lost on a "darkling plain" (Matthew Arnold, *Dover Beach*). They do not worry about whether they have souls, or whether these will survive their death. They do not reach poignant moments of truth.

Animal particularities are mute; humans can articulate their individual biographies. A person's narrated story line—with a normative fiction setting a gap between the real and the ideal, and introspectively orienting the real—produces a *persona,* a lived presence to which each self has privileged access. There is an immediately given self, always in encounter with opportunity and threat. We experience romance and tragedy. This idiographic inwardness becomes a proper-named Presence, an "I," an ego. Such an "I" confronts others as "Thou."[40] This is the elation of auto/bio/graphy, not yet intellectual in the child, often not in the adult, but always existential and impulsive from our psychic depths.

Neuroscience has imaged much of the brain, only to realize that it was imaging brains or, more accurately, blood flow in brains, and not thoughts articulated in the minds of persons. There has been little or no success in correlating the flow of mental representations (as when the story unfolds in a novel) with the details of neural architecture, even though one can map some of the synaptic connections and reconnections. What will neuroscientists think when, imaging their own thinking brains, they ask one another how it is that one species has gained the capacity to do this, discuss the significance of such neuroscience, and watch the brain images of their discussion? Neuroscientists too are existential selves, historical persons with careers, each a subjective "I" in the midst of "Thous," even when they make "it-objects" of their brains.

The capacity for one person to take the mind of another, mind-reading as it were, produces in humans their capacity to be insulted and belittled, or to be respected and treated with dignity. Not only can we learn from others, but we can learn what they think of us—not just how they treat us (animals can learn that), but their point of view toward us. I can take up the ideational perspective of others, but that means I can infer their ideational perspective toward me. Relationships become interpersonal.

Such a "person" can suffer affliction by verbal insult (including omissions), of which animals are incapable, although animals can be ostracized. A human being can self-reflect about his or her status and encountered behavior in the view of others. "I am being treated poorly here, perhaps because I am poor." "I wonder if I should complain, or just be glad to get minimal emergency room service." "I was wrong about that woman being a nurse; she's a doctor. The nurses are more respectful than are the doctors. They treat me like a real person." Animals have no such capacities.

Bertrand Russell analyzes how, with language, humans can experience themselves biographically and present that biographical self to others. Animals can do neither. "A dog cannot relate his autobiography; however eloquently he may bark, he cannot tell you that his parents were honest though poor."[41] But a person can tell you that; indeed, for many persons, the fact that they and their parents have been honest, though poor, is the linchpin of their dignity.

With humans, the medical therapist is likely to work with a patient's face, hands, genitalia with more awareness of personhood, as would not be the case for a veterinarian with animals—think of hands versus paws, for instance. The human face has evolved progressively refined features of self-expression, with more than thirty finely tuned muscles of facial expression and vocal control. This facilitates the subtle communication of moods, desires, intentions, personality, character. Animals too pick up subtle behavioral cues, as when they play, or when they recognize that a predator is hungry. But humans take a slur of profanity as an affront to their dignity—unless the remark is said with a sly smile, which can turn it into a compliment.

Within minutes of birth infants turn their heads and eyes toward faces, and within days they discriminate between the face of the mother and that of a stranger. Humans have a spectacular capacity to recognize faces; a person can distinguish his wife or his brother from any of the other six billion persons on Earth. Soon after birth, animals may imprint on parents; perhaps the human capacities arose from such animal precedents, initially selected for their survival value. Animals too notice eyes, and they react as if there is somebody there, even if they have no theory of mind. But such capacities for being present and for detecting presence in others—myself a person here, another person there—have in humans escalated into qualitatively different domains.

Animals do not have a sense of mutual gaze in the sense of joint attention, of "looking with." "Nonhuman primates in their natural habitats…do not point or gesture to outside objects for others; do not hold objects up to show them to others; do not try to bring others to locations so that they can observe things there; do not actively offer objects to other individuals by holding them out."[42] They do not negotiate the presence of an existential self, interacting interpersonally with other such agents, in the process of thinking about and pursuing goals in the world. Animals do see others in pursuit of the food, mates, or territories they wish to have; but they do not know that other minds are there, much less other spirits. This capacity for referencing others as distinct, intentional, existential selves like ourselves gives rise to an enhanced sense of the worth of such fellow humans, parallel to our own worth.

The principal focus of many discussions of human dignity is autonomy. A violation of such autonomy shuts down this distinctively human openness for particular life-imagination, construction, and responsibility. Violations of human dignity typically involve unjustified constraints on such chosen ideas, beliefs, attitudes, feelings. This may be by abuse, vilification, and ridicule, or by overlooking and neglect. Psychotropic drugs can be used to impose conformity and obedience. Medical treatment or hospital care can be insensitive to such freedom, so far as it remains in the patient.

Dignity is a threshold concept, at first. All humans have it, and no animals—at least not with those characteristics analyzed here. But it is also a relative concept. Some behaviors are more dignified than others; some activities are beneath our dignity. Here the phenomenological sense of self-identity enters, in the sense of a goal or norm to which we hold ourselves accountable. We find it difficult to say that some animal's behavior was undignified. But human beings, enacting their embodied lives, have the capacity to treat their own behavior, cognition, and careers as objects of contemplation for what they are in themselves; there is a dialectic of reflection and action. This makes possible "style" in presenting self to others, as when one makes an effort to dress, speak, and behave with dignity.

Animals may fit into their social hierarchies; they can be keenly aware of their relations with conspecifics. They take up roles. Coyotes may have a hierarchy problem in the pack, but a coyote does not have an ego problem, wondering if its behavior is beneath its dignity, or if it has been treated without dignity by the alpha male. Humans evolved to have dignity when they evolved to be able to entertain the concept of dignity (and to acknowledge dignity by way of respect, recognition, courtesy), as chimpanzees cannot.

Such self-presentation can become overstudied and artificial, so that dignity can collapse. We dislike those who project images. Dignity operates often best at subliminal levels; but, on occasion, it can be brought to mind and refined. It is always near enough the surface to be readily affronted. Inherent dignity may be latent, an endowment; but expressed dignity always requires some considered self-control, an achievement. We are always keeping up a broken wholeness. Animals may exemplify the potential of their species with more or less success, but we do not know of any parallels of such considered and controlled dignity in animal behavior.

## Ethical Uniqueness

Ethics is distinctively a product of the human genius, a phenomenon of our social behavior. To be ethical is to reflect on considered principles of right and wrong and to act accordingly, in the face of temptation. This is a possibility in all and only human life, so that we expect and demand that persons behave morally and hold them responsible for doing so. This is true even when, alas, they are tragically diminished in capacity and we cannot presume to hold them to what they ought to have been, or perhaps once were, at least aspirationally. Such an emergence of ethics is as remarkable as any other event we know; in some form or other ethics is pervasively present in every human culture, whether honored in the observance or in the breach. This fact looms large in human dignity.

In this, humans are unique; there is nowhere in animal behavior the capacity to be reflectively ethical. After a careful survey of behavior, Helmut Kummer concludes, "It seems at present that morality has no specific functional equivalents among our animal relatives."[43] Peter Singer's *Ethics* has a section called "Common Themes in Primate Ethics," including a section on "Chimpanzee Justice," and he wants to "abandon the assumption that ethics is uniquely human."[44] But many of the behaviors examined (helping behavior; dominance structures) are more pre-ethical than ethical; he has little or no sense of holding chimpanzees morally culpable or praiseworthy.

Frans de Waal finds precursors of morality, but concludes:

> Even if animals other than ourselves act in ways tantamount to moral behavior, their behavior does not necessarily rest on deliberations of the kind we engage in. It is hard to believe that animals weigh their own interests against the rights of others, that they develop a vision of the greater good of society, or that they feel lifelong guilt about something they should not have done. Members of some species may reach tacit consensus about what kind of behavior to tolerate or inhibit in their midst, but without language the principles behind such decisions cannot be conceptualized, let alone debated.[45]

As before with "culture" and with "teaching," finding "ethics" in nature is partly a matter of discovering previously unknown animal behavior, but mostly a matter of redefining and stretching what the word "ethics" means to cover behavioral adjustments in social groups.

Christopher Boehm finds that in some primate groups not only is there dominance hierarchy, but there are controls to keep such hierarchy working because this produces arrangements that the primates can live with, improving their overall success. Chimpanzees fight with each other over food and mates; but fighting is unpleasant, so the chimps will allow the dominant to break up such fights. If, however, the dominant becomes overly aggressive, the chimps will gang up on the dominant, who can control one but not several arrayed against him. The result is more "egalitarian behavior."[46] Perhaps such behaviors are the precursors out of which such maxims as "treat equals equally; treat unequals equitably" once emerged, but it must be equally clear that such chimps are orders of magnitude away from deliberate reflection on how to treat others fairly, respecting their rights, much less their dignity.

After her years of experience with chimpanzees, and though she found among them pair bonding, grooming, and the pleasure of the company of others, Jane Goodall wrote: "I cannot conceive of chimpanzees developing emotions, one for the other, comparable in any way to the tenderness, the protectiveness, tolerance, and spiritual exhilaration that are the hallmarks of human love in its truest and deepest sense. Chimpanzees usually show a lack of consideration for each other's feelings which in some ways may represent the deepest part of the gulf between them and us."[47]

Higher animals realize that the behavior of other animals can be altered, and they do what they can to shape such behavior. So relationships evolve that set behavioral patterns in animal societies—dominance hierarchies, for example, or ostracism from a pack or troop. But it is not within the animal capacity to become a reflective agent interacting with a society of similar reflective agents, knowing that other actors, like oneself, are (if normal) able to choose between options and bear responsibility for their behavior. Nor is there among nonhuman animals any cultural or ideological heritage to defend.

Animals lack awareness that there are mental others whom one might hold responsible. Or to whom one might be held responsible. This precludes any critical sense of justice, or in general of values that could and ought to be fairly shared because they are enjoyed by others who, like oneself, are the existential subjects of their own lives. Even more, this lack precludes respecting the dignity of others as part of moral responsibility. Such consideration is not a possibility in their private worlds, nor is a morally binding social contract such as that in inter-human ethics. Yet all this, undeniably, has emerged within the human genius.

Persons set up a reflective gap between the real and the ideal. The human must be moral, however brokenly the ideal mixes with the real, and in that consists the human dignity. So we find in persons an agent who must be oriented by a belief system, as animals are not, and that leaves us, in the end, with the question of how to authorize such a belief system. Ethics is essential to the human genius; we cannot realize our dignity without it. To put this provocatively, not only are the animals pre-ethical, but even humans when operating as scientists are pre-ethical. For centuries we have been welcoming scientific insights into our apparent uniqueness, into how our human nature evolved out of animal nature. But in the end we find that science not only struggles to understand how amoral nature evolved the moral animal, but finds itself incompetent to analyze how even now *Homo sapiens* has duties, how to set up and resolve that reflective tension between real and ideal.

Science and conscience have a complex, elusive relationship. Science needs conscience but cannot justify it. The *is-ought* divide continues, past, present, and future. Humans crossed it during their evolutionary history and now live in moral territory. That is dignity by heritage and endowment. But such endowment potential has to be made actual, generation after generation, in each new age, in each human life, lest we lose our dignity. After four hundred years of science and enlightenment, the value questions in the 21st century remain as sharp and as painful as ever. Not the least of such questions is how to recognize and to respect human dignity. Much in our future depends on the answer.

# Notes

[1] Immanuel Kant, *The Metaphysics of Morals* (1797), Part II: "The Metaphysical Principles of Virtue," in Kant, *Ethical Philosophy*, trans. James W. Ellington (Indianapolis, Indiana: Hackett, 1983), p. 127.
[2] United Nations General Assembly, *Universal Declaration of Human Rights*, General Assembly Resolution 217 A (III), 10 December, 1948 (New York: United Nations General Assembly Official Records, 1948), available online at www.un.org/Overview/rights.html.
[3] Indeed, some complain that human dignity is a vague and ill-defined concept, so much so that people on all sides of disputes about it claim the term for their own view. See Ruth Macklin, "Dignity is a Useless Concept," *BMJ* 327 (2003): 1419-1420; Doron Shultziner, "Human dignity—functions and meanings," *Global Jurist Topics* 3 (2003), 1-21; Timothy Caulfield and Audrey Chapman, "Human Dignity as a Criterion for Science Policy," *PLoS Medicine (Public Library of Science)* 2 (2005): 736-738, available online at dx.doi.org/10.1371/journal.pmed.0020244.
[4] Peter J. Richerson and Robert Boyd, *Not by Genes Alone: How Culture Transformed Human Evolution* (Chicago: University of Chicago Press, 2005), pp. 126, 195.
[5] *Chimpanzee Cultures*, ed. Richard W. Wrangham, William C. McGrew, Frans B. M. de Waal, and Paul G. Heltne (Cambridge, Massachusetts: Harvard University Press, 1994), p. 2.
[6] Alex Thornton and Katherine McAuliffe, "Teaching in Wild Meerkats," *Science* 313 (2006): 227-229.
[7] Tim M. Caro and Marc D. Hauser, "Is There Teaching in Nonhuman Animals?" *Quarterly Review of Biology* 67 (1992): 151-174.
[8] Nigel R. Franks and Tom Richardson, "Teaching in Tandem-running Ants," *Nature* 439 (2006): 153.
[9] Bennett G. Galef, Jr., "The Question of Animal Culture," *Human Nature* 3 (1992): 157-178, p. 161; similarly in Gretchen Vogel, "Chimps in the Wild Show Stirrings of Culture," *Science* 284 (1999): 2070-2073.
[10] Richard Byrne, *The Thinking Ape: Evolutionary Origins of Intelligence* (New York: Oxford University Press, 1995), pp. 141, 146, 154.
[11] Michael Tomasello, Ann Cale Kruger, and Hilary Horn Ratner, "Cultural Learning," *Behavioral and Brain Sciences* 16 (1993): 495-552, pp. 504-505.
[12] Michael Tomasello, *The Cultural Origins of Human Cognition* (Cambridge, Massachusetts: Harvard University Press, 1999), p. 21.
[13] Daniel J. Povinelli, Jesse M. Bering, and Steve Giambrone, "Toward a Science of Other Minds: Escaping the Argument from Analogy," *Cognitive Science* 24 (2000): 509-541, p. 509; Daniel J. Povinelli and Jennifer Vonk, "Chimpanzee Minds: Suspiciously Human?" *Trends in Cognitive Sciences* 7 (2003): 157-160.
[14] Marc D. Hauser, *The Evolution of Communication* (Cambridge, Massachusetts: MIT Press, 1996); Donald R. Griffin, *Animal Minds*, 2nd ed. (Chicago: University

of Chicago Press, 2001).

[15] Terrence W. Deacon, *The Symbolic Species: The Co-evolution of Language and the Brain* (New York: Norton, 1997), p. 21.

[16] Mark Twain, *Following the Equator and Anti-imperialist Essays* (New York: Oxford University Press, 1996[1897]), p. 256.

[17] Blaise Pascal, *Pensées*, trans. William F. Trotter (New York: Dutton, 1958[1670]), pensée no. 347, p. 97.

[18] Stephen R. Anderson, *Doctor Dolittle's Delusion: Animals and the Uniqueness of Human Language* (New Haven, Connecticut: Yale University Press, 2004), pp. 2-8.

[19] Ibid., p. 11.

[20] Ibid., p. 318.

[21] Ian Tattersall, *Becoming Human: Evolution and Human Uniqueness* (New York: Harcourt Brace, 1998), p. 3.

[22] Richard Potts, "Sociality and the Concept of Culture in Human Origins," in *The Origins and Nature of Sociality*, ed. Robert W. Sussman and Audrey R. Chapman (New York: Aldine de Gruyter, 2004), p. 263.

[23] Morten H. Christiansen and Simon Kirby, "Language Evolution: The Hardest Problem in Science?" in *Language Evolution*, ed. Morten H. Christiansen and Simon Kirby (New York: Oxford University Press, 2003), pp. 1-15.

[24] Kuniyoshi L. Sakai, "Language Acquisition and Brain Development," *Science* 310 (2005): 815-819, p. 817.

[25] Joaquín M. Fuster, *Cortex and Mind: Unifying Cognition* (New York: Oxford University Press, 2003), p. 53.

[26] J. Craig Venter, et al., "The Sequence of the Human Genome," *Science* 291 (2001): 1304-1351, pp. 1347-1348.

[27] José Ortega y Gasset, "History as a System," in *Philosophy and History: Essays Presented to Ernst Cassirer*, ed. Raymond Klibansky and Herbert J. Paton (New York: Harper and Row, 1963[1936]), p. 313.

[28] Michael A. Merzenich, "The Power of Mutable Maps," in Mark F. Bear, Barry W. Connors, and Michael Paradiso, *Neuroscience: Exploring the Brain*, 2nd ed. (Baltimore, Maryland: Lippincott Williams & Wilkins, 2001), p. 418.

[29] Thomas Elbert, et al., "Increased Cortical Representation of the Fingers of the Left Hand in String Players," *Science* 270 (1995): 305-307.

[30] Christo Pantev, et al., "Increased Auditory Cortical Representation in Musicians," *Nature* 392 (1998): 811-814.

[31] Eleanor A. Maguire, et al., "Navigation-Related Structural Change in the Hippocampi of Taxi Drivers," *Proceedings of the National Academy of Sciences of the United States of America* 97 (2000): 4398-4403.

[32] Andrea Mechelli, et al., "Structural Plasticity in the Bilingual Brain," *Nature* 431 (2004): 757.

[33] Bogdan Draganski, et al., "Changes in Grey Matter Induced by Training," *Nature* 427 (2004): 311-312.

[34] Bear, Connors, and Paradiso, op. cit., p. 418.

[35] Alvaro Pascual-Leone, et al., "The Plastic Human Brain Cortex," *Annual Review*

*of Neuroscience* 28 (2005): 377-401, p. 377.

[36] John D. Barrow, *The Infinite Book* (New York: Pantheon Books, 2005), p. 19; cf. Mike Holderness, "Think of a Number," *New Scientist* 170 (2001): 45, and Owen Flanagan, *Consciousness Reconsidered* (Cambridge, Massachusetts: MIT Press, 1992), p. 3.

[37] Tomasello, *Cultural Origins*, p. 11.

[38] Bear, Connors, and Paradiso, op. cit., p. 434.

[39] Jennifer A. Mather and Roland C. Anderson, "Personalities of Octopuses (*Octopus rubescens*)," *Journal of Cognitive Psychology* 107 (1993): 336-340.

[40] Martin Buber, *I and Thou*, trans. Walter Kaufmann (New York: Charles Scribner's Sons, 1970).

[41] Bertrand Russell, *Human Knowledge: Its Scope and Limits* (New York: Simon & Schuster, 1948), p. 60.

[42] Tomasello, *Cultural Origins*, p. 21.

[43] Helmut Kummer, "Analogs of Morality Among Nonhuman Primates," in *Morality as a Biological Phenomenon*, ed. Gunther S. Stent (Berkeley, California: University of California, 1980), pp. 31-47, at p. 45.

[44] Peter Singer, *Ethics* (New York: Oxford University Press, 1994), p. 6.

[45] Frans de Waal, *Good Natured: The Origins of Right and Wrong in Humans and Other Animals* (Cambridge, Massachusetts: Harvard University Press, 1996), p. 209.

[46] Christopher Boehm, *Hierarchy in the Forest: The Evolution of Egalitarian Behavior* (Cambridge, Massachusetts: Harvard University Press, 1999).

[47] Jane van Lawick-Goodall, *In the Shadow of Man* (Boston: Houghton Mifflin, 1971), p. 194.

# 7

# Human Dignity and the Future of Man

## Charles Rubin

We are accustomed to the fact that modern science and technology allow people to lead healthier, wealthier and even happier lives by reducing disease and disability and opening up new opportunities for thought and action. Furthermore, we expect the future to look like the past in this respect, perhaps even more so as our knowledge of nature expands. So it is hardly surprising to find that expected advances in biotechnology focus on gene therapies to correct heritable defects,[1] or that nanotechnology promises tiny machines that could monitor our health or repair cell damage from the inside,[2] or that artificial intelligence and robotics are being developed to enhance the mobility of those with missing or non-functioning limbs.[3] What is surprising is that, in some quarters, speculation about the uses of these technologies embraces the ardent hope that human beings will soon arrange to replace themselves with a vastly improved "Mark II" version. Even a healthy human being, these enthusiasts reason, is subject to all kinds of limits that we can imagine overcoming. Why be satisfied with senses that perceive in the limited range of our own?[4] Why accept that we must sleep, eat and excrete as we now do?[5] Why be content with the clumsy media of spoken or written language for learning and for the exchange of our thoughts?[6] Why not be fully happy all the time rather than intermittently and imperfectly?[7] Why not become a computer program that could travel the stars at the speed of light?[8] Why ever die?[9]

For a small but growing number of writers and thinkers—who refer to themselves as transhumanists,[10] extropians,[11] or singularitarians,[12]—the answers to these questions are more or less obvious, and the solutions are to be found in future science and technology. They do not see themselves as idle day-dreamers; for they believe that the force of necessity stands behind their hopes for self-directed evolution to some better form of life not subject to present limitations. They claim that our ever-increasing knowledge of how nature works puts us on a very slippery slope. The nanotechnology that might be used to repair a damaged eye, or the robotics that might replace a lost limb, could just as readily be used to enhance our vision or increase our strength beyond "normal." And a technology that can be used to enhance an existing capacity will likely add entirely new abilities.[13] Thus, human beings are on the verge of a "transhuman" transformation that will, because of the ever-accelerating rate of technological development, at no greatly distant date lead us to a "posthuman" future in which intelligence far beyond our own will be embodied in forms we can barely begin to imagine. Perhaps minds will one day be downloaded as "software" into far more durable, flexible and capable machines.[14] Perhaps future lives will be lived in virtual realities, or in hybrid realms where the distinction between "virtual" and "real" will have become meaningless.[15] Some day the individual consciousnesses of our "mind children" may be able to mix and meld, even with the consciousnesses of other animals, into a group mind.[16] The search for ever greater computational power could lead our descendants to overcome the speed of light in order to "saturate the universe with our intelligence."[17] They might use a neutron star as an "immense simulator" modeling Earth at the atomic scale, able to run its history backward and forward, providing for "wholesale resurrection" of the "long dead."[18] If human beings as we know them survive at all in this new world—and it is hard to say why we would, given the wonders that are held up before us if we consent to abandon our mere humanity—it will be as mere epigones and curiosities.

In the face of these thinkers' fantastic hopes and visions of the future, it might appear that a notion of "human dignity" would prove useful in restraining their excesses and bringing their most extravagant thinking back down to earth. Yet, interestingly, the transhumanists themselves claim to be friends and defenders of human dignity—at least as they understand it. But the more seriously we take their conception of human dignity, the more problematic it becomes. On the other hand, as we shall see, its very defects point the way to something more solid. Let us therefore examine the transhumanist conception of human dignity: where it comes from and where it leads; how it undermines itself; and what sounder notion of dignity emerges from the wreckage.

# I

First of all, the transhumanist advocates of *de facto* human extinction follow the lead of thinkers like Bacon and Descartes in believing themselves to be the true defenders of human dignity against all the indignities imposed on us by the naturally given: disease, deprivation, decay, and death. They see the story of humanity as the triumphant tale of an organism unwilling to accept these limitations on their own terms and progressively gaining greater power to confront and eventually overcome them. We are, on their view, the resourceful beings who can become ever increasingly the masters and possessors of nature, including our own nature. We are consummate problem solvers who have come to understand how much better things would have been if someone had asked *us* how they should be arranged, and who can solve the ultimate problem of our own defective natures.[19]

From this point of view, rectifying the flaws in our design is simply the next logical step in what human beings as such have always done. Indeed, it is precisely this rejection of resignation, this capacity for perpetual problem-solving and self-overcoming, that makes human beings worthy of respect in the first place, that gives us our *dignity*. For otherwise, we are no more deserving of dignity than any other randomly evolved living configuration of matter that has come down the pike.

A certain kind of skeptic might answer that to introduce any moral valuation into this description of what we are—to reason from the fact that we *are* beings who can take charge of our own destiny to the conclusion that we *should* do so, and that our dignity *consists* in our doing so—would be to violate the distinction between facts and values, one of the bedrock assumptions of modern natural science and of much contemporary moral philosophy. In a universe of matter, motion and chance, one is not permitted to derive an "ought" from an "is"; put simply, there is no such thing as natural right. But transhumanism has an answer of sorts to this scruple. For in demonstrating our worth by using our intelligence to improve on nature, we introduce conscious purpose into a universe that was formed without it. The brute facts of randomly configured nature thus give way before the values imposed on matter by intellect, and through science we make the "is" into what it "ought" to be.

It is important to understand that the universe thus remanufactured would be unlikely to strike any human being presently alive as more comprehensibly good or right than that in which we live today, if only because it would be so totally alien to anything we know. To their credit, the transhumanists acknowledge this point. For many of them, the transformation to posthumanity represents a huge discontinuity, a historical "singularity."* The capacities of our posthuman, self-optimizing successors will exceed our own by orders of magnitude comparable to the gulf between humans and bacteria. It follows that present humanity would be as incapable of comprehending the posthuman world of the future as bacteria are of comprehending ours.[20†]

It appears, then, that while in the near term transhumanists are content to rely on technology to make our lives better in ways that conform to our all too human desires, for the longer term the

---

* Vernor Vinge is usually credited with this insight. His presentation of it differs significantly from the manner of presentation by Kurzweil, e.g., in his recognition that for humans the outcome could be "…pretty bad. The physical extinction of the human race is one possibility…. Yet physical extinction may not be the scariest possibility. Again, analogies: Think of the different ways we relate to animals. Some of the crude physical abuses are implausible, yet…." Vernor Vinge, "Vernor Vinge on the Singularity" (1993), online at www.mindstalk.net/vinge/vinge-sing.html.

† Vinge, for his part, thinks the singularity may not be so incomprehensible; a posthuman world "could well be still comprehensible to a broad-minded human with enough time and desire to learn." Yet he makes the significant qualification that "there could be things our minds aren't big enough to grasp, ideas we don't have the memory to hold the parts of; there could be Powers capable of thinking faster than we do." That surely suggests effective incomprehensibility so long as humans are mortal and limited as they presently are. See www.mindstalk.net/vinge/antising.html.

extraordinary good to be achieved by the transformation of ourselves and our world must be taken more or less on faith.* That might sound reassuring to those who expect that, over the next years and decades, technological advances will continue to ease our lot without radically altering our nature. For them it is enough to know that we are steadily curing more illnesses, or growing more wheat per acre, or extracting more miles per gallon. From this pragmatic point of view, the propensity to speculate about distant prospects will make any discussion of transhumanist radicalism seem like a harmless (though useless) diversion.

But once the transhumanist challenge has been laid down and the road to posthumanity marked out, what is the ground for dismissing it in this way? To assert now that we know what will be technologically impossible in the future is a well-recognized fool's argument. To ignore what look like distant and unlikely prospects ("sufficient unto the day...") is to risk *assuming* that the transhumanists are wrong. But the transhumanists will reply that the accelerating rate of technological change could well mean that their desired future is less distant than it seems,† and they may well be right. More important, those who too hastily dismiss the transhumanist agenda run the risk of *assuming* that the transhumanists are wrong about the slippery slope that runs from therapy to enhancement to transformation of human nature. It may be naïve to assume that, in the absence of scientific/technical "stopping points" along the way, there will be moral ones to restrain us in our march toward self-reinvention.

---

* Contrary to Kurzweil, e.g., who claims that "being a Singularitarian is not a matter of faith but one of understanding" (Kurzweil, *Singularity*, 370, full citation in endnote 12 below). What the Singularitarian understands is that it is "our destiny now to evolve into the vast intelligence of the Singularity" (Kurzweil, op. cit., p. 298). A great deal of effort is made to show how the development of posthumanity is necessary by those who also regard it as highly desirable. Such arguments, and their persuasive power, are well presented in Joel Garreau, *Radical Evolution: The Promise and Peril of Enhancing Our Minds, Our Bodies—and What it Means to be Human* (New York: Doubleday, 2005).

† The point of Garreau's "the Curve" (Garreau, op. cit., pp. 47-77) and of Kurzweil's "Law of Accelerating Returns" (Kurzweil, op. cit., pp. 7-14) is that the speed of technological development is increasing exponentially; new technology allows the next generation to develop that much faster. So, for example, by 2030 Kurzweil expects totally immersive virtual realities, brains enhanced by nanobots, and direct sharing of sensory experience.

There is in fact no guarantee that any moral considerations restraining present-day technological development will hold sway in the future—all the more so given already powerful intellectual trends that deny the very possibility of rational moral judgment in the first place.[21] Even today the warning signs are apparent; there is already powerful and growing resistance to any attempt to direct and restrict science and technology "on moral grounds." Beyond that, the transhumanists catch a glimpse of something that the pragmatically-minded observer of the scientific scene is likely to miss. The transhumanists have fully assimilated the lesson of J. B. S. Haldane's reading of the moral meaning of technological progress in his famous 1923 essay, "Daedalus, or Science and the Future." Haldane's Nietzschian lesson can be summed up simply: Science creates new moral orders as it enlarges our capacities for thought and action; when it comes to discoveries and inventions, what starts as perversion ends as ritual. But science is also inherently destructive of those new moral orders as well, always pushing beyond to some new possibility.[22]

This argument may well prove wrong, but it is far from simple to refute. Neither is it terribly alien to the relativism that is practically the default mode of moral belief for a great many educated Westerners. This relativism, allied with the commercial, military and intellectual forces that so effectively drive technological development today, makes saying "no" to any new thing very difficult. So the fact that the transhumanists are openly agitating for the extinction and supersession of the present human species may be just the sort of thing that could spur a search for clarity about the real meaning of "human dignity." Otherwise—just as the transhumanists expect—there are so many good and enticing things to be achieved on the road to posthumanity, including longer, healthier, wealthier lives filled with undreamt-of opportunities and choices, that merely by allowing people the freedom to do as they please we may pave the way to a redesigned humanity without ever directly intending to.[23]

We have seen so far how—by defining human dignity in terms of ceaseless self-overcoming—the transhumanists open the door to an incomprehensible human future. In so doing, they deprive the term "dignity" of any determinate moral meaning. Nevertheless, the conjectured "happiness" of our descendants proves serviceable to the transhumanists for cultivating a low opinion of human beings as we now are. If (they assure us) there were all that much to be said for humanity "Mark I," their advocacy of our obsolescence would be far less vociferous. But, as Nick Bostrom informs us,

> Nature's gifts are sometimes poisoned and should not always be accepted. Cancer, malaria, dementia, aging, starvation, unnecessary suffering, cognitive shortcomings are all among the presents that we wisely refuse. Our own species-specified natures are a rich source of much of the thoroughly unrespectable and unacceptable—susceptibility for disease, murder, rape, genocide, cheating, torture, racism.[24]

Given the many flaws and vulnerabilities of man as we know him, were we to fail to strive or fail in our striving to escape our plight and overcome our defective nature, we would eventually be squashed like bugs, in some sense deservedly, by some random cosmic catastrophe like a stray comet hitting Earth, or by the self-destructive human behaviors rooted in our own outmoded evolutionary design. There is no God-created or God-supported providential order. Blind nature does not care for our well-being and did not make us perfect for all time; the very forces of nature that gave rise to us will eventually destroy us.

So the transhumanist conception of human dignity that takes its bearings from what we can be goes hand in hand with a contemptuous attitude toward what we actually are. School children have long been instructed as to the modest value of the heap of chemicals that make up our body; pound for pound we are worth far less than many varieties of inanimate matter (never mind that we are the ones doing the valuing). More recently they have also been enlightened as to just how much DNA we share with chimps or even frogs, so as to inculcate the lesson that we are not so different from other living things, despite what prideful "species-ism" might tell us. The transhumanists would no doubt applaud such lessons pointing out the commonness and ordinariness of human nature, for they are merely the flip side of their view that the core of dignity is the rebellion against nature. But the conviction that there is nothing special about man threatens to make all our supposedly dignified striving look merely like boastfulness and species self-deception. Give bacteria the right medium, and their numbers will expand too. Viewed from the outside, what human civilizations do is really not that different from what invasive living things do whenever they are given a chance, that is to say, modify and adapt to their environments so as to produce ever more favorable conditions for expanding numbers. Nor should that thought surprise us, as it is but a consequence of the "decentering" of humanity in the cosmic scheme of things that played such a central part in the development of modern science. Compare Alan Gregg's famous speculation (in 1955) that "The world has cancer and the cancer is man"[25] with Haldane's yet earlier remark (in 1927) that "At worst our earth is only a very small septic area in the universe, which could be sterilized without very great trouble, and conceivably is not even worth sterilizing."[26] Essentially the same thought is to be found in the recent film *The Matrix* (1999), where Agent Smith describes the human race as a virus, a disease, a cancer of the planet.\*

In this way, the logic of the new transhumanist dignity turns back on itself. Are we uniquely striving, or are we merely typically invasive? What does it mean to say that our dignity resides in the fact that by nature we strive to overcome our nature? What seems to come through most clearly is that the misery of what we are should drive us to be something else. Or to put it another way, the human dignity defended by advocates of scientific and technological transcendence is a cattle-prod humanitarianism that has contempt for what we are in the name of the unfathomable things we could become.

## II

The new transhumanist dignity arises first and foremost from self-conscious negation. That marks it off quite clearly from older meanings

---

\* Agent Smith: "I'd like to share a revelation I had, during my time here. It came to me when I tried to classify your species. I realized that you're not actually mammals. Every mammal on this planet instinctively develops a natural equilibrium with the surrounding environment, but you humans do not. You move to an area and you multiply until every natural resource is consumed. The only way you can survive is to spread to another area. There is another organism on this planet that follows the same pattern. Do you know what it is? A virus. Human beings are a disease, a cancer of this planet. And we are the cure." *The Matrix* (directed by Andy and Larry Wachowski, Warner Bros. and Village Roadshow Pictures, 1999).

of dignity, which revolved around affirmations of what was owed to particular kinds or classes of human beings. One had dignity if one was of "the dignity," one of the usually small class whose conventional or natural distinction from others made them worthy of due regard or respect from others and of honor from their own. At first glance, the new transhumanist dignity follows in the democratic footsteps already suggested by the very phrase "human dignity," which surely would have sounded paradoxical to those who believed their dignity set them apart from everyone else. Evidently the hoped-for truth that human beings as such possess dignity is not *immediately* evident to human beings as such. It is perhaps conceptually easiest to overcome the aristocratic origins of dignity if "human dignity" comes to be understood as a revealed truth about God's equal regard for all human beings. Alternatively, one can have recourse to a notion of dignity built on certain inalienable rights that we possess by nature. But for reasons already articulated, neither of these sources of inherent human dignity (God or nature) is available to the transhumanist.

Is there a transhumanist foundation for democratized dignity? Actually, there is more reason to suspect that transhuman dignity is in some loose sense aristocratic in the older fashion. In the future, "the dignity" will be the enhanced and the redesigned, and any mere unimproved humans who manage to remain will likely be treated with pity and condescension.* Indeed, for some transhumanists, humanity's ability to reconstruct itself introduces a new kind of *noblesse oblige*. The dignity of self-creation requires us to strive to expand the circle of those freed from the misery and unhappiness of natural contingency, including not only our fellow humans but also members of animal species not hitherto endowed with dignity at all. For these transhumanists who have taken philanthropy to the next level, we have a moral obligation to engage in "uplift" efforts, at least to free other animals from fear and deprivation, and perhaps even to redesign them in such a way as to place them on the path of infinite self-improvement.[27]

---

* See Garreau's account of what it may be like for a second grader of today to go to law school in fifteen years with "enhanced" fellow students: "Her new friends are polite when she can't keep up with their conversations, as if she were handicapped. They can't help but condescend to her, however, when she protests that embedded technology is not natural for humans." Garreau, *Radical Evolution*, p. 8.

Nevertheless, despite this sense of obligation to enhance the dignity of their fellows, both within the human race and beyond, the transhumanists are reluctant to own up forthrightly to aspirations to become elite and beneficent supermen; much of their rhetoric is devoted to establishing their democratic credentials. The effort is largely, though not completely, successful because of their wholehearted adoption of the democratic principle of "doing as you like." If creative self-overcoming is the source of our dignity, there will be an infinite variety of ways to be dignified. There are no absolute standards governing what one's given nature is to be replaced by. News reports of a recent transhumanist gathering featured an individual who calls himself Cat Man. By the crude methods now available, he has been tattooed and surgically altered so as to vaguely resemble a cat; he is evidently on the lookout for a workable tail.[28] If Cat Man is dignified, then Dog Man and Deer Man can hardly be far behind. We see in transhumanism the libertarian relativism that follows naturally from this obsession with freedom (or that prompts it), where the spirit of enhancement and modification is essentially "anything goes" so long as it is freely chosen (some would add "and safe and effective"). Nobody is to be forced to be enhanced, nobody is to be forced not to be enhanced.[29] Individual choice—mere will—is the final arbiter, with due deference to the liberal principle of not harming others (at least against their wills).

So the worth of an individual is shown in the perpetual overcoming of the self in whatever manner the self wishes, a paradoxical position likely to result either in restless dissatisfaction or principled unhappiness. Furthermore, more is at stake than literal "self" overcoming. As it is undignified to accept what nature produces by chance, it is crucial to the transhumanist agenda that parents be encouraged to design their own children genetically. If it remains an open question whether the children, like their parents presumably contemptuous of the given, will be grateful to their parents for designing them, at least they will at some point be able to exercise their own powers of reconstruction, if the transhumanists have their way. Then again, perhaps those who want to design their progeny will look for someone more tractable.

And yet there is also a deeper paradox here, for the modern scientific materialism on which the hopes of these transformations depend is hard to enlist in the cause of "free choice." We are, they tell us, bound by the same natural laws that bind all other matter. The brain is a very complex computation machine, but a machine nonetheless. While there are scientists who attempt to find room in the interstices of physics for freedom,[30] it is hard to see how transhumanists—committed as they are to materialism—can see freedom and even self-consciousness as anything other than "user illusion."[31] Some indeed explicitly call into question the existence of a core, choosing "self."[32] From this point of view, the dignity owed to an individual consists in the exercise of a free choice that is likely not free, in order to negate and refashion a self that is likely not a self.

So even as the transhumanist vision of dignity envisages an ever-ascending chain of self-overcoming beings that suggests a new aristocratic order, it also fragments our sense of self and splinters the human race into a multitude of isolated self-overcomers, lest a shared choice not appear to be my authentic expression of self-overcoming. That is a significant departure from the old understanding of dignity, aristocratic or democratic, which expressed and embodied dignity in actual public and private relations. The act of negation from which the new transhumanist dignity arises comes from an impulse that is entirely aspirational. In technologized and democratized form, the dignity that is sought characterizes no real persons or relationships, but rather is based on imaginative negation of the characteristics of real persons and relationships. While dignity in this sense certainly avoids the danger of becoming a source of inertia in ossified or even oppressive social and political systems, the price of being so progressive is that it can never flourish comfortably in any enduring here and now.

Which is presumably the point, given that there is, according to the transhumanists, so little of value in the actual here and now. But we are again forced to conclude that the new transhumanist dignity is in effect nothing more than a leap of faith. Transhumanists would deny that, of course, pointing out that human ingenuity in the past has often solved problems once thought insurmountable. Were it not so, we would "still be picking lice off each other's backs."[33] Yet, while transhumanists are only too happy to provide reassurance that their critics are presenting nothing but imaginary horribles, their future of unknowable posthuman dignity can hardly even be said to be grounded in imagination. (Indeed, there is a body of transhumanist criticism of *merely* imaginative science fiction visions of the future such as *Star Trek*.[34]) For, unlike serious fiction writers, the transhumanists want to dismiss inconvenient lessons of experience or history that might restrain speculative hopes about novel technical possibilities. That is why, contrary to its intention, the vision of the future inherent in the new transhumanist dignity cannot genuinely be called progressive. We can judge something as progress when it brings us closer to some goal, but transhumanism at the deepest level is goal-less. Hence it can really promise only change.

## III

The new transhumanist dignity starts from an important question. What does it mean that human beings can engage in self-overcoming as a species and as individuals? And it is certainly not wrong in that connection to question the beneficence of the naturally given. But a notion of dignity whose default mode is to negate whatever is present in the name of an unspecifiable future is not really attempting serious answers to these questions. What we have found to be *missing* from the new transhumanist dignity, however, suggests an outlook on human dignity that could support serious reflection to counterbalance the inhuman possibilities inherent in the relentless march of science and technology. Such serious reflection would provide a basis for addressing whether the undoubted changes the future holds for us can be called genuine progress, and not merely change.

As we have seen, the new transhumanist dignity is minimally concerned with moral judgment of what people do with themselves, or how they do it, judging instead according to what transcends the given and what does not. But human dignity ought in fact to be a term of finer discrimination, requiring that people be treated in accordance with *what is due to them*. When we deny the moral relevance of the conventional distinctions that in aristocratic ages marked out "the dignity," we readily fall into the trap of denying the moral relevance of any and all observable distinctions among human beings. The recognition that such a thing as "human dignity" exists, however, ought to imply that *as human beings* we deserve to be given *our due*—and that is, as any reader of *Charlotte's Web* knows, something not routinely extended to other animals. Human dignity implies that we are morally responsible beings, worthy of judging what others do and are, and of being judged for what we do and are. Thus the equal possession of dignity by human beings provides the opportunity for moral discrimination among them. Accordingly, for human beings, the recognition of equal dignity does not have the same result as love. Doubtless there is something owed to people simply in light of their being human, but beyond that minimum some actions and choices are more worthy of regard, more dignified, than others. For example, people who expose and revel in their disgraceful secrets on television are not so worthy of our regard, are not as dignified or honorable, as are quiet benefactors of mankind.

To speak of things like honor, regard, and dignity in this way may seem to some at best anachronistic and at worst repressive. In our time, entirely apart from any transhumanist aspirations, there are well-meaning people in the comfortable circumstances of post-industrial liberal democracies who—while acknowledging the social pathologies of our easygoing culture—are afraid that holding people to our moral standards would be a remedy worse than the disease. We don't want to "impose our views on others," we seek to be "open-minded." This misplaced (and likely inconsistent) reticence is the main practical challenge that any notion of human dignity that goes beyond mutual, nonjudgmental niceness will have to face.

Such skeptics need to be reminded that taking human freedom and dignity seriously is perfectly consistent with laws, rights, customs and norms, religious or otherwise, that constrain the *consequences* of individual or collective judgments of moral behavior. Individual, social or legal disapproval of something as dishonorable does not automatically mean tyrannical repression. Furthermore, between the obvious extremes of self-debasement and greatness of soul, there will often enough be vigorous debate about the virtues and vices that define dignified and undignified behavior—which is just as it should be in a diverse modern society. But for human dignity to be meaningful, this debate will also have to be understood to be meaningful, not just the expression of incommensurable preferences or tastes. Finally, in the manner of the "natural aristocracy" that Jefferson hoped would arise under democratic conditions, the dignity owed to individuals is not to be defined by some class characteristic shared automatically by every member of the group. We may consider human beings to be of equal dignity by birth, and yet still believe that by action and accomplishment some are more honorable than others.

In the second place, as human dignity ought to be grounded in an understanding of what is owed to us as human beings and as individuals, it must be framed by what we essentially are as human beings. Human beings living as they ought, thought Aristotle, are neither beasts nor gods.[35] We are, the Psalmist says, a little lower than the angels;[36] and with the proposition that men are not angels the authors of *The Federalist Papers* are in agreement,[37] without boasting in Kantian fashion that they have built a political system that will work perfectly well for a population of devils.[38] However one wishes to understand the metaphysics of such various statements of "human in-betweenness," they can be taken to point to human dignity as properly residing in a realm between the best and worst that we can imagine of ourselves. As much as it may be part of being human to aspire nobly to transcend this middling state, the honest truth about such transcendence, whether in traditional religious form or in scientistic transhuman form, is that at a certain point it "passeth understanding."

With such limits in mind, we can still hope for and strive for better. But we will also avoid that contempt for what we are that results from thinking that we *know* something far better to be possible (when in fact we can only have faith in it). Human dignity ought to be humanly understandable, at any rate, and conformable to the limited capacities of imperfect beings. Here again, we brush up against the controversial question of how to shape a life that makes the most of the limits, strengths, and weaknesses that define us. But, as the ability to use speech or reason to engage in such controversy is part of what makes us human, to engage in it is far more an expression of human dignity than to avoid it through the dogmatic belief that anything goes.

That human dignity needs to be understood in terms of giving people their due already strongly suggests that it is relational, unlike the isolating exercise of the will that characterizes the new transhumanist dignity. To put it another way, while human dignity requires a moment of freedom with respect to our ability to make moral choices, that moment is mediated through real relations, institutions, customs and mores, and we may judge such things by their success or failure at promoting proper regard for one another. Of necessity these relationships will vary from close to distant, but as such they moderate the pretentiousness of notions of "human dignity" which begin and end with concerns for the fate of the "human species" as such. While the rubric of human dignity does call forth some attention to this highest level of generality, for that realm to be its sole expression risks the impotent abstraction of the "telescopic philanthropy" so well illustrated by the character of Mrs. Jellyby in Charles Dickens's *Bleak House*, whose unsuccessful efforts on behalf of those far away made her oblivious to the needs of her own family.

This embodiment of human dignity in real relations does not have to be comprehensive, let alone (as some transhumanists claim) totalitarian, in order to be meaningful.[39] We can expect that there will be outliers, deviants, criminals, and creative envelope-pushers of all stripes who will not conform to the culturally, politically, socially, and legally expressed common judgments of human dignity. Cat Man can be permitted to be Cat Man without having to be respected *for being Cat Man*; we can tolerate him while pitying his self-defacing self-promotion. This tolerance is worth preserving, since it expresses that aspect of human dignity, which is found in freedom. In fact, human dignity properly understood will doubtless provide ample grounds for concerns about hypocrisy, properly understood as the tribute vice plays to virtue. But knowing in advance that people will break boundaries does not mean that the effort to contain their influence should be abandoned, any more than the fact that people continue to kill each other invalidates, in principle or practice, our many efforts against homicide.[40]

That real human dignity involves judgment and relationships is the source of the most powerful argument against it. For by being relational, the door is open for dignity to be based on how people seem to be rather than how they actually are; and because it involves judgment, dignity may be accorded to qualities that do not in fact deserve to be honored. To "solve" these problems by reconstructing dignity so that it involves neither judgment nor relation, however, is to throw out the baby with the bath water. Instead, acknowledging the problematic status of human dignity is part and parcel of understanding the human limits within which it must operate (e.g., that we do poorly at seeing into the hearts of others and even into our own) and the human possibilities on which it builds (e.g., that we can deliberate about the noble and the base).

This richer characterization of human dignity can at best begin to counterbalance, and certainly not cure, all the problems and perils that our increasing power over nature will create. Doubtless the world 200 or 2,000 years hence will be at least as different from our own as ours is from the world of 200 or 2,000 years ago. If history is any guide, that world will be more dangerous in some respects, less dangerous in others; some possibilities will have widened, others narrowed. In some realms, the changes over these past centuries might well be called a progressive enhancement of human dignity, while in others change has come at a terrible cost. Human dignity in the terms suggested here is a way of thinking toward a future that, however different, will likely exhibit some of the same morally unsettled continuity. We can look back 200 years, or 2,000 years, and still see a human world, a world of people whose actions and motivations, pleasures and pains, triumphs and tragedies are recognizably akin to our own. Human dignity properly conceived may help us make choices that will mold a future in which the fundamental things still apply.*

---

* The author thanks the Scaife Foundation, which supported the leave during which this essay was written, and Adam Schulman and Leslie Rubin for their substantive and editorial advice.

# Notes

1 *Engineering the Human Germline*, ed. Gregory Stock and John Campbell (New York: Oxford University press, 2000).
2 K. Eric Drexler, *Engines of Creation: The Coming Era of Nanotechnology* (New York: Anchor Books, 1990), pp. 104-116.
3 David Brown, "Bionic Woman Grabs the Future: Controls Artificial Arm by Thoughts," *The Pittsburgh Post-Gazette*, September 15, 2006, p. A-3.
4 Ray Kurzweil, *The Age of Spiritual Machines: When Computers Exceed Human Intelligence* (New York: Penguin, 1999), p. 221.
5 Simon Young, *Designer Evolution: A Transhumanist Manifesto* (Amherst, New York: Prometheus Books, 2006), p. 28.
6 Ramez Naam, *More Than Human: Embracing the Promise of Biological Enhancement* (New York: Broadway Books, 2005), pp. 189-205.
7 David Pearce, "The Hedonistic Imperative," online at www.hedweb.com/hedethic/hedonist.htm.
8 Hans Moravec, *Mind Children: The Future of Robot and Human Intelligence* (Cambridge, Massachusetts: Harvard University Press, 1988), pp. 114-121.
9 Moravec, loc. cit.
10 Nick Bostrom, "The Transhumanist FAQ: A General Introduction (Version 2.1)," online at www.transhumanism.org/resources/FAQv21.pdf.
11 Max More, "Principles of Extropy Version 3.11" (2003), online at www.extropy.org/principles.htm.
12 Ray Kurzweil, *The Singularity Is Near: When Humans Transcend Biology* (New York: Viking, 2005), p. 369.
13 See, for example, Naam, op. cit., pp. 2-3.
14 Moravec, op. cit., pp. 107-108.
15 Kurzweil, *The Age of Spiritual Machines*, p. 240.
16 Moravec, op. cit., pp. 115-116.
17 Kurzweil, *Singularity*, pp. 356-366.
18 Moravec, op. cit., pp. 122-123.
19 Kurzweil, *Singularity*, pp. 1-5; Young, op. cit., pp. 27-29; Nick Bostrom, "Transhumanist Values" (2003), section 2, online at www.transhumanism.org/index.php/WTA/more/transhumanist-values/.
20 The analogy is to be found in Kurzweil, *Singularity*, pp. 297-298.
21 Han Jonas, "Technology and Responsibility: Reflections on the New Tasks of Ethics," in *Philosophical Essays: From Ancient Creed to Technological Man* (Chicago: University of Chicago Press, 1980), p. 18.
22 J. B. S. Haldane, "Daedalus, or Science and the Future," in Krishna R. Dronamraju, ed., *Haldane's Daedalus Revisited* (Oxford: Oxford University Press, 1995), pp. 23-50.
23 Naam, op. cit., pp. 3-9; Young, op. cit., pp. 66, 251, 294.
24 Nick Bostrom, "In Defense of Posthuman Dignity," online at www.nickbostrom.com/ethics/dignity.html. Also published in *Bioethics* 19 (2005): 202-214.

[25] Alan Gregg, "A Medical Aspect of the Population Problem," *Science* 121 (1955): 681-682, p. 682.
[26] J. B. S. Haldane, "The Last Judgment," in *Possible Worlds* (London: Chatto and Windus, 1927), p. 288.
[27] David Pearce, "Hedonistic Imperative," Chapter 4, Objection 29, online at www.hedweb.com/hedethic/hedon4.htm.
[28] Wesley J. Smith, "The Catman Cometh: Among the Transhumanists," *The Weekly Standard*, June 26, 2006, p. 20.
[29] One finds degrees of libertarianism among transhumanists. Compare, for example, the account in Young, op. cit., pp. 292-295, with James Hughes, *Citizen Cyborg: Why Democratic Societies Must Respond to the Redesigned Human of the Future* (Cambridge, Massachusetts: Westview Press, 2004), pp. 164-180. Kurzweil charmingly notes that in any case those who choose enhancement will inherit the Earth, as those who reject it die off. See Kurzweil, *Singularity*, p. 322.
[30] See for example, Steven Wolfram, *A New Kind of Science* (Champaign, Illinois: Wolfram Media, 2002), pp. 750-753, or Stuart Hameroff and Roger Penrose, "Orchestrated Objective Reduction of Quantum Coherence in Brain Microtubules: The 'Orch OR' Model for Consciousness" (1996), online at www.quantumconsciousness.org/penrose-hameroff/orchOR.html.
[31] Tor Norretranders, *The User Illusion: Cutting Consciousness Down to Size* (New York: Penguin, 1999).
[32] Naam, op. cit., p. 59. This problem is not unique to transhumanism and is arguably an inevitable consequence of the way modern natural science understands human beings. See Tzvetan Todorov, *Imperfect Garden: The Legacy of Humanism* (Princeton, New Jersey: Princeton University Press, 2002).
[33] Bostrom, "Posthuman Dignity," p. 205.
[34] Nick Bostrom, "The Transhumanist FAQ." See also Chris Wren, "Star Trek's Greatest Weakness" (2006), online at www.cyborgdemocracy.net/2006_05_07_archive.html.
[35] Aristotle, *Politics* 1253a29.
[36] *Psalms* 8:5.
[37] James Madison, "The Federalist #51," in Jacob E. Cooke, ed., *The Federalist* (Cleveland, Ohio: Meridian Books, 1961), p. 349.
[38] Immanuel Kant, "Perpetual Peace: A Philosophical Sketch," in *Kant's Political Writings*, ed. Hans Reiss (Cambridge: Cambridge University Press, 1970), pp. 112-113.
[39] Kurzweil, *Singularity*, pp. 395, 406, 407.
[40] Francis Fukuyama, *Our Posthuman Future: Consequences of the Biotechnology Revolution* (New York: Farrar, Straus & Giroux, 2002), p. 11.

# 8

# Dignity and Enhancement

## Nick Bostrom

Does human enhancement threaten our dignity, as some prominent commentators have asserted? Or could our dignity perhaps be technologically enhanced? After disentangling several different concepts of dignity, this essay focuses on the idea of dignity as a quality, a kind of excellence admitting of degrees and applicable to entities both within and without the human realm. I argue that dignity in this sense interacts with enhancement in complex ways which bring to light some fundamental issues in value theory, and that the effects of any given enhancement must be evaluated in its appropriate empirical context. Yet it is possible that through enhancement we could become better able to appreciate and secure many forms of dignity that are overlooked or missing under current conditions. I also suggest that, in a posthuman world, dignity as a quality could grow in importance as an organizing moral/aesthetic idea.

## The Meanings of Dignity and Enhancement

The idea of dignity looms large in the postwar landscape of public ethics. Human dignity has received prominent billing in numerous national and international declarations and constitutions. Like some successful politicians, the idea of dignity has hit upon a winning formula by combining into one package gravitas, a general feel-good quality, and a profound vagueness that enables all constituencies to declare their allegiance without thereby endorsing any particular course of action.

The idea of dignity, however, also has behind it a rich historical and philosophical tradition. For many of the ancients, dignity was a kind of personal excellence that only a few possessed to any significant degree. Marcus Tullius Cicero (106–43 BC), a Roman following in the footsteps of the Athenian Stoics, attributed dignity to all men, describing it as both a characteristic (human rationality) and a requirement (to base one's life on this capacity for rationality).[1] In Medieval Christianity, the dignity of man was based on the belief that God had created man in His image, allowing man to share some aspects of His divine reason and might.[2] Theologians thought they saw man's dignity reflected in his upright posture, his free will, his immortal soul, and his location at the center of the universe. This dignity was viewed as an essential characteristic of the human being, possessed by each one of us, independent of social rank and personal excellence.

In the philosophy of Immanuel Kant, the intrinsic dignity of man was decoupled from theological assumptions about a divine heritage of the human species. According to Kant (here partly echoing the Stoics), all persons have dignity, a kind of absolute value that is incomparable to any price or instrumental utility.* Kant held that dignity is not a quantitative notion; we cannot have more or less of it. The ground of the dignity of persons is their capacity for reason and moral agency. In order to respect this dignity, we must always treat another person as an end and never solely as a means. In order to avoid affronting our own dignity, we must also refrain from treating ourselves merely as a tool (such as by groveling to others, or selling ourselves into slavery) and from acting in ways that would undermine our rational agency (such as by using intoxicants, or committing suicide).†

---

* This grounding of dignity in personhood and rational moral agency leaves out small children and some humans with mental retardation. This might be viewed as a major problem (that Kant largely ignored).

† The Stoics claimed that we *ought* to commit suicide if we know that our rational

The term "human dignity" did not feature in any European declarations or constitutions in the 18th and 19th centuries. Dignity is to be found for the first time, albeit more or less in passing, in the German constitution drawn up in 1919 by the Weimar National Assembly, and its next appearance is in the corporate-fascist Portuguese constitution of 1933. Only in the aftermath of the Second World War does the concept's heyday begin. It appears in about four constitutions in the period 1900–1945 and in more than thirty-seven from 1945 to 1997.[3] It is also prominent in the UN *Charter* of 1945, in the *Universal Declaration of Human Rights* of 1948, and in numerous later declarations, proclamations, and conventions.

Within applied ethics, the concept of dignity has been particularly salient in medical ethics and bioethics.[4] It has been used to express the need for informed consent in medical research on human subjects. It has also been invoked (on both sides of the argument) in debates about end-of-life decisions and assisted euthanasia, and in discussions of organ sales and organ donations, assisted reproduction, human-animal chimeras, pornography, torture, patenting of human genes, and human cloning. Recently, the idea of dignity has also been prominent in discussions of the ethics of human enhancement, where it has mostly been invoked by bioconservative commentators to argue against enhancement.[5]

If we examine the different uses that have been made of the idea of dignity in recent years, we can distinguish several different concepts. Before we can talk intelligibly about "dignity," we must disambiguate the term. I propose the following taxonomy to regiment our dignity-talk:

*Dignity as a Quality*: A kind of excellence; being worthy, noble, honorable. Persons vary in the degree to which they have this property. A form of Dignity as a Quality can also be ascribed to nonpersons. In humans, Dignity as a Quality may be thought of as a virtue or an ideal, which can be cultivated, fostered, respected, admired, promoted, etc. It need not, however, be identified with moral virtue or with excellence in general.*

---

agency is at risk. Kant's dignity-based argument against suicide is more complex but less persuasive.

* For Aristotle, excellence and virtue went together; his term for this was *to kalon*, the noble. Earlier, however, in what we might call "Homeric ethics," there was not

*Human Dignity* (*Menschenwürde*): The ground upon which—according to some philosophers—rests the full moral status of human beings. It is often assumed that at least all normal human persons have the same level of human dignity. There is some disagreement about what precisely human dignity consists in, and this is reflected in disagreements about which individuals have human dignity: Only persons (as Kant maintained)? Or all human individuals with a developed nervous system who are not brain-dead? Or fetuses in the womb as well? Might some nonhuman primates also have this kind of dignity?[6]

Two other related ideas are:

*Human Rights*: A set of inalienable rights possessed by all beings that have full moral status. One might hold that human dignity is the ground for full moral status. Human rights can be violated or respected. We might have a strict duty not to violate human rights, and an imperfect duty to promote respect for human rights.

(*Dignity as*) *Social Status*: A relational property of individuals, admitting of gradation. Multiple status systems may exist in a given society. Dignity as Social Status is a widely desired prudential good. Our reasons for seeking social status are not distinctly moral, but the standards and conditions that determine the allocation of social status are topics for ethical critique. Some social status is earned, but traditionally it was also thought that some individuals have a special intrinsic Dignity as Social Status, such as an aristocrat or a Brahmin.* Even though the Latin root word (*dignitas*) originally referred to a social status commanding respect, it might be best to refer to this property simply as Social Status to forestall confusion, reserving the word "dignity" for other uses.

Each of these concepts is relevant to ethics, but in different ways.†

---

such a close identification of virtue with honor or excellence. (I'm grateful to Guy Kahane for this point.)

\* In respect of referring to a property partly acquired and partly inherent, the original concept of Dignity as Social Status might be thought of as intermediary between the concept of Dignity as a Quality and the concept of Human Dignity.

† See also Lennart Nordenfelt, "The Varieties of Dignity," *Health Care Analysis* 12 (2004): 69-81, for discussion of different types of dignity. Three of his dignity-concepts can be roughly mapped onto Dignity as a Quality, Human Dignity, and Dignity as Social Status. In addition, Nordenfelt also discusses a notion of *Dignity of Identity*, "the dignity we attach to ourselves as integrated and autonomous per-

In this paper, I shall focus on Dignity as a Quality and the ways in which this concept interacts with that of human enhancement.[7]

Before discussing its relations to enhancement, we shall need a richer characterization of Dignity as a Quality. I will draw on the sensitive linguistic and phenomenological analysis provided by Aurel Kolnai.\*

On the idea of Dignity as a Quality of that which is dignified, Kolnai notes:

> Dignity means Worth or Worthiness in some "absolute," autonomized and objectivized, as it were "featural" sense.... [Yet it] has *descriptive content*.... It is, in this respect, on a par with any of the basic moral virtues such as justice, truthfulness, benevolence, chastity, courage, etc., including even integrity or conscientiousness, none of which is synonymous with Moral Goodness or Virtue as such, and each of which, notwithstanding its possible built-in reference to Morality (and moral evaluation) as such, is susceptible to contentual description.[8]

On this understanding, Dignity as a Quality is a thick moral concept: it contains both descriptive and evaluative components, and may not be in any simple way reducible to more basic moral predicates. Dignity as a Quality also has certain aesthetic overtones. The

---

sons, persons with a history and persons with a future with all our relationships with other human beings" (p. 75). See also Adam Schulman's introduction to this volume and Doron Shultziner, "Human dignity—functions and meanings" (cited in endnote 3). One might also use "dignity" to refer to some combination of social status and self-esteem. For example, Jonathan Glover describes how stripping victims of their dignity (in this sense) is a common prelude to even greater atrocities; see Jonathan Glover, *Humanity: a Moral History of the Twentieth Century* (London: Jonathan Cape, 1999).

\* Kolnai, "Dignity" (cited in endnote 6). The Hungarian-born moral and political philosopher Aurel Kolnai (1900-1973) was, according to Karl Popper and Bernard Williams, one of the most original, provocative, and sensitive philosophers of the 20th century. His writings have suffered some neglect and are not very widely known by philosophers working in the analytic tradition today. His explication of the concept of Dignity as a Quality is especially interesting because it seems to capture an idea that is motivating many contemporary bioconservative critiques of human enhancement.

term might have its own unique contribution to make to our normative vocabulary, but it should not be identified with Morality. If possessing Dignity as a Quality is a virtue, it is one out of many. The concept is hardly a promising candidate for the central and pivotal role in an ethical system that the idea of Human Dignity plays in Kantian philosophy and in some international declarations.*

We can proceed further by describing the appropriate responses to Dignity as a Quality. These seem to incorporate both aesthetic and moral elements. According to Kolnai, the term subtly connotes the idea of verticality, albeit tempered by also connoting a certain idea of reciprocity:

> Can we attempt at all to assign, to adumbrate at least, a distinctive response to Dignity (or "the dignified")? Whatever such a response might be, it must bear a close resemblance to our devoted and admiring appreciation of beauty (its "high" forms at any rate) on the one hand, to our reverent approval of moral goodness (and admiration, say, for heroic virtue) on the other. Dignity commands empathic respect, a reverential mode of response, an "upward-looking" type of the *pro* attitude: a "bowing" gesture if I may so call it.[9]

Next, let us consider what features call for such responses. What characteristics are typically dignified? While not claiming to produce an exhaustive list, Kolnai suggests the following:

> First—the qualities of composure, calmness, restraint, reserve, and emotions or passions subdued and securely controlled without being negated or dissolved.... Secondly—the qualities of distinctness, delimitation, and distance; of something that conveys the idea of being intangible, invulnerable, inaccessible to destructive or corruptive or subversive interference.... Thirdly, in consonance therewith, Dignity also tends to connote the features of self-contained serenity, of a certain inward and toned-down but yet translucent and perceptible power of self-assertion.... With its firm stance and

---

* The related concept of *to kalon*, however, does have such a foundational role in Aristotle's ethics.

solid immovability, the dignified quietly defies the world.[10]

Finally, regarding the bearers of such dignity, Kolnai remarks:

> [T]he predicates...are chiefly applicable to so-called "human beings," i.e. persons, but again not exclusively so: much dignity in this sense seems to me proper to the Cat, and not a little, with however different connotation, to the Bull or the Elephant.... Is not the austere mountainous plateau of Old Castile a dignified landscape...? And, though man-made, cannot works of art (especially of the "classic," though not exactly "classicist," type) have a dignity of their own?[11]

The term "enhancement" also needs to be explicated. I shall use the following rough characterization:

*Enhancement:* An intervention that improves the functioning of some subsystem of an organism beyond its reference state; or that creates an entirely new functioning or subsystem that the organism previously lacked.

The function of a subsystem can be construed either as *natural* (and can be identified with the evolutionary role played by the subsystem, if it is an adaptation), or as *intentional* (in which case the function is determined by the contribution that the subsystem makes to the attainment of relevant goals and intentions of the organism). The functioning of a subsystem is "improved" when the subsystem becomes more efficient at performing its function. The "reference state" may usually be taken to be the normal, healthy state of the subsystem, i.e., the level of functioning of the subsystem when it is not "diseased" or "broken" in any specific way. There is some indeterminacy in this definition of the reference state. It could refer to the state that is normal for some particular individual when she is not subject to any specific disease or injury. This could either be age-relative or indexed to the prime of life. Alternatively, the reference state could be defined as the "species-typical" level of functioning.

When we say "enhancement," unless we further specify these and other indeterminacies, we do not express any very precise thought. In what follows, however, not much will hinge on exactly how one may choose to fill in this sketch of a definition of enhancement.

## Greater Capacities

We can now begin our exploration of the relations between dignity and enhancement. If we recall the features that Kolnai suggests are associated with Dignity as a Quality—composure, distinctness, being inaccessible to destructive or corruptive or subversive interference, self-contained serenity, etc.—it would appear that these could be promoted by certain enhancements. Consider, for example, enhancements in executive function and self-control, in concentration, or in our ability to cope with stressful situations; further, consider enhancements of mental energy that would make us more capable of independent initiative and that would reduce our reliance on external stimuli such as television; consider perhaps also enhancement of our ability to withstand mild pains and discomforts, and to more effectively self-regulate our consumption of food, exercise, and sleep. All these enhancements could heighten our Dignity as a Quality in fairly direct and obvious ways.

Other enhancements might reduce our Dignity as a Quality. For instance, a greatly increased capacity for empathy and compassion might (given the state of this world) diminish our composure and our self-contained serenity, leading to a reduction of our Dignity as a Quality. Some enhancements that boost motivation, drive, or emotional responsiveness might likewise have the effect of destabilizing a dignified inner equilibrium. Enhancements that increase our ability rapidly to adapt to changing circumstances could make us more susceptible to "destructive or corruptive or subversive interference" and undermine our ability to stand firm and quietly defy the world.

Some enhancements, therefore, would increase our Dignity as a Quality, while others would threaten to reduce it. However, whether a particular enhancement—such as a strongly amplified sensitivity to others' suffering—would in fact diminish our dignity depends on the context, and in particular on the character of the enhanced individual. A greatly elevated capacity for compassion is consistent with an outstanding degree of Dignity as a Quality, provided that the compassionate person has other mental attributes, such as a firm sense of purpose and robust self-esteem, that help contain the sympathetic perturbations of the mind and channel them into effective compassionate action. The life of Jesus, as described in the

Bible, exemplifies this possibility.

Even if some enhancement reduced our Dignity as a Quality, it would not follow that the enhanced person would suffer a net loss of virtue. For while Dignity as a Quality might be a virtue, it is not the only virtue. Thus, some loss of Dignity as a Quality could be compensated for by a gain in other virtues. One could resist this conclusion if one believed that Dignity as a Quality is the only virtue rather than one among many. This is hardly a plausible view given the Kolnai-inspired understanding of Dignity as a Quality used in this paper.* Alternatively, one might hold that a certain threshold of Dignity as a Quality is necessary in order to be able to possess any other virtues. But even if that were so, it would not follow that any enhancement that reduced our Dignity as a Quality would result in a net loss of virtue, for the enhancement need not reduce our Dignity as a Quality below the alleged threshold.

## The Act of Enhancement

Our Dignity as a Quality would in fact be greater if some of our capacities were greater than they are. Yet one might hold that *the act of enhancing* our capacities would in itself lower our Dignity as a Quality. One might also hold that *capacities obtained by means of some artificial enhancement* would fail to contribute, or would not contribute as much, to our Dignity as a Quality as the same capacities would have done had they been obtained by "natural" means.

For example, the ability to maintain composure under stressful conditions might contribute to our Dignity as a Quality if this capacity is the manifestation of our native temperament. The capacity might contribute even more to our Dignity as a Quality if it is the fruit of spiritual growth, as the result of a long but successful psychological journey that has enabled us to transcend the trivial stressors that plague everyday existence. But if our composure is brought about by our swallowing a Paxil,† would it still reflect as

---

\* By contrast, e.g., to the Aristotelian concept of *to kalon*.
† Paroxetine, a selective serotonin reuptake inhibitor (SSRI) used to treat symptoms of depression and anxiety.

favorably on our Dignity as a Quality?*

It would appear that our maintaining composure under stress will fully count toward our Dignity as a Quality only if we are able to view it as an *authentic* response, a genuine reflection of our autonomous self. In the case of the person who maintains composure only because she has taken Paxil, it might be unclear whether the composure is really a manifestation of her personality or merely of an extraneous influence. The extent to which her Paxil-persona can be regarded as her true persona would depend on a variety of factors.[12] The more permanently available the anxiolytic is to her, the more consistent she is in using it in the appropriate circumstances, the more the choice of taking it is her own, and the more this choice represents her deepest wishes and is accompanied by a constellation of attitudes, beliefs, and values on which availing herself of this drug is part of her self-image, the more we may incline to viewing the Paxil-persona as her true self, and her off-Paxil persona as an aberration.

If we compare some person who was born with a calm temperament to a one who has acquired the ability to remain calm as a result of psychological and spiritual growth, we might at first be tempted to think that the calmness is more fully a feature of the former. Perhaps the composure of a person born with a calm temperament is more stable, long-lasting, and robust than that of a person whose composure results from learning and experience. However, one could argue that the latter person's Dignity as a Quality is, *ceteris paribus*, the greater (i.e., even setting aside that this person would likely have acquired many other attributes contributing to his Dignity as a Quality during the course of his psychological trek). The reasoning would be that a capacity or an attribute that has become ours because of our own choices, our own thinking, and our own experiences, is in some sense more authentically ours even than a capacity or attribute

---

* For this example to work properly, we should assume that the psychological states resulting are the same in each case. Suppose one thinks that there is a special dignity in *feeling* stressed out yet managing to *act* cool through an exertion of self-control and strength of character. Then the thought experiment requires that we *either* assume that the feeling of stress would be absent in all three cases (native temperament, psychological growth, Paxil), *or else* assume that (again in each of the cases) the feeling of stress would be present and the subject would succeed in acting cool thanks to her self-control (which might again have come about in either of the ways).

given to us prenatally.

This line of reasoning also suggests that a trait acquired through the deliberate employment of some enhancement technology could be more authentically ours than a trait that we possessed from birth or that developed in us independently of our own agency. Could it be that not only the person who has acquired a trait through personal growth and experience, but also one who has acquired it by choosing to make use of some enhancement technology, may possess that trait more authentically than the person who just happens to have the trait by default? Holding other things constant—such as the permanency of the trait, and its degree of integration and harmonization with other traits possessed by the person—this would indeed seem to be the case.

This claim is consistent with the belief that coming to possess a positive trait as a result of personal growth and experience would make an *extra* contribution to our Dignity as a Quality, perhaps the dignity of effort and of the overcoming of weaknesses and obstacles. The comparison here is between traits, capacities, or potentials that we are given from birth and ones that we could develop if we were given access to enhancement technologies.*

A precedent for the view that our self-shaping can contribute to our Dignity as a Quality can be found in Pico della Mirandola's *Oration on the Dignity of Man* (1486):

> We have given you, O Adam, no visage proper to yourself, nor endowment properly your own, in order that whatever place, whatever form, whatever gifts you may, with premeditation, select, these same you may have and possess through your own judgment and decision. The nature of all other creatures is defined and restricted within laws which We have laid down; you, by contrast, impeded by no such restrictions,

---

* The claim I make here is thus also consistent with the view put forward by Leon Kass that the "naturalness" of the means matters. Kass argues that in ordinary efforts at self-improvement we have a kind of direct experience or "understanding in human terms" of the relation between the means and their effects, one that is lacking in the case of technological enhancements; see Leon R. Kass, "Ageless Bodies, Happy Souls: Biotechnology and the Pursuit of Perfection," *The New Atlantis* 1 (Spring 2003): 9-28.

may, by your own free will, to whose custody We have assigned you, trace for yourself the lineaments of your own nature.... We have made you a creature neither of heaven nor of earth, neither mortal nor immortal, in order that you may, as the free and proud shaper of your own being, fashion yourself in the form you may prefer.[13]

While Mirandola does not distinguish between different forms of dignity, it seems that he is suggesting both that our Human Dignity consists in our capacity for self-shaping and also that we gain in Dignity as a Quality through the exercise of this capacity.

It is thus possible to argue that the act of voluntary, deliberate enhancement *adds* to the dignity of the resulting trait, compared to possessing the same trait by mere default.

## The Enhancer's Attitude

At this point we must introduce a significant qualification. Other things being equal, defiance seems more dignified than compliance and adaptation. As Kolnai notes, "pliability, unresisting adaptability and unreserved self-adjustment are prototypal opposites of Dignity." Elaborating, Kolnai writes:

> It might be argued that the feature sometimes described as the "meretricious" embodies the culmination of Un-Dignity.... What characterizes the meretricious attitude is the intimate unity of abstract self-seeking and qualitative self-effacement. The meretricious type of person is, ideally speaking, at once boundlessly devoted to the thriving of his own life and indifferent to its contents. He wallows in his dependence on his environment—in sharp contrast to the dignity of a man's setting bounds to the impact of its forces and undergoing their influence in a distant and filtered fashion—and places himself at the disposal of alien wants and interests without organically (which implies, selectively) espousing any of them.... [He] escapes the tensions of alienation by precipitate fusion and headlong surrender, and evades self-transcendence by

the flitting mobility of a weightless self.[14]

So on the one hand, the "self-made" man or woman might gain in Dignity as a Quality from being the author (or co-author) of his or her own character and situation. Yet on the other hand, it is also possible that such a person instead gains in Un-Dignity from their self-remolding. The possibility of such Un-Dignity, or loss of Dignity as a Quality, is an important concern among some critics of human enhancement. Leon Kass puts it uncompromisingly:

> [The] final technical conquest of his own nature would almost certainly leave mankind utterly enfeebled. This form of mastery would be identical with utter dehumanization. Read Huxley's *Brave New World*, read C. S. Lewis's *Abolition of Man*, read Nietzsche's account of the last man, and then read the newspapers. Homogenization, mediocrity, pacification, drug-induced contentment, debasement of taste, souls without loves and longings—these are the inevitable results of making the essence of human nature the last project of technical mastery. In his moment of triumph, Promethean man will also become a contented cow.[15]

The worry underlying this passage is, I think, the fear of a total loss of Dignity as a Quality, and its replacement with positive Un-Dignity.

We should distinguish two different ways in which this could result. The more obvious one is if, in selecting our enhancements, we select ones that transform us into undignified people. The point here is that these people would be undignified no matter how they came about, whether as a result of enhancement or through any other process. I have already discussed this issue, concluding that some enhancements would increase our Dignity as a Quality, other enhancements would risk reducing it, and also that whether a particular enhancement would be a benefit, all things considered, cannot usually be decided by looking only at how it would affect our dignity.

A more subtle source of Un-Dignity is one that emanates from the very activity of enhancement. In this latter case, the end state is not necessarily in itself undignified, but the process of refashioning ourselves that brings us there reduces our Dignity as a Qualit argued above that a dignified trait resulting from deliberate enhancement can in favorable circumstances contribute more to our Dignity as a Quality than the same trait would if it had happened to be ours by default. Yet I think it should also be acknowledged that in *unfavorable* conditions, the act of self-transformation could be undignified and might indeed express the "meretricious" attitude described by Kolnai.

When is the activity of self-transformation dignity-increasing and when is it dignity-reducing? The Kolnai quote suggests an answer. When self-transformation is motivated by a combination of "abstract self-seeking and qualitative self-effacement," when it is driven by alien wants and interests that have not been organically and selectively endorsed by the individual being enhanced, when it represents a surrender to mere convenience rather than the autonomous realization of a content-full personal ideal, then the act of enhancement is not dignified and may be positively undignified—in exactly the same way that other actions resulting from similar motivations may fail to express or contribute to our Dignity as a Quality.*

Let us use an example. Suppose that somebody takes a cognition-enhancing drug out of mere thoughtless conformity to fashion or under the influence of a slick advertising campaign. There is then nothing particularly dignified about this act of enhancement. There might even be something undignified about it inasmuch as a person who has Dignity as a Quality would be expected to exert more autonomous discretion about which substances she puts in her body, especially ones that are designed to affect her mental faculties. It might still be the case that the person after having taken the cognitive enhancer will gain in Dignity as a Quality. Perhaps the greater power and clarity of her thinking will enable her henceforth better to resist manipulative advertisements and to be more selective in her embrace of fads and fashions. Nonetheless, in itself, the enhancement act may be Un-Dignified and may take away something from her Dignity as

---

* The act of enhancement could also be undignified under some other conditions. For example, one might think that if an intervention involves immoral conduct, or if it involves the use of "tainted means" (such as medical procedures developed using information obtained in cruel experiments), this would tend to make the intervention undignified. Again, however, this problem is not specific to enhancement-related acts.

a Quality. The problem is that her motivation for undergoing the enhancement is inappropriate. Her attitude and the behavior that springs from it are Un-Dignified.

Here we would be remiss if we did not point out the symmetric possibility that *refraining* from making use of an opportunity for enhancement can be Un-Dignified in exactly the same way and for the same reasons as it can be Un-Dignified to make use of one. A person who rejects a major opportunity to improve her capacities out of thoughtless conformity to fashion, prejudice, or lazy indifference to the benefits to self and others that would result, would thereby reduce her Dignity as a Quality. Rejection and acceptance of enhancement are alike in this respect: both can reflect an attitude problem.

## Emotion Modification as a Special Hazard?

"Enhancements" of drives, emotions, mood, and personality might pose special threats to dignity, tempting us to escape "the tensions of alienation by precipitate fusion and headlong surrender." An individual could opt to refashion herself so as to be content with reality as she finds it rather than standing firm in proud opposition. Such a choice could itself express a meretricious attitude. Worse, the transformation could result in a personality that has lost a great portion of whatever Dignity as a Quality it may have possessed before.

One can conceive of modifications of our affective responses that would level our aspirations, stymie our capacity for emotional and spiritual growth, and surrender our ability to rebel against unworthy life conditions or the shortcomings of our own characters. Such interventions would pose an acute threat to our Dignity as a Quality. The fictional drug "soma" in *Brave New World* is depicted as having just such effects. The drug seems to dissolve the contours of human living and striving, reducing the characters in Huxley's novel to contented, indeterminate citizen-blobs that are almost prototypical of Un-Dignity.

Another prototypical image of Un-Dignity, one from the realm of science, is that of the "wire-headed" rat that has had electrodes inserted into its brain's reward areas.[16] The model of a self-stimulating rat, that will relentlessly press its lever—foregoing opportunities for mating, rest, or even food and drink—until it either collapses from fatigue or dies, is not exactly one that commands a "reverential mode of response" or an "upward-looking type of the *pro* attitude." If we picture a human being in place of the rat, we would have to say that it is one Un-Dignified human, or at any rate a human engaged in a very Un-Dignified activity.*

Would life in such an Un-Dignified state (assuming for the sake of argument that the pleasure was indefinitely sustainable and ignoring any wider effects on society) be preferable to life as we know it? Clearly, that depends on the quality of the life that we know. Given a sufficiently bleak alternative, intracranial electrical stimulation certainly seems much preferable; for example, for patients who are slowly dying in unbearable cancer pain and for whom other methods of palliation are ineffective.† It is even possible that for such patients, wire-heading and similar interventions increase their Dignity as a Quality (not to mention other components of their well-being).[17] Some estimable English doctors were once in the habit of administering to cancer patients in their last throes an elixir known as the Brompton cocktail, a mixture of cocaine, heroin and alcohol:

> Drawing life to a close with a transcendentally orgasmic bang, and not a pathetic and god-forsaken whimper, can turn dying into the culmination of one's existence rather than its present messy and protracted anti-climax.... One is conceived in pleasure. One may reasonably hope to die in it.[18]

Bowing out in such a manner would not only be a lot more fun, it seems, but also more *dignified* than the alternative.

But suppose the comparison case is not unbearable agony but a typical situation from an average person's life. Then becoming like

---

* The Stoics generalized this point, maintaining that "sensual pleasure is quite unworthy of the dignity of man and that we ought to despise it and cast it from us." See Cicero, *De officiis*, trans. Walter Miller (Cambridge, Massachusetts: Harvard University Press, 1913), book 1, chapter 30. The virtue and dignity of asceticism and the converse sinfulness and debasement of flesh-pleasing have also been recurring themes in some religious traditions.

† Intracranial stimulation is used for this purpose in humans; Krishna Kumar, Cory Toth, et al., "Deep Brain Stimulation for Intractable Pain: A 15-Year Experience," *Neurosurgery* 40 (1997): 736-746.

a wire-headed rat, obsessively pressing a lever to the exclusion of all other activities and concerns, would surely entail a catastrophic loss of Dignity as a Quality. Whether or not such a life would nevertheless be preferable to an ordinary human life (again assuming it to be sustainable and ignoring the wider consequences)—depends on fundamental issues in value theory. According to hedonism such a life would be preferable. If the pleasure were great enough, it might also be preferable according to some other accounts of well-being. On many other value theories, of course, such a wire-headed life would be far inferior to the typical human life. These axiological questions are outside the scope of this essay.*

Let us refocus on Dignity as a Quality. A life like that of a wire-headed rat would be radically deprived of Dignity as a Quality compared to a typical human life. But the wire-heading scenario is not necessarily representative—even as a caricature—of what a life with some form of emotional enhancement would be like. Some hedonic enhancements would not transform us into passive, complacent, loveless, and longing-less blobs. On the contrary, they could increase our zest for life, infuse us with energy and initiative, and heighten our capacity for love, desire, and ambition. There are different forms of pleasurable states of mind—some that are passive, relaxed, and comfortable, and others that are active, excited, enthusiastic, and joyfully thrilling. The wire-headed rat is potentially a highly misleading model of what even a simply hedonically enhanced life could be like. And emotional enhancement could take many forms other than elevation of subjective well-being or pleasure.

If we imagine somebody whose zest for and enjoyment of life has been enhanced beyond the current average human level, by means of some pharmaceutical or other intervention, it is not obvious that we must think of this as being associated with any loss of Dignity as a Quality. A state of mania is not dignified, but a controlled passion for life and what it has to offer is compatible with a high degree of

---

* To assume that Dignity as a Quality has any intrinsic value would already be to renounce strict hedonism. However, even if one denies that Dignity as a Quality has intrinsic value, one might still think that it has other kinds of significance—for example, it might have instrumental value, or it might have value insofar as somebody desires it, or the concept of Dignity as a Quality might express or summarize certain common concerns.

Dignity as a Quality. It seems to me that such a state of being could easily be decidedly more dignified than the ho-hum affective outlook of a typical day in the average person's life.

Perhaps it would be slightly preferable, from the point of view of Dignity as a Quality, if the better mood resulted from a naturally smiling temperament or if it had been attained by means of some kind of psychological self-overcoming. But if some help had to be sought from a safe and efficacious pill, I do not see that it would make a vast difference in terms of how much Dignity as a Quality could be invested in the resulting state of mind.

One important factor in the Dignity as a Quality of our emotions is the extent to which they are appropriate responses to aspects of the world. Many emotions have an evaluative element, and one might think that for such an emotion to have Dignity as a Quality it must be a response to a situation or a phenomenon that we recognize as deserving the evaluation contained in the emotion. For example, anger might be dignified only on occasions where there is something to be angry about and where the anger is directed at that object in recognition of its offensiveness. This criterion could in principle be satisfied not only by emotions arising spontaneously from our native temperament but also by emotions encouraged by some affective enhancement. Some affective enhancements could expand our evaluative range and create background conditions that would enable us to respond to values with regard to which we might otherwise be blind or apathetic. Moreover, even if some situations objectively call for certain emotional responses, there might be some indeterminacy such that any response within a range could count as objectively appropriate. This is especially plausible when we consider baseline mood or subjective well-being. Some people are naturally downbeat and glum; others are brimming with cheer and good humor. Is it really the case that one of these sentiments is objectively appropriate to the world? If so, which one? Those who are sad may say the former; those who are happy, the latter. I doubt that there is a fact of the matter.

It appears to me that the main threat to Dignity as a Quality from emotional enhancement would come not from the use of mood-brighteners to improve positive affect in everyday life, but from two other directions. One of these is the socio-cultural dimension, which

I shall discuss in the next section. The other is the potential use of emotional "enhancements" by individuals to clip the wings of their own souls. This would be the result if we used emotional enhancers in ways that would cause us to become so "well-adjusted" and psychologically adaptable that we lost hold of our ideals, our loves and hates, or our capacity to respond spontaneously with the full register of human emotions to the exigencies of life.

Critics of enhancement are wont to dwell on how it could erode dignity. They often omit to point out how enhancement could help raise our dignity. But let us pause and ask ourselves just how much Dignity as a Quality a person has who spends four or five hours every day watching television? Whose passions are limited to a subset of eating, drinking, shopping, gratifying their sexual needs, watching sports, and sleeping? Who has never had an original idea, never willingly deviated from the path of least resistance, and never devoted himself seriously to any pursuit or occupation that was not handed him on the platter of cultural expectations? Perhaps, with regard to Dignity as a Quality, there is more distance to rise than to fall.

## Socio-Culturally Mediated Effects

In addition to their direct effects on the treated individuals, enhancements might have indirect effects on culture and society. Such sociocultural changes will in turn affect individuals, influencing in particular how much Dignity as a Quality they are likely to develop and display in their lives. Education, media, cultural norms, and the general social and physical matrix of our lives can either foster or stymie our potential to develop and live with Dignity as a Quality.

Western consumerist culture does not seem particularly hospitable to Dignity as a Quality. Various spiritual traditions, honor cultures, Romanticism, or even the Medieval chivalric code of ethics seem to have been more conducive to Dignity as a Quality, although some elements of contemporary culture—in particular, individualism—could in principle be important building blocks of a dignified personality. Perhaps there is a kind of elitism or aristocratic sensibility inherent in the cultivation of Dignity as a Quality that does not sit easily with the mass culture and egalitarian pretensions of modernity.

Perhaps, too, there is some tension between the current emphasis on instrumentalist thinking and scientific rationality, on the one hand, and the (dignified) reliance on stable personal standards and ideals on the other. The perfect Bayesian rationalist, who has no convictions but only a fluid network of revisable beliefs, whose probability she feels compelled to update according to a fixed kinematics whenever new evidence impinges on her senses, has arguably surrendered some of her autonomy to an algorithm.*

How would the widespread use and social acceptance of enhancement technologies affect the conditions for the development of individual Dignity as a Quality? The question cannot be answered *a priori*. Unfortunately, neither can it currently be answered a posteriori other than in the most speculative fashion. We lack both the theory and the data that would be required to make any firm predictions about such matters. Social and cultural changes are difficult to forecast, especially over long time spans during which the technological bases of human civilizations will undergo profound transformations. Any answer we give today is apt to reveal more about our own hopes, fears, and prejudices than about what is likely to happen in the future.

When Leon Kass asserts that homogenization, mediocrity, pacification, drug-induced contentment, debasement of taste, and souls without loves and longings are the inevitable results of making human nature a project of technical mastery, he is not, as far as I can glean from his writings, basing this conviction on any corroborated social science model, or indeed on any kind of theory, data set, or well-developed argument. A more agnostic stance would better match the available evidence. We can, I think, conceive of scenarios in which Kass's forebodings come true, and of other scenarios in which the opposite happens. Until somebody develops better arguments, we shall be ignorant as to which it will be. Insofar as both scenarios are within reach, we might have most reason to work to realize one in which enhancement options do become available and are used in

---

* I say this as a fan of the Bayesian way. Another view would be that we do not have any coherent notion of autonomy that is distinct from responding to one's reasons, in which case the perfect Bayesian rationalist might—at least in her epistemic performance—be the epitome of dignity. That view would be more congruent with many earlier writers on dignity, including Kant.

ways that increase our Dignity as a Quality along with other more important values.

## The Dignity of Civilizations

Dignity as a Quality can be attributed to entities other than persons, including populations, societies, cultures, and civilizations. Some of the adverse consequences of enhancement that Kass predicts would pertain specifically to such collectives. "Homogeneity" is not a property of an individual; it is a characteristic of a group of individuals. It is not so clear, however, what Dignity as a Quality consists in when predicated to a collective. Being farther from the prototype application of the idea of dignity, such attributions of Dignity as a Quality to collectives may rely on value judgments to a greater extent than is the case when we apply it to individuals, where the descriptive components of the concept carry more of the weight.

For example, many moderns regard various forms of *equality* as important for a social order to have Dignity as a Quality. We may hold that there is something undignified about a social order which is marked by rigid status hierarchies and in which people are treated very unequally because of circumstances of birth and other factors outside their control. Many of us think that there is something decisively Un-Dignified about a society in which beggars sit on the sidewalk and watch limousines drive by, or in which the conspicuous consumption of the children of the rich contrasts too sharply with the squalor and deprivation of the children of the poor.

An observer from a different era might see things differently. For instance, an English aristocrat from the 17th century, placed in a time machine and brought forward into contemporary Western society, might be shocked at what he would see. While he would, perhaps, be favorably impressed by our modern comforts and conveniences, our enormous economic wealth, our medical techniques and so forth, he might also be appalled at the loss of Dignity as a Quality that has accompanied these improvements. He steps out of the time machine and beholds vulgarized society, swarming with indecency and moral decay. He looks around and shudders as he sees how the rich social architecture of his own time, in which everybody, from the King down to the lowliest servant, knew their rank and status, and in which people were tied together in an intricate tapestry of duties, obligations, privileges, and patronage—how this magnificently ordered social cathedral has been flattened and replaced by an endless suburban sprawl, a *homogenized* society where the spires of nobility have been demolished, where the bonds of loyalty have been largely dissolved, the family pared down to its barest nucleus, the roles of lord and subject collapsed in those of consumer and purveyor, the Majesty of the Crown usurped by a multinational horde of Burger Kings.

Whether or not our imaginary observer would judge that on balance the changes had been for the better, he would most likely feel that they had been accompanied by a tragic loss, and that part of this loss would be a loss of Dignity as a Quality, for individuals but especially for society. Moreover, this loss of societal Dignity would reside in some of the same changes that many of us would regard as gains in societal Dignity as a Quality.

We strike up a conversation with our time-traveling visitor and attempt to convince him that his view about Dignity as a Quality is incorrect. He attempts to convince us that it is our view that is defective. The disagreement, it seems, would be about value judgments and, to some extent, about aesthetic judgments. It is uncertain whether either side would succeed in persuading the other.

We could imagine other such trans-temporal journeys, perhaps bringing a person from ancient Athens into the Middle Ages, or from the Middle Ages into the Enlightenment Era, or from the time when all humans were hunter-gatherers into any one of these later periods. Or we could imagine these journeys in the reverse, sending a person back in time. While each of these time travelers would likely recognize certain *individuals* in all the societies as having Dignity as a Quality, they might well find all the *societies* they were visiting seriously lacking in Dignity as a Quality. Even if we restrict ourselves to the present time, most of us probably find it easier to identify Un-Dignity in societies that are very different from our own, even though we have been taught that we ought not to be so prejudiced against the customs of foreign cultures.

The point I wish to make with these observations is that, if you or I were shown a crystal ball revealing human society as it will be a few centuries from today, it is likely that the society we would see would appear to us as being in important respects Un-Dignified compared to our own. This would seem to be the default expectation even apart from any technological enhancements which might by then have entered into common use. And therein lies one of those fine ironies of history. One generation conceives a beautiful design and lays the ground stones of a better tomorrow. Then they die, and the next generation decides to erect a different structure on the foundation that was build, a structure that is more beautiful in their eyes but that would have been hideous to their predecessors. The original architects are no longer there to complain, but if the dead could see they would turn in their graves. *O tempora, o mores,* cry the old, and the bones of our ancestors rattle their emphatic assent!

It is possible to take a more optimistic view of the possibilities of secular change in the societal and cultural realms. One might believe that the history of humankind shows signs of moral progress, a slow and fluctuating trend toward more justice and less cruelty. Even if one does not detect such a trend in history, one might still hope that the future will bring more unambiguous amelioration of the human condition. But there are many variables other than Dignity as a Quality that influence our evaluation of possible cultures and societies (such as the extent to which Human Dignity is respected, to name but one). It may be that we have to content ourselves with hoping for improvements in these other variables, recognizing that Dignity as a Quality, when ascribed to forms of social organization rather than individuals, is too indeterminate a concept—and possibly too culture-relative—for even an optimist to feel confident that future society or future culture will appear highly dignified by current lights.

I will therefore not discuss by what means one might attempt to increase the Dignity as a Quality of present or future society, except to note that enhancement could possibly play a role. For example, if homogenization is antithetical to a society having Dignity as a Quality, then enhancements that strengthen the ability of individuals to resist group pressure and that encourage creativity and originality, and maybe even a degree of eccentricity, could help not only individuals to attain more Dignity as a Quality but also society, thanks to the cultural diversification that such individuals would create.

## A Relational Component?

Let us return to the Dignity as a Quality of individuals. One might attribute Dignity as Quality to an individual not only because of her intrinsic characteristics but, arguably, also because of her relational properties. For example, one might think that the oldest tree has a Dignity as a Quality that it would not possess if there were another tree that was older, or that the last of the Mohicans had a special Dignity as a Quality denied to the penultimate Mohican.

We humans like to pride ourselves on being the smartest and most advanced species on the planet. Perhaps this position gives us a kind of Dignity as a Quality, one that could be shared by all humans, including mediocrities and even those who fall below some nonhuman animals in terms of cognitive ability. We would have this special Dignity as a Quality through our belonging to a species whose membership has included such luminaries as Michelangelo and Einstein. We might then worry that we would risk losing this special dignity if, through the application of radical enhancement technologies, we created another species (or intelligent machines) that surpassed human genius in all dimensions. Becoming a member of the second-most advanced species on the planet (supposing one were not among the radically enhanced) sounds like a demotion.

We need to be careful here not to conflate Dignity as a Quality with other concepts, such as social rank or status. With the birth of cognitively superior posthumans, the rank of humans would suffer (at least if rank were determined by cognitive capacity). It does not follow that our Dignity as a Quality would have been reduced; that is a separate question. Perhaps we should hold, rather, that our Dignity as a Quality would have been increased, on grounds of our membership in another collective—the Club of Tellurian Life. This club, while less exclusive than the old Club of Humanity, would boast some extremely illustrious members after the human species had been eclipsed by its posthuman descendants.

There might nevertheless be a loss of Dignity as a Quality for individual human beings. Those individuals who were previously at the top of their fields would no longer occupy such a distinguished position. If there is a special Dignity as a Quality (as opposed to merely social status) in having a distinguished position, then this dignity would be transferred to the new occupants of the pinnacles of excellence.

We cannot here explore all the possible ways in which relational properties could be affected by human enhancement, so I will draw attention to just one other relational property, that of uniqueness. Reproductive cloning is not a prototypical enhancement, but we can use it to raise a question.* Does a person's uniqueness contribute something to her Dignity as a Quality? If so, one might object to human cloning on grounds that it would result in progeny who—other things being equal—would have less Dignity as a Quality than a sexually conceived child. Of course, we should not commit the error of genetic essentialism or genetic determinism; but neither should we make the opposite error of thinking that genes don't matter. People who have the same genes tend to be more similar to one another than people who are not genetically identical. In this context, "uniqueness" is a matter of degree, so a set of clones of an average person would tend to be "less unique" than most people.†

Naturally occurring identical twins would be as genetically similar as a pair of clones. (Natural identical twins also tend to share the same womb and rearing environment, which clones would not necessarily do.) Since we do not think that natural twins are victims of a significant misfortune, we can conclude that *either* the loss of one's degree of uniqueness resulting from the existence of another individual who is genetically identical to oneself does not entail a significant loss of Dignity as a Quality, *or* losing some of one's Dignity as a Quality is not a significant misfortune (or both).

One might still worry about more extreme cases. Consider the possibility of not just a few clones being created of an individual, but many millions. Or more radically, consider the possibility of the creation of millions of copies of an individual who would all be much more similar to one another than monozygotic twins are.‡ In

---

* One could argue that reproductive cloning would be an enhancement of our reproductive capacities, giving us the ability to reproduce in a way that was previously impossible.
† Unless, perhaps, cloning were so rare that being a clone would itself mark one out as a highly unusual and "unique" kind of person.
‡ Human "uploading" is one possible future technology that might lead to such a scenario; see Hans Moravec, *Mind Children: the Future of Robot and Human Intelligence* (Cambridge, Massachusetts: Harvard University Press, 1988). Another

these imaginary cases, it seems more plausible that a significant loss of Dignity as a Quality would occur among the copied individuals. Perhaps this would be a *pro tanto* reason against the realization of such scenarios.

## Dignity Outside the Human World: Quiet Values

Dignity as a Quality is not necessarily confined to human beings and collectives of human beings:

> The redwoods, once seen, leave a mark or create a vision that stays with you always. No one has ever successfully painted or photographed a redwood tree. The feeling they produce is not transferable. From them comes silence and awe. It's not only their unbelievable stature, nor the color which seems to shift and vary under your eyes, no, they are not like any trees we know, they are ambassadors from another time. They have the mystery of ferns that disappeared a million years ago into the coal of the carboniferous era…. The vainest, most slaphappy and irreverent of men, in the presence of redwoods, goes under a spell of wonder and respect…. One feels the need to bow to unquestioned sovereigns.[19]

It is easy to empathize with the response that John Steinbeck describes, and it fits quite well with Kolnai's account of the characteristic response to dignity.

Another example:

> [One] of my colleagues [recounts a story] about once taking his young son to a circus in town, and discovering a lone protestor outside the tent silently holding aloft a sign that read "REMEMBER THE DIGNITY OF THE ELEPHANTS." It hit him like a lightning bolt, he said. The protester's point is surely an intelligible one, though we could debate whether it is genuinely reason enough to avoid all types of circuses.[20]

---

would be the creation of many copies of the same sentient artificial intelligence.

We need a name for the property that we feel we are responding to in examples like the above, and "Dignity as Quality" fits the bill. We might also apply this concept to certain actions, activities, and achievements, perhaps to certain human relationships, and to many other things, which I shall not explore here.

The Dignity as a Quality that we attribute to nonhumans (or more accurately, to non-persons) is of a different type from that which we attribute to human beings. One way to characterize the difference is by using a distinction introduced by Stephen Darwall.[21] Darwall describes two different kinds of attitude, both of which are referred to by the term "respect." The first kind he calls *recognition respect*. This attitude consists in giving appropriate consideration or recognition to some feature of its object in deliberating about what to do, and it can have any number of different sorts of things as its object. The other kind, which he calls *appraisal respect*, consists in an attitude of positive appraisal of a person either as a person or as engaged in some particular pursuit. The appropriate ground for appraisal respect is that a person has manifested positive characteristics or excellences that we attribute to his character, especially those that belong to him as a moral agent.

For example, when we say that Human Dignity must be respected, we presumably mean that it must be given recognition respect. We owe this respect to all people equally, independently of their moral character or any special excellences that they might have or lack. By contrast, when say that we should respect Gandhi for his magnanimity, we are probably referring to appraisal respect (although his magnanimity should also in certain contexts be given recognition respect). Similarly, if someone has a high degree of Dignity as a Quality (perhaps Gandhi again), this also calls for appraisal respect.

The kind of Dignity as a Quality that we attribute to non-agents does not call for appraisal respect, since only agents have moral character. Thus we can distinguish between Dignity as a Quality in the narrow sense, as a property possessed only by (some) agents and that calls for appraisal respect, and Dignity as a Quality in a wider sense, which could be possessed by any number of types of object, and which calls for recognition respect only. We do not have to literally *admire* or *give credit to* the redwoods for having grown so tall and having lived so long; but we can still recognize them as possessing certain features that we should take into account in deliberating about what we do to them. In particular, if we are truly impressed by their Dignity as a Quality (in the wide sense), then we ought to show our recognition respect for their dignity—perhaps by not cutting them down for their timber, or by refraining from urinating on them.

Dignity as a Quality, in this wide sense, is ubiquitous. What is limited, I would suggest, is not the supply but our ability to appreciate it. Even inanimate objects can possess it. For a mundane example, consider the long, slow, sad decline of a snowman melting in the backyard. Would not an ideally sensitive observer recognize a certain Dignity as a Quality in the good Snowman, Esq.?

The ethical fades here into the aesthetic (and perhaps into the sentimental), and it is not clear that there exists any sharp line of demarcation. But however we draw our conceptual boundaries, our normative discourse would be impoverished if it could not lend expression to and genuinely take into account what is at stake in cases like these. Perhaps we could coin the category of *quiet values* to encompass not only Dignity as a Quality in this extended sense, but also other small, subtle, or non-domineering values. We may contrast these quiet values with a category of *loud values*, which would be more starkly prudential or moral, and which tend to dominate the quiet values in any direct comparison. The category of loud values might include things like alleviation of suffering, justice, equality, freedom, fairness, respect for Human Dignity, health and survival, and so forth.*

It is not necessarily a fault of applied ethics, insofar as it aims to influence regulation and public policy, that it tends to focus exclusively on loud values. If on one side of the scales we put celebrating the Dignity as a Quality of Mr. Snowman, and on the other we put providing a poverty-stricken child with a vaccination, the latter will always weigh more heavily.

---

* It is, of course, a substantive normative question in which of these categories to place a given value. For example, Nietzsche might have held Dignity as a Quality to be a loud value, and he might have thought that equality was of no value at all. One big question, even if one does not share Nietzsche's view, is how we ought to treat Dignity as a Quality from an impartial standpoint. Is it better to have a few supremely dignified persons surrounded by many with little dignity, or better to have a modicum of dignity widely spread?

Nevertheless, there may be a broader significance to the quiet values. While individually weak, in aggregate they are formidable. They are the dark matter of value theory (or, for all ye business consultants among my readers, *the long tail of axiology*). Fail to uphold a quiet value on one occasion, and nothing noticeable is lost. But extirpate or disregard all the quiet values all the time, and the world turns into a sterile, desolate, impoverished place. The quiet values add the luminescence, the rich texture of meaning, the wonder and awe, and much of the beauty and nobility of human action. In major part, this contribution is aesthetic, and the realization of this kind of value might depend crucially on our subjective conscious responses. Yet, at least in the idea of Dignity as a Quality, which is our focal concern here, the moral and the aesthetic blend into one another, and the possibility of responding to the realm of quiet values (or helping it into existence through acts of creative imagination and feeling) can have moral implications.

## The Eschatology of Dignity

Kolnai describes a certain mode of utopian thinking as inimical to Dignity as a Quality:

> Perhaps [certain people] believe that by the ensuring through a collective agency of everybody's "Human Dignity" (including a sense of individual self-assertion and self-fulfillment) everyone will also acquire Dignity as a Quality or, what comes to the same thing, the concept of "Dignity as a Quality" will lose its point—a view prefigured by the first great apostle of Progress, Condorcet, who confidently foresaw a rationally and scientifically redrawn world in which there would be no opportunity for the exercise of heroic virtue nor any sense in revering it.
>
> The core of Un-Dignity, as I would try to put it succinctly, is constituted by an attitude of refusal to recognize, experience, and bear with, the tension between Value and Reality; between what things ought to be, should be, had better be or are desired to be and what things are, can be

and are allowed to be.*

This raises the question of whether there would be any role left to play for Dignity as a Quality if the world, thanks to various political, medical, economical, and technological advances, reached a level of perfection far beyond its present troubled state. The question becomes perhaps especially acute if we suppose that the transhumanist aspiration to overcome some of our basic biological limitations were to be realized. Might the tension between Value and Reality then be relaxed in such a way that Dignity as a Quality would become meaningless or otiose?

Let us make a leap into an imaginary future posthuman world, in which technology has reached its logical limits. The superintelligent inhabitants of this world are *autopotent*, meaning that they have complete power over and operational understanding of themselves, so that they are able to remold themselves at will and assume any internal state they choose. An autopotent being could, for example, easily transform itself into the shape of a woman, a man, or a tree. Such a being could also easily enter any subjective state it wants to be in, such as a state of pleasure or indignation, or a state of experiencing the visual and tactile sensations of a dolphin swimming in the sea. We can also assume that these posthumans have thorough control over their environment, so that they can make molecularly exact copies of objects and implement any physical design for which they have conceived of a detailed blueprint. They could make a forest of redwood trees disappear, and then recreate an exactly similar forest somewhere else; and they could populate it with dinosaurs or dragons—they would have the same kind of control of physical reality as programmers and designers today have over virtual reality, but with the ability to imagine and create much more detailed (e.g. biologically realistic) structures. We might say that the autopotent superintelligences are living in a "plastic world" because they can easily remold their environment exactly as they see fit.

Now, it might be that in any technological utopia that we have any realistic chance of creating, all individuals will remain constrained

---

* Kolnai, "Dignity," p. 262. Kolnai adds that the "core of Un-Dignity" does *not* include "either submission to the existing order of things and the virtue of patience, or a sustained endeavor for reform, improvement and assuagement."

in important ways. In addition to the challenges of the physical frontiers, which might at this stage be receding into deep space as the posthuman civilization expands beyond its native planet, there are the challenges created by the existence of other posthumans, that is, the challenges of the social realm. Resources even in Plastic World would soon become scarce if population growth is exponential, but aside from material constraints, individual agents would face the constraints imposed on them by the choices and actions of other agents. Insofar as our goals are irreducibly social—for example to be loved, respected, given special attention or admiration, or to be allowed to spend time or to form exclusive bonds with the people we choose, or to have a say in what other people do—we would still be limited in our ability to achieve our goals. Thus, a being in Plastic World may be very far from omnipotent. Nevertheless, we may suppose that a large portion of the constraints we currently face have been lifted and that both our internal states and the world around us have become much more malleable to our wishes and desires.

In Plastic World, many of the moral imperatives with which we are currently struggling are easily satisfiable. As the loud values fall silent, the quiet values become more audible.* With most externally imposed constraints eliminated by technological progress, the constraints *that we choose to impose on ourselves* become paramount.

In this setting, Dignity as a Quality could be an organizing idea. While inanimate objects cannot possess Human Dignity, they can be endowed with a kind of Dignity as a Quality. The autopotent inhabitants of Plastic World could choose to cultivate their sensibility for Dignity as a Quality and the other quiet values. By choosing to recognize these values and to treat the world accordingly, they would be accepting some constraints on their actions. It is by accepting such constraints that they could build, or rather *cultivate,* their Plastic World into something that has greater value than a daydream. It is also by accepting such constraints—perhaps only by doing so— that it would be possible for them to preserve their own Dignity as a Quality. This dignity would not consist in resisting or defying the

---

* This is not to say that the quiet values would actually be heard or heeded if and when the loud values fall silent. Whether that would happen is difficult to predict. But an ideal moral agent would begin to pay more attention to the quiet values in such circumstances and would let them play a greater role in guiding her conduct.

world. Rather, theirs would be a dignity of the strong, consisting in self-restraint and the positive nurturance of both internal and external values.*

---

* For their comments, I'm grateful to Robin Hanson, Rebecca Roache, Anders Sandberg, Julian Savulescu, and to participants of the James Martin Advanced Research Seminar (20 October 2006, Oxford) and the Enhance Workshop (27 March 2007, Stockholm) where earlier versions of this paper were presented. I am especially indebted to Guy Kahane for discussions and insights, many of which have been incorporated into this paper, and to Rebecca Roache for research assistance. I would also like to thank Tom Merrill for helpful editorial suggestions.

## Notes

[1] Franz Josef Wetz, "The Dignity of Man," in *Anatomy Art—Fascination Beneath the Surface* (catalogue of the exhibition) ed. Gunther von Hagens (Heidelberg: Institute for Plastination, 2000), pp. 239-258.
[2] Ibid., p. 242.
[3] See Doron Shultziner, "Human dignity—functions and meanings," *Global Jurist Topics* 3 (2003): 1-21, citing Teresa Iglesias, "Bedrock Truths and the Dignity of the Individual," *Logos* 4 (2001): 114-134.
[4] Some think this salience is undeserved: e.g., Ruth Macklin, "Dignity is a Useless Concept," *British Medical Journal* 327 (2003): 1419-1420, and Dieter Birnbacher, "Human cloning and human dignity," *Reproductive BioMedicine Online* 10, Supplement 1 (2005): 50-55. See also Richard E. Ashcroft, "Making sense of dignity," *Journal of Medical Ethics* 31 (2005): 679-682, and Timothy Caulfield and Roger Brownsword, "Human dignity: a guide to policy making in the biotechnology era?" *Nature Reviews Genetics* 7 (2006): 72-76.
[5] E.g., Leon R. Kass, *Life, Liberty and the Defense of Dignity: The Challenge for Bioethics* (San Francisco, California: Encounter Books, 2002).
[6] These first two meanings are discussed in Aurel Kolnai, "Dignity," *Philosophy* 51 (1976): 251-271, p. 259.
[7] For an earlier discussion of mine on the relation between enhancement and human dignity, see Nick Bostrom, "In Defence of Posthuman Dignity," *Bioethics* 19 (2005): 202-214.
[8] Kolnai, op. cit., pp. 251-252.
[9] Ibid., p. 252.
[10] Ibid., pp. 253-254.
[11] Ibid., p. 254.
[12] Cf. Peter D. Kramer, *Listening to Prozac* (New York: Viking, 1993).
[13] Giovanni Pico della Mirandola, *Oration on the Dignity of Man* (1486), trans. Elizabeth Livermore Forbes, in *The Renaissance Philosophy of Man*, ed. Ernst Cassirer, Paul Oskar Kristeller, and John Herman Randall (Chicago: University of Chicago Press, 1948), available online, edited and with an introduction by P. James Clark, at www.angelfire.com/wizard/regulus_antares/pico_della_mirandola.htm.
[14] Kolnai, op. cit., pp. 265-266.
[15] Kass, op. cit., p. 48.
[16] Aryeh Routtenberg and Jacob Lindy, "Effects of the availability of rewarding septal and hypothalamic stimulation on bar pressing for food under conditions of deprivation," *Journal of Comparative and Physiological Psychology* 60 (1965): 158-161.
[17] For a discussion of the relations between dignity and suffering, see Daryl Pullman, "Human dignity and the ethics and aesthetics of pain and suffering," *Theoretical Medicine* 23 (2002): 75-94.
[18] David Pearce, "When Is It Best To Take Crack Cocaine?" *LA Weekly*, July 6-12, 2001.

[19] John Steinbeck, *Travels with Charley: In Search of America* (New York, Viking Press, 1962), pp. 168*ff*.
[20] Craig Duncan, "Respect for Dignity: A Defense," online manuscript, 10/06 draft, p. 5; see www.ithaca.edu/faculty/cduncan/respect.doc.
[21] Stephen Darwall, "Two Kinds of Respect," *Ethics* 88 (1977): 36-49. What follows is a simplified description of Darwall's account that skirts some of its finer points.

# Commentary on Bostrom
## Charles Rubin

In his essay for this volume, Nick Bostrom acknowledges that the consequences of emerging technologies for what he, following Aurel Kolnai, calls "Dignity as Quality" are hard to predict and even harder to judge. What Bostrom doesn't seem to notice is that Kolnai himself would almost certainly have opposed the transhumanist agenda and that the very essay Bostrom draws upon provides ample grounds for doubting the wisdom of transhumanism's ultimate goals. Rather than supporting his case, the attempt to enlist Kolnai in his cause reveals instead how Bostrom fails to appreciate that genuine human dignity, like all human excellence, requires that we acknowledge and accept certain natural necessities, even those we sometimes struggle against.

Kolnai (1900-73) would seem to be an odd source for the case for transhumanism. A Hungarian-born philosopher who converted to Catholicism after reading G. K. Chesterton, Kolnai spent much of his career as an expatriate. Trained in phenomenology by Husserl, Kolnai articulated a politics of "Christian imperfectionism" and a powerful anti-utopianism, a politics not at all well suited to a thoroughgoing project to remake human nature.[1] In particular, the essay "Dignity," to which Bostrom refers, provides no grounds for thinking that our dignity, in the sense Kolnai is most interested in, could be enhanced by an increase in our power—indeed, quite the opposite.

Unlike most writers on dignity, Kolnai is at pains to distinguish the dignity he cares about—"dignity as quality"—from the related notions of human dignity and human rights. "Dignity as quality" is primarily a characteristic that elicits from us reverence and awe, "a 'bowing' gesture if I may so call it" (252).[2] Kolnai is at pains to avoid reducing "dignity as quality" to a merely moral claim, such as "the so-called rights of man" (257). He is skeptical of the natural basis of such rights, and he thinks that the moral imperative implied in them obscures our appreciation of "dignity as quality." As for the notion of human dignity, he finds it to be a hybrid concept halfway between the prescriptive character of rights and the descriptive character of "dignity as quality" (258).

"Dignity as quality" in this sense would seem to be tailor-made for Bostrom's purposes, since it transcends merely human dignity and can be attributed to elephants, cats, bulls, and even landscapes (254). As Bostrom might well ask, if a cat can have dignity, why not Cat Man? If nonhuman beings can have it, why not transhuman beings?

Furthermore, we would be remiss if we failed to acknowledge that Kolnai's discussion of these matters is itself fraught with ambiguity and uncertainty, some of which may have seemed to Bostrom to point in his direction. In particular Kolnai's skepticism about there being a true natural basis of natural rights spills over into questions he raises about the place of "dignity as quality" in human life. But despite this skepticism, Kolnai seems genuinely to wonder whether there is a moral order congruent with being human, for which human beings are not simply responsible but which makes sense of human dignity even if it does not resolve all ambiguities. "Dignity as quality" is an effort to give an account of dignity without starting from an answer to this question. Kolnai proceeds instead by elucidating the lived experience of the phenomenon of dignity. But Kolnai chooses not to evade the issue of the ultimate ground of dignity altogether.

Bostrom, on the other hand, leaves all Kolnai's nuance and uncertainty aside. To be sure, Bostrom makes the anodyne observation that any given potential enhancement to human life may or may not turn out to enhance human dignity. Yet when he turns to the logical culmination of his defense of enhancement, his concluding "leap into an imaginary future posthuman world," Bostrom fails to confront many passages in Kolnai that warn against just such a world and that suggest that its fundamental assumptions could not help but make it undignified. For example, Kolnai finds Condorcet's "rationally and scientifically redrawn world" to be a place where "there would be no opportunity for the exercise of heroic virtue nor any sense in revering it" (262). Why should we not think that Kolnai would see Bostrom's Plastic World as just another "Utopian Delusion" like Condorcet's?

Here again, Kolnai goes some way toward Bostrom's point of view when he writes that "an elementary, not to say elemental, feature of dignity…[is] clarifying, developing, pursuing, and making valid personal tastes and choices" (261). Bostrom thinks, of course, that posthuman capacities can only widen the realm of such activity. And yet, for Kolnai, this aspect of dignity exists within a larger framework of "what is most important," which is "not to 'get what one likes' but to be able to endure what one 'gets' without necessarily assenting to it or growing to 'like' it" (262). The dignified attitude thus has an element of resignation quite antithetical to the very plasticity of Plastic World. Why should autopotent human beings ever concern themselves with the constraints of "an existing order of things" or the "tension between Value and Reality" (262)? Yet refusal to "recognize, experience, and bear with" that tension is for Kolnai "the core of Un-dignity" (262).

Bostrom suggests that his posthumans will be "Bayesian rationalists" who have "no convictions but only a fluid network of revisable beliefs." While such qualities may appear to allow a dignified-sounding "self-transcendence," it is hard to distinguish such rationalism from what Kolnai calls a meretricious "flitting mobility of a weightless self" (266). While Bostrom might well be right that a posthuman being will have "spectacular success" at "creating around himself a world for his own use," he fails to note that Kolnai thinks such self-creation is precisely what will lead to dignity as quality being "crowded out" (266).

We might also pose to Bostrom the question George Orwell asked in *The Road to Wigan Pier* about H. G. Wells's portrayal of the physical traits of the man of the future. In a highly mechanized society, Orwell wondered, why should we expect to find human beings of the godlike physique and fitness Wells describes? It seems to Orwell far more likely that, as the necessity for physical fitness declines, one would find "little fat men,"[3] a point that early 21st-century Americans can hardly gainsay. Of course, we might reply to Orwell that we will choose to constrain ourselves: physical fitness is better for our health, a fun hobby besides! And yet somehow rigorous programs of diet and exercise are hardly the norm. Many more indulge the freedom of separating high caloric consumption from intense physical activity and are on the lookout for the magic pill that will free them from the consequences of such indulgence.

In Plastic World dignity will become a quality as rare as is physical excellence in a mechanized world. Perhaps the best we can expect is that, just as we today admire intensive physical cultivation in boutique settings, e.g., sports, there will be a super-intelligent audience in Plastic World for "dignity games." After all, we see in contemporary America a taste for "Masterpiece Theatre" renditions of vanished worlds of honor and gentlemanliness. The inhabitants of Plastic World, we might imagine, will enjoy highly ritualized moral encounters, appreciated by some for the display of antiquated excellence and by most for the frisson of horrific insight they provide into a barbaric past.

According to Kolnai, true dignity (and its opposite) arises only in how we come to terms with things not of our own choice or making. But if that is the case, there can be no dignity in the world of autopotent posthumans, who know no restraint or constraint not of their own making. Unlike Kolnai, Bostrom is confident that posthuman inhabitants of plastic world will exhibit the "dignity of the strong." Out of their autopotency they will choose to restrain themselves in accordance with "quiet values." In human terms we know what that might mean: the mercy of the king or conqueror, the act of noblesse oblige. But in the world we have known hitherto, the dignity of such acts still depends on external constraints felt by the strong, such as the binding power of religious obligation, the existence of powerful social hierarchies, even the mere sense of prudence that restraint is good today because one never knows what tomorrow will bring. Will "quiet values" produce any like reasons to compel the strong in plastic world to show self-restraint? Bostrom never worries that the strong might not want to restrain themselves in Plastic World, or that there might be a real ugliness in the human will that will only be exposed once we are freed of natural constraints.

By Kolnai's lights, then, it seems likely that Bostrom has fallen into a utopian trap, a classic expression of which can be found in Shakespeare's *The Tempest*. The old courtier Gonzalo expatiates on the ideal commonwealth he would create if he were king, concluding paradoxically that there would be "No sovereignty." The not merely cynical Antonio comments, "The latter end of his commonwealth forgets the beginning" (*The Tempest* 2.1.160, 162-3.) Likewise, Bostrom begins by having us seek the power of gods, though in the "latter end" he paradoxically expects us to refrain from using our godlike powers to the maximum.

# Notes

[1] David Wiggins and Bernard Williams, "Aurel Thomas Kolnai (1900-1973)," in *Ethics, Values, and Reality: Selected Papers of Aurel Kolnai* (Indianapolis, Indiana: Hackett, 1978), ix-xxv.
[2] All references to Kolnai in the text are to Aurel Kolnai, "Dignity," in *Philosophy* 51 (1976): 251-271.
[3] George Orwell, *The Road to Wigan Pier* (New York: Harcourt Brace Jovanovich, 1958), p. 193.

# Part III.
# Dignity and Modern Culture

# 9

# Human Dignity and Public Discourse

## Richard John Neuhaus

Dr. Adam Schulman's thoughtful overview (in the introduction to this volume) of the problems posed by bioethics and human dignity begins with a succinct description of what might be called the state of the question. His words bear repeating:

> Human dignity—is it a useful concept in bioethics, one that sheds important light on the whole range of bioethical issues, from embryo research and assisted reproduction, to biomedical enhancement, to care of the disabled and the dying? Or is it, on the contrary, a useless concept—at best a vague substitute for other, more precise notions, at worst a mere slogan that camouflages unconvincing arguments and unarticulated biases?

To begin the discussion by reference to what is "useful" or "useless" does not necessarily imply a thoroughgoing utilitarian calculus, but it does invite the question, Useful or useless to what end? The statement of the state of the question says that "useful" means that it sheds important light on various bioethical issues, while "useless" means that it is less useful than "more precise notions" or, worse, that it is misleading and deceptive. Clearly, "light"—i.e., wisdom, knowledge, truth, guidance—is what we desire. Since the subject is bioethics, the kind of light we are looking for is ethical or moral light.

We need not enter into the debate over whether there is a qualitative difference between the ethical and moral. It is argued by some that the *ethical* deals with right and wrong while the *moral* deals with good and evil, with right and wrong being defined by us while good and evil are discovered in the way things really are. With respect to the actions addressed by bioethics, perhaps all can agree that the goal is to *do the right thing*, with most claiming that the right thing is the moral thing. In the history of Western civilization's reflection on ethics and morality, the most elementary maxim is, "Do good and avoid evil." For purposes pertinent to the questions addressed by bioethics, this can also be phrased as "Do right and avoid wrong." The first principle of practical (moral) reason, in obedience to that maxim, is to direct one's will in accord with the human good.

To be sure, it is argued by some that in some circumstances it is permissible to do evil—a "necessary evil," as it is called—in order to do the right thing, meaning in order to achieve the right result. This touches on the divide between the utilitarian and deontological lamented by Dr. Schulman. From one viewpoint, it is at least doubtful that an act is evil if it is indeed necessary to achieving a good (i.e., doing the right thing). From another viewpoint, assuming that good and evil are antithetical, it is allowed that good may result from an act or course of action that will foreseeably result in a circumstance that it would be wrong to intend, but the good result is *despite* and never *because* of the doing of evil. The relevance of this brief excursus on the distinction between ethics and morality, including the distinction between right and wrong, on the one hand, and good and evil, on the other, will become evident in due course.

The stated subject is the usefulness of the concept "human dignity." The better phrase is "the dignity of the human person." "Human dignity" may suggest the collective and include efforts such as taking technological charge of the evolution of the human species. "The dignity of the human person" places the accent on the individual, albeit, to be sure, the individual situated in community. The dignity of the human person may entail an important, although limited, measure autonomy. Dignity as autonomy features strongly in, for instance, arguments for "death with dignity." Morally, however, the dignity of the human person is affirmed most importantly not in the assertion of one's autonomy but in the protection of others who are most subject to having their dignity violated. Therefore, in bioethics as in medicine more generally, the first rule is "Do no harm." That first rule enjoins us to protect and maintain something that is recognized as good in its being.

That first rule is perceived by some to be a restriction on scientific and technological progress, and it is intended to be exactly that. More precisely, it is a frankly moral placing of limits on what some, driven by what is aptly described as the scientific or technological imperative, deem to be progress. Morality is not to be pitted against genuine progress, and we should be grateful for all the advances that have been made and no doubt will be made in "the relief of man's estate" (Bacon). But it is precisely the business of ethical and moral reason to make normative judgments regarding present and proposed measures aimed at such relief. This is true with respect to the dignity of the human person and with respect to more ambitious proposals aimed not so much at relieving as at transforming "man's estate." In this connection, Dr. Schulman's citing of C. S. Lewis's *The Abolition of Man* is entirely to the point.

Understanding of the questions before us has not been well served by the ill-defined discipline of bioethics. Militating against the task of normative moral judgment is not only the scientific and technological imperative, with all the fame and glory attending "breakthrough" achievements, but also the weight of inestimable financial interests. Think, for instance, of what those who can pay will pay for a significant extension of their life span or for the "perfect baby." It is only somewhat cynical to observe that institutions with the greatest vested interest in dubious advances have recruited the best bioethicists that money can buy.

One must acknowledge that bioethics as an intellectual institution is, in significant part, an industry for the production of rationalized—sometimes elegantly rationalized—permission slips in the service of the technological imperative joined to the pursuit of fame and wealth. Which is not to deny that such permission slips are also issued in the service of what some believe to be the relief of suffering and the enhancement of man's estate. Even when bioethics is conducted with intellectual and moral integrity, a question must be raised about the nature of the authority of those who are called bioethicists. This touches on politics and political legitimacy in addressing bioethical controversies.

Dr. Schulman notes the complaint that the idea of the dignity of the human person in international agreements and declarations in the aftermath of World War II "does not offer clear and unambiguous guidance in bioethical controversies." He says, correctly, that in such statements "the meaning, content, and foundations of human dignity are never explicitly defined. Instead, the affirmation of human dignity in these documents reflects a political consensus among groups that may well have quite different beliefs about what human dignity means, where it comes from, and what it entails. In effect, 'human dignity' serves here as a placeholder for 'whatever it is about human beings that entitles them to basic human rights and freedoms.'" He adds, "This practice makes a good deal of sense."

It makes a great deal of sense indeed. In a world indelibly marked and marred by the Holocaust, the Gulag Archipelago, Mao's Great Leap Forward, and myriad other crimes against humanity, a political consensus as a placeholder against great evils, no matter how intellectually rickety its structure, is not to be scorned. In *A World Made New: Eleanor Roosevelt and the Universal Declaration of Human Rights*,[1] Harvard law professor Mary Ann Glendon describes the ways in which the drafters of the declaration were keenly aware that their goal was a political consensus, not a philosophical or moral treatise on human nature and the rights and dignities attending human nature. Given the enormous cultural, religious, intellectual, and ideological diversity of those involved, a political consensus was a great achievement. While rights and freedoms are positively asserted, they are largely defined negatively against the background of evils to which the declaration says, in effect, "Never again!" Thus was the morally elementary rule "Do no harm" given new specificity.

Nor should it be thought that a political consensus is somehow inferior to a coherent treatise on the moral and philosophical foundations of human dignity. In a world that continues to be characterized by what Saint Augustine called *libido dominandi*—the unbridled lust for power and glory—politics is an instrument for the straint of great evil. In ethics, and in bioethics specifically, "politics" is frequently seen as an alien intrusion upon or a poor substitute for the search for "clear and unambiguous guidance." But the search for guidance through the controversies besetting us is precisely a political task.

Aristotle's *Nicomachean Ethics* and his *Politics* are both discourses on morality. From them we can derive this definition of politics: *Politics is free persons deliberating the question, How ought we to order our life together?* The "ought" in that suggested definition clearly indicates that politics is—in its nature, if not always in its practice—a moral enterprise. Our political vocabulary—what is fair or unfair, what is just or unjust, what serves the common good—is inescapably a moral vocabulary. Contra David Hume and many others, an *ought* can be derived from an *is*, and typically is so derived in the ordinary experience of individuals and communities. Neither agreement nor consensus is required on all the details of "whatever it is about human beings that entitles them to basic human rights and freedoms."

The political consensus of the *Universal Declaration,* although very important, undoubtedly rests upon a philosophically thin account of the dignity of the human person. That is in large part because the "international community" is not a community. It is not, in Aristotle's sense of the term, a *polis* in which free persons deliberate the question, How ought we to order our life together? Of course, there are many and interesting debates about whether the United States or its several states qualify as a *polis*. Without going into the details of those debates, it is beyond dispute that our constitutional order presents itself as a political community deliberating its right ordering on the basis of the political sovereignty of "the people" exercised through the specified means of representative democracy. The foundational principle here is the statement of the Declaration of Independence that just government is derived from the consent of the governed.

The question of the dignity of the human person is rightly understood as a political question. It is inescapably a political question. The resolution (always provisional and open to revision) of the great majority of political disputes does not ordinarily require delving into the foundational truths explored by philosophy, ethics, and theology. Our political discourse is guided, and frequently misguided, by custom, habits, and tacit understandings. Proponents of "natur~1 1 theory" rely heavily on moral reasoning attuned to "those things that we cannot not know." And of course other theories are advanced, both because they are held to be true and because they are thought to be useful for purposes of political persuasion.

In general, however, our political life is not heavily burdened by theory, or at least not by the explication of theory. That is because knowing and judging the good things of human life is not so burdened. In the realm of bioethics, however, and specifically with respect to the dignity of the human person, such explication is sometimes required. An obvious example is abortion, and the many issues inseparably tied to abortion. The most consequential political event of the past half century in the United States was the Supreme Court's *Roe* and *Doe* decisions of January 1973. Numerous political analysts have described how those decisions have dramatically reconfigured the nation's cultural and political life. And of course those decisions are intimately tied to many other "hot button" issues in bioethics. As an act of "raw judicial power" (Justice Byron White in dissent), *Roe v. Wade* removed a preeminently political, which is to say moral, question from public deliberation. The abortion decisions were a profoundly anti-political act and are accurately described as instances of the judicial usurpation of politics. And, of course, by attempting to remove the question, the Court turned it into something very much like the vortex of American politics.

The moral question is not, as the court majority supposed, about when a human life begins. That is a biological and medical question on which there is no serious dispute. The moral question can be put this way: At what point in its existence ought we, and for what reasons ought we, to recognize that a human life should be protected in law?

On this issue, if no other, Peter Singer has it right. As the noted Princeton advocate of infanticide said in a letter to the *New York Times* rebuking Mario Cuomo for his confused thinking about abortion, "The crucial moral question is not when human life begins, but when human life reaches the point at which it merits protection . . . Unless we separate these two questions—when does life begin, and when does it merit protection?—we are unlikely to achieve any clarity about the moral status of embryos."[2]

That moral question is also and unavoidably a political question.

One might make the case that it is the most fundamental of political questions. If politics is deliberating how we ought to order our life together, there can hardly be a more basic question than this: Who belongs to the "we"? Although ostensibly removing it from politics, the abortion decisions forced into the political arena an issue that was thought to have been settled in the centuries of civilizational tradition of which our polity is part. Namely, that it is morally wrong and rightly made unlawful deliberately to kill unborn children.

If a principle is established by which some indisputably human lives do not warrant the protections traditionally associated with the dignity of the human person—because of their size, dependency, level of development, or burdensomeness to others—it would seem that there are numerous candidates for the application of the principle, beginning with the radically handicapped, both physically and mentally, not to mention millions of the aged and severely debilitated in our nation's nursing homes. It may be objected that *of course* we as a people are not about to embark upon such a program of extermination. To think we might do so is simply bizarre.

As a culturally and politically contingent fact, that is true. But under the regime of *Roe*, a regime extended to embryonic stem cell research and other bioethical controversies, we have no "clear and unambiguous" agreed-upon rule precluding such horrors. We do have in our constituting texts, notably in the Declaration of Independence, a commitment to natural rights; and we do have deeply entrenched in our culture and politics a concept of the dignity of the human person.

The question is: Who belongs to the community for which we as a community accept responsibility, including the responsibility to protect, along with other natural rights, their right to life? This is a preeminently political question. It is not a question to be decided by bioethicists. Bioethicists, by virtue of their disciplined attention to this and related questions, are in a position to help inform political deliberations and decisions about these matters, but they are rightly and of necessity to be decided politically. They are rightly so decided because our constitutional order vests political sovereignty in the people who exercise that sovereignty through prescribed means of representation. They are of necessity so decided because in this society the views of moral philosophers—whether trained as such in the academy or acting as such on the bench—are not deemed to be determinative. Witness the democratic non-ratification of the Supreme Court's imposition of the unlimited abortion license.

To say that such decisions are rightly decided politically is not to say that the resulting decisions will always be morally right. Those who disagree with the decisions that are made must make their case in the political arena. The product of bioethics may be prescriptive in theory—resulting in "clear and unambiguous" guidelines—but, in this constitutional order, it has to be persuasive in practice. In fact, of course, disagreements among moral philosophers, including bioethicists, are as strong as those found in the general public, and probably stronger.

In the happy absence of philosopher kings, everybody enters the process of debate, deliberation, and decision equipped only with the powers of persuasion. Obviously, not everybody enters on equal terms, since powers of persuasion, access to the means of persuasion, and audiences inclined to be persuaded to one position or another are far from equal. This is a highly unsatisfactory circumstance in which the achievement of "clear and unambiguous" rules is rare and a "political consensus" resting on a moral point of reference as a "placeholder" may be deemed a great achievement.

The dignity of the human person—construed not, or not primarily, as the assertion of the rights of the autonomous but as the obligation to protect those whose autonomy is very limited—is such a point of reference. It is complained that those who defend that point of reference have an unfair advantage in that it is so widely shared in our culture. They are engaged, it is said, not in moral or ethical argument but in politics. As suggested earlier, however, politics *is* moral argument about how we ought to order our life together. After the June 1953 uprising in East Germany, the secretary of the Writers Union distributed leaflets declaring that the people had lost the confidence of the government and it would take redoubled efforts to win it back. To which the playwright Bertolt Brecht is supposed to have responded, "Would it not be easier in that case for the government to dissolve the people and elect another?" Our present day bioethicists, moral philosophers, and judges sometimes appear to want to heed Brecht's advice and dissolve the people that they have and who have proven so recalcitrant to their expertise.

The people who are the American *polis* are deeply attached to the concept of the dignity of the human person. For those who have a moral adherence to this constitutional order and the means it provides for addressing the *res publica*, that is a factor of considerable significance. Yet there are those who contend that such popular attachments are prejudices or unreflective biases that have no legitimate place in authentically *public* discourse. Well known is the proscription, commonly associated with John Rawls, of "comprehensive accounts" from authentically public discourse. The proscription is most rigorously asserted when such comprehensive accounts are perceived to be "religious" in nature.

The moral authority of those who would make the rules for what is to be admitted and what is to be excluded from public discourse is far from being clear to many students of these arguments and is totally baffling to the people who are the public. The perfectly understandable suspicion is that there is a self-serving dynamic in the efforts of some to appoint themselves the gatekeepers and border patrol of the public square, admitting some arguments and excluding others. The proscription of comprehensive accounts—especially when they are religious or associated with a religious tradition—gives a monopoly on the public square to accounts that are non-religious or anti-religious in character. Such accounts are, in fact, no less comprehensive, as has been persuasively argued by, among others, Alasdair MacIntyre in *Whose Justice? Which Rationality?*[3] Conflicts that are described as being between reason and tradition are typically conflicts between different traditions of reason, each invoking its own authorities.

In the comprehensive accounts that would proscribe other comprehensive accounts, especially if they are perceived as "religious" in nature, the operative assumption is typically atheism. This is not to say that all who support such proscriptions are atheists. It is to say that, in their moral reasoning, they are *methodological* atheists. Only those arguments are to be admitted to public deliberation that proceed *as if* God does not exist. This is a non-rational prejudice in which the great majority of Americans do not acquiesce. Whether by invoking Pascal's Wager or some other argument, they believe it is a great deal more rational to proceed as if God does exist. In any event, they do so proceed. The politically sovereign people are free to acknowledge, and generally do acknowledge, a sovereignty higher than their own, and to give public expression to that acknowledgment.

For most purposes in the ordering of our common life, it is neither necessary nor wise to invoke an account of moral reality beyond what is required for the resolution of the issue at hand. Explicitly moral arguments are not to be expanded or multiplied beyond necessity. On most issues, a sustainable measure of political equilibrium can be achieved by appeal to a widely shared and "thin" account of moral reality that is far less than comprehensive. This is frequently not the case, however, in questions related to bioethics.

People who are themselves devoutly religious may in the public square advance arguments that are not distinctively religious in character. This is notably the case with proponents of natural law theory. They proceed on the basis that human beings are naturally endowed with a rational capacity to discern the truth, including the moral truth, of things. In public argument, they generally prescind from religious or theological claims, contending that agreement on the ultimate sources and ends of human reason is not necessary to the exercise of human reason.

Contrary to the critics of natural law theory, the theory and its practice is not discredited by the observation that many, if not most, of its practitioners do in fact have definite ideas on sources and ends. Nor is it discredited by being widely perceived as a distinctively Catholic theory. Its proponents can readily respond that a distinctively Catholic contribution to our common life is to have preserved a universal understanding of reason that is, being universal, in no way peculiarly Catholic. It is an understanding that has strong roots in the Aristotelian view of politics and public discourse under discussion here.

Not all Americans are as abstemious as natural law theorists when it comes to unfurling in public argument their ultimate and comprehensive truth claims. For the great majority of Americans, religion and morality are inextricably intertwined. Public arguments involve different publics or different parts of the public. To those publics who are presumed to share their comprehensive account of reality in its fullness, proponents of this position or that will make the arguments that they think will be most effective in persuading. This is inevitable, and those who have a problem with it have a problem with democracy. (Obviously, many thoughtful people, from ancient times to the present, have had and do have grave reservations about democracy.)

There is, of course, a necessary concern about unbridled populism, raw majoritarianism, and the dangers of demagoguery. The framers of our constitutional order were keenly aware of these problems. Thus our system of representation, checks and balances, staggered elections, vetoes, overrides, judicial review, and other mechanisms conducive to more sober deliberation of how we ought to order or life together. While this intentionally complex order slows the course of turning arguments into law and public policy, it in no way restricts the arguments that can be made.

Demagogic agitation for specific laws or policies is sometimes employed, for instance, by identifying one's policy preferences with the will of God. Such appeals are usually limited to audiences where it is thought they might be persuasive. There is also the demagoguery of appeals to the more general public that—for instance in the controversy over embryonic stem cell research—cruelly exploit human suffering and exaggerated or unfounded hopes for cures. Demagoguery will be always with us. Our constitutional order is not a machine that runs of itself. It depends upon the cultivation of restraint, civility, and disciplined reason, which are always in short supply. And we do well to keep in mind that the wisest of our public philosophers, from Tocqueville onward, cautioned not only against the tyranny of the majority but also against the tyranny of the minority. Today that caution is pertinent to the minority that would impose a rule that authentically public discourse must be methodologically atheistic.

Restraint, civility, and disciplined reason are seriously undermined by the hostility to "comprehensive accounts" in our public discourse—especially if they are perceived to be religious in nature. In most intellectual enterprises, and not least in ethics, there is a propensity to emulate the methodologies and exactitude associated with the physical sciences. Philosopher Thomas Nagel writes:

> This reductionist dream is nourished by the extraordinary success of the physical sciences in our time, not least in their recent application to the understanding of life through molecular biology. It is natural to try to take any successful intellectual method as far as it will go. Yet the impulse to find

an explanation of everything in physics has over the last fifty years gotten out of control. The concepts of physical science provide a very special, and partial, description of the world that experience reveals to us. It is the world with all subjective consciousness, sensory appearances, thought, value, purpose, and will left out. What remains is the mathematically describable order of things and events in space and time.... We have more than one form of understanding. Different forms of understanding are needed for different kinds of subject matter. The great achievements of physical science do not make it capable of encompassing everything, from mathematics to ethics to the experiences of a living animal.[4]

The concept of the dignity of the human person was arrived at, and is today sustained, by such a different form of understanding. It is a form of understanding that is carefully reasoned, frankly moral and, for most people who affirm it, is in fact, if not by theoretical necessity, inseparable from a comprehensive account that is unapologetically acknowledged as religious. The hostility to admitting this account to public discourse is longstanding. Indeed, it has long been argued by some that moral referents should be eliminated altogether from law and public policy, that ours is a strictly procedural polity devoted only to means and prescinding from ends, and especially from overtly moral ends. Oliver Wendell Holmes famously wrote that it would be a great benefit "if every word of moral significance could be banished from the law altogether, and other words adopted which should convey legal ideas uncolored by anything outside the law."[5]

But, of course, it was by ideas and experiences outside the law that the concept of the dignity of the human person was enshrined in the law. The word "enshrined" is used advisedly, indicating the sacred sources of that dignity. In religious thought, and in Christian thought specifically, the dignity of the human person has become the touchstone of ethical reflection. Pope John Paul II wrote on several occasions that the entirety of Catholic social doctrine rests on the understanding of the dignity of the human person.[6] The *Catechism of the Catholic Church* devotes no less than 23 pages to explaining the concept and its implications. It is an explanation that in its essentials is embraced also by non-Catholic Christians, as is evident, for instance, in the recent statement of Evangelicals and Catholics Together, "That They May Have Life."[7] It is a concept firmly grounded in the Jewish tradition and—although not without troubling ambiguities—in that of Islam.[8]

That concept, on which almost all Americans rely, with varying degrees of reflectiveness and consistency, in deliberating how we ought to order our life together can be briefly summarized: A human being is a person possessed of a dignity we are obliged to respect at every point of development, debilitation, or decline by virtue of being created in the image and likeness of God. Endowed with the spiritual principle of the soul, with reason, and with free will, the destiny of the person who acts in accord with moral conscience in obedience to the truth is nothing less than eternal union with God. This is the dignity of the human person that is to be respected, defended, and indeed revered.

That is beyond doubt a very comprehensive account of the dignity of the human person. I have referred to the political sovereignty of "the people" in our constitutional order. The location of sovereignty—the authority to which the *polis* holds itself finally accountable—has in the post–World War II been, one might say, personalized. Ours is a period that Karl Barth, the most influential Protestant theologian of the past century, described as one of "disillusioned sovereignty."[9] The great disillusionment is with the sovereignty of the state.

If one asked almost all Enlightenment thinkers what is sovereign, they would not have answered "reason" or "the individual" or "science." The unhesitating answer would be "the state." The darkest and most relentless depiction of the modern political project was offered by Thomas Hobbes. He taught that the incarnate and resurrected God-man who lives and governs is to be replaced in the temporal world by a mortal god (*deus mortalis*)—a machine-like man, mythologically known as the Leviathan. Engraved on the title page of the 1651 edition of his book by that title is *Job* 41:24: *Non est potestas super terram quae comparetur ei*—"There is upon the earth no power like his."[10] After Auschwitz and the Gulag Archipelago, none can read those words without a moral shudder.

There is on earth Leviathan's like and, indeed, his sovereign: the human person. The concept of the dignity of the human perso be a "placeholder" in international covenants, but in the American political experiment, when public discourse is not arbitrarily constricted by methodological atheism, it is, with respect to bioethics and other matters of great moral moment, a concept richly and rationally elaborated and claiming overwhelming public support. It is, in sum, a concept that is indispensable to the political task of deliberating and deciding how we ought to order our life together.

## Notes

[1] Mary Ann Glendon, *A World Made New: Eleanor Roosevelt and the Creation of the Universal Declaration of Human Rights* (New York: Random House, 2001).

[2] Peter Singer, letter to the editor, *The New York Times*, June 23, 2005, responding to Mario Cuomo, "Not on Faith Alone," Op-Ed column, *The New York Times*, June 20, 2005.

[3] Alasdair MacIntyre, *Whose Justice? Which Rationality?* (Notre Dame, Indiana: University of Notre Dame Press, 1988).

[4] Thomas Nagel, "The Fear of Religion," a review of Richard Dawkins's *The God Delusion*, in *The New Republic*, October 23, 2006.

[5] Oliver Wendell Holmes, "The Path of the Law," in *Collected Legal Papers* (New York: Harcourt Brace, 1920), p. 179.

[6] Luke Gormally, "Pope John Paul II's Teaching on Human Dignity and its Implications for Bioethics," in Christopher Tollefson, ed., *Pope John Paul II's Contribution to Catholic Bioethics* (Dordrecht, Netherlands: Kluwer Academic Publishers, 2004).

[7] "That They May Have Life," *First Things*, October, 2006.

[8] For a discussion of different religious understandings, see David Novak's *Natural Law in Judaism* (Cambridge: Cambridge University Press, 1998) and C. S. Lewis's discussion of the Tao in *The Abolition of Man* (Oxford: Oxford University Press, 1943).

[9] Cited by Russell Hittinger in "Human Nature and States of Nature in John Paul II's Theological Anthropology," in Daniel N. Robinson, Gladys M. Sweeney, and Richard Gill, eds., *Human Nature in Its Wholeness* (Washington, D.C.: Catholic University of America Press, 2006), pp. 14-15.

[10] Cited by Hittinger, ibid., p. 280, n. 16. I am indebted to Professor Hittinger for directing me to unfamiliar literature on the historical development of the idea of the dignity of the human person.

# 10

# Modern and American Dignity

## Peter Augustine Lawler

Modern society—or at least its more sophisticated parts—is distinguished by its concern for individual dignity. Individuals demand to exist for themselves. They refuse to be reduced to useful and expendable means for ends that are not their own. Increasingly, modern government is based on the dignified principle that the individual can't be understood to exist for a community, a country, an ideology, a God, or even a family. We think it undignified to believe that earthly or real human beings exist for heavenly or imaginary ones, as we believe religions once led us to believe. We also think it undignified to regard today's individuals as existing for human beings of the future, as did the millenarian ideologies that disappeared with the 20th century. Protecting my dignity, from this view, means protecting what the moral fanatics are all too ready to sacrifice—my particular life, my particular being, myself.[1] My purpose here is to explore some of the modern dimensions of the dignified "I," and so to show how indispensable, wonderful, and strange the idea of personal dignity is for us Americans. One reason for this exploration is to show how technology and biotechnology are both reflections of and challenges to our proper understanding of our ineradicable human dignity.

## The Christian Understanding of Human Freedom

Our understanding of the dignity of the individual or the person originates, I think, with Christianity, particularly with St. Augustine. We find it in Augustine's criticism of the civil and natural theologies—the respectable theologies—of the Greeks and the Romans for misunderstanding who the human being is. Civil theology—the gods of the city or political community—is based on the premise that human beings are essentially citizens or part of a city. But that's not true. Human longings point beyond one's own country and can't be satisfied by any kind of political dedication or success. It's finally undignified or untruthful for a Roman to identify himself or his fate with Rome. Augustine didn't deny there was a certain nobility or dignity of citizens who subordinated their selfish interests for their country's common good. But even or especially the best Romans were looking in the wrong place for genuine personal security and significance or immortality. They were looking in the wrong place for personal meaning or transcendence or perfection.[2]

The polytheism of civil theology was also undignified insofar as it was an offense against the human mind. It required that educated men degrade themselves by feigning belief in unbelievable gods and engage in a futile effort to fend off moral deterioration as their country became more sophisticated. Such efforts were also degrading to others; they opposed the particular human being's efforts to free himself from what are finally selfish communal illusions. Civil theology, by defining us as citizens and nothing more, hides from us the dignity that all human beings share in common.

Sophisticated Greeks and Romans, Augustine adds, rejected the gods of their country for nature's God, the God of the philosophers. But that growth in theological sophistication in the direction of impersonal monotheism was only ambiguously progress. All reasonable theology is monotheistic; the orderly universe and essentially equal human beings must be governed by a single God. But Augustine still saw two problems with nature's God. First, he is too distant or too impersonal to provide any real support for the moral duties of particular human beings; dignified personal action or personal existence can't be based on a God that is finally not a "who" but a "what." Second, natural theology is based on the premise that the human being is a part of nature and nothing more. So it can't account for the realities of human freedom and dignity.

The God of the philosophers is meant as a replacement for civil theology and later becomes a competitor to Biblical theology. The philosopher orients himself toward the truth about God by liberating his mind from all the moral, political, and religious illusions that allow human beings confidently to experience themselves as at home in the world as whole persons. He frees himself from the illusions that give most people some sense of dignity or significance. The philosopher discovers that the human mind is at home in the world, and so that God must be the perfection of our intellectual capacity to comprehend all that exists.

We grasp our true dignity—the dignity of our minds—only by seeing that the mind necessarily depends on a body that exists for a moment nowhere in particular and then is gone. So my being at home as a mind depends on my radical homelessness or insignificance as a whole, embodied being. Any being that is genuinely eternal—such as a star—couldn't possibly know anything at all. Only a being who is absolutely mortal—or, better, absolutely contingent as a living being—could know both the truth about the stars and the truth about the insignificance of himself. Nature's God can establish the dignity of human minds, but only at the expense of denying the dignity of all human lives to the extent they aren't genuinely governed by thought.[3]

Understanding ourselves as wholly natural beings means surrendering any sense of real personal dignity to impersonal natural necessity, to a God who is a principle, not a person. But according to Augustine, human beings are more than merely natural beings. They long to be seen, in their particular, distinctive, infinitely significant freedom, by a personal God Who knows them as they truly are. Natural theology can't account for equally free, unique, indispensable, and irreplaceable beings under God, or for human persons who can distinguish themselves not only from the other animals and God but from each other.

Natural theology also can't account for, much less point to the satisfaction of, the longing of each particular human being really to be. Each human being longs to be and is an exception to the general, necessitarian laws that account for the rest of creation. Each of us has the freedom and dignity that comes with personal transcendence: The laws of nature can't account for our free will, for either our sinfulness or our virtue, for our love of particular persons (including the personal God), for the misery of our personal contingency and mortality without a personal, loving God, for our capacity to sense, even without revelation, that we were made for eternal life through our ineradicable alienation in this world, and for our literal transcendence of our biological existence as whole persons through God's grace.

## The Dignity of the Individual

The Augustinian criticism of both natural and civil theology on behalf of the particular person's or individual's dignity retains its force in the post-Christian climate of modern thought. The individual's claim for transcendent and dignified freedom actually intensifies as faith in the Biblical God recedes. What we faithfully trusted God to do for us we now have to do for ourselves. Our claim is also more insistent because it can now be based in our manly pride; my infinite significance no longer depends on my feigning humble self-surrender to an omnipotent God Who cares for me in particular.

The human individual described by John Locke and the other liberal philosophers regards himself as free, unique, and irreplaceable. I'm so full of dignity or inestimable worth that the whole world should center on what's best for me. The individual has the right to use his freedom to transform his natural condition, to act against the nature that's indifferent or hostile to his particular existence. And he has the right to oppose freely every effort of other human beings—even or especially priests and kings—to risk or even deploy his life for purposes other than his individual ones. His dignity isn't given to him by God or nature; it is found in his freedom, in his singular capability to exercise rights.[4]

We can call rights natural insofar as we acknowledge that we didn't make ourselves capable of making ourselves free. Freedom from nature is a quality mysteriously possessed by members of our species alone, and that mystery deepens, of course, when we doubt that the Bible can even begin to explain it. But that means, paradoxically, that our singular natural quality is our free or transcendent ability to transform nature to give to ourselves what nature did not give us. There is, in fact, no life according to nature that is worthy of my particular freedom and dignity. From the individual view, the natural life that the undignified species are stuck with living is nasty, brutish, and short, not to mention untranscendent or unfree.*

There was an attempt to revive natural theology or "Nature's God" in the modern world. But it was disabled from the beginning by a basic contradiction: the modern view of nature, like the one of the Greeks and Romans, is of an impersonal principle that governs all that exists. But that view that we're completely or eternally governed by fixed principles of eternal natural necessity really can't capture the existence of the free individual—the being who has the right to use his reason and his will to free himself from his natural limitations.

"Nature's God" returns us to the ancient thought that the world is the home of the human mind, and the Americans today who most firmly believe in such a God might be the physicists who believe that their minds have cracked the cosmic code. But can the mind really grasp as a whole a world in which the individual is distinguished in his self-consciousness and his freedom from everything else? The physicist may be able to comprehend the mind or the body of the physicist, but not the whole human person who, among other things, engages in physical inquiry. That's one reason why the more characteristically modern view is that the mind is for transforming nature to make the individual genuinely at home or secure. Insofar as Nature's God is taken seriously, it mostly undermines the individual's sense of his irreplaceable and unique dignity. If, as Tom Wolfe explains, the dignity of the individual (which we can see with our own eyes) is taken seriously, then we can't help but conclude that the integrity of the natural world—or the rule of nature's God—came to an end with the mysterious emergence of the free and self-conscious individual.[5]

For the modern individualist, the truth remains that our dignified pretensions still point in the direction of a personal God, but, for

---

* The discussion of transcendence here is indebted to Harvey C. Mansfield, *Manliness* (New Haven, Connecticut: Yale University Press, 2006). The present essay as a whole is an Augustinian reflection on manliness or a manly reflection on St. Augustine. What is it that causes human beings to claim the dignity of irreplaceable personal significance? Does that claim make any sense beyond human assertion?

him, only a blind sucker relies upon such an imaginary projection. For Locke, it makes some sense to speak of a Creator as the source of the visible universe and of our mysterious liberty. But it's foolish to think of oneself as a creature or as fundamentally dependent on a providential God who guarantees us eternal life. Locke's Creator is not personal or present-tense enough really to do anything for particular individuals.

Our dignity, from this individual view, comes from facing up to the truth about how un-provided-for our condition as individuals is. My existence is radically contingent and mortal. But I have the resources to improve upon my condition, to act intelligently and responsibly on my own behalf. The dignity of the individual flows from his authentic self-consciousness, from what sets him apart from his natural, political, and familial environment. All the other animals act unconsciously to perpetuate their species. To the extent that we are dignified in our difference from them, we don't. The other particular animals aren't conscious of their temporary, utterly vulnerable, and irreplaceable existences. They're utterly replaceable because they don't know they're irreplaceable. I know others will come along a lot like me, but they won't be me. The evidence of my dignity is in my acting in response to my self-consciousness, my thought about myself. It's in my truthful and resolute efforts to continue to be me.

I feel indignation toward anyone who denies the truth about my self-consciousness and my freedom, my being. I feel especially righteous indignation toward those who would morally criticize or constrain me by imagining me to be other than I really am. That's because I'm convinced of the fundamental rightness of my free and responsible efforts to sustain my individual existence—my existence as a self-conscious, free, and body-dependent being—as long as possible.[6] I'm indignant enough freely to endanger my life to secure my freedom. I know enough to know that free beings can't pursue even wimp ends with consistently wimp means. So I know I may be stuck with displaying my dignity by risking my life on behalf of my right to life.

Sometimes indignantly insisting on my rights to life and liberty can seem undignified: I might say I have the right to sell my allegedly surplus kidney for the right price, because my body is my property, to be used as I think best. But surely it is undignified to regard my body—part of me—as merely part of my net worth of dollars. And surely a man or woman with a strong sense of personal worth—and so with a strong desire to display the nobler virtues of courage and generosity—would always want to do more than merely secure his or her biological existence. The individual responds that I'm going to be courageous or generous on my own terms; such risky virtue is not to be required of me. And an obsession with the needlessly risky virtues is for losers who don't understand themselves. Dead people have no real dignity or significance at all.

The real evidence, the individual notices, is on the side of identifying dignity with the protection of rights. Leon Kass reminds us that "liberal polities, founded on this doctrine of equal natural rights, do vastly less violence to human dignity than do their illiberal (and often moralistic and perfection-seeking) antagonists."[7] The 20th century's monstrous offenses against human dignity—so monstrous that they can't be described as mere violations of rights[8]—came from those who denied the real existence of individuals and their rights. Particular human beings were ideologically reduced to fodder for their race, class, or nation, for murderous and insane visions of humanity's non-individualistic future. Every attempt to restore civil theology in the modern world—from the Rousseau-inspired dimensions of the French Revolution onward—morphed into insane frenzies of unprecedented cruelty aiming to eradicate the alienation that inevitably accompanies our freedom. In a post-Christian context, we can't really defend personal dignity by neglecting individual rights.

## Dignity vs. Nature

A sensible understanding of "inalienable rights" might be the protections given to or required by self-conscious mortals, to beings stuck in between the other animals and God. But the modern individual characteristically doesn't rest content with locating his dignity in his acceptance of the intractable limitations of his embodiment. The modern individual—the modern self—aims to be autonomous, to use the mind as an instrument of liberation from or transcendence of dependence on material or natural necessity. From this view, modern individualism is not that different from the 20th century's historical or ideological projects to radically transform the human condition. The difference is that the individual never loses his focus on his own freedom, his rights; communism, fascism, and so forth were all diversions from what we really know, impossible efforts to transfer my truthful sense of my individual significance to some impersonal or ideological cause. The Europeans regard those efforts as the last and worst vestiges of civil theology. That's why they've apparently decided to abandon both religious and political life on behalf of a humanitarian concern for individual dignity.[9]

But the modern self is even more than a humanitarian or a humanist; he's the very opposite of a materialist in his own case. My mind is free to transform my body. The modern self identifies itself with the mind (I think, therefore I am) liberating itself through technology and enlightened education from the undignified drudgery of material necessity and from the tyranny of the unconscious. The mind frees the self from both material and moral repression for self-determination.[10] Our struggle for the rational control that would secure our dignity really does point in the direction of transhumanism.* We aim to use technology and biotechnology to overcome our human limitations as embodied beings. We aim at the self-overcoming of time, infirmity, death, and all the cruel indignities nature randomly piles upon us. Our dignity, from this view, depends on the orders we're really capable of giving to ourselves, meaning to our natures. Our dignity is in our awareness that what we're given by nature is worthless unless we bring it under our conscious control. So the individual doesn't really aim to secure himself as a biological being, because he's fully aware that he's more or other than a biological being. His biological dependence has already been lessened by his freedom, and he recognizes no limits to how much his mind might take command over his body and bodies. Nature has been and will be increasingly shaped and limited by his free action on behalf of his individual being. Impersonal natural evolution is being supplanted by personal or conscious and volitional evolution.

---

* See the essay by Charles Rubin in this volume.

## Dignity vs. Anxious Contingency

The trouble, of course, is that, for the foreseeable future, the pursuit of transcendence of our biological being is bound to fail every particular human individual in the end. The individual now makes only quite ambiguous and finally radically unsatisfactory progress toward indefinitely continuing to be. So our best efforts do little to free us from the anxious sense of contingency that comes with self-consciousness—the undignified perception that we're meaningless accidents that exist for a moment between two abysses. The more secure our efforts make us, it may be, the more anxious or disoriented we feel. The more we push back the necessity of death, the more accidental death becomes. And so the more not being an accident governs our lives. If, despite our best efforts, all we succeed in doing is making our lives more accidental or pitiful, it's hard to say that our technological successes have made our individual existences more secure or dignified.[11]

That's why Hobbes says that people become particularly restless and troublesome—unreasonable and dignity-obsessed—in times of peace. Freed somewhat from their rather dignified struggle against natural necessity, they can't avoid reflection on the inevitability of their long-run failure. No matter what I do, I won't be important or dignified for long, because I won't be around for long, or at least long enough. As long as death remains as an accidental possibility and an eventual certainty, my dignity defined as autonomy remains constantly in question. Modern individuals, as Tocqueville explains, are restlessly time- and death-haunted in the midst of prosperity, unable really to enjoy what seem to be the most fortunate circumstances in the history of their species. Just below the surface of our proud pragmatism lurks, as Solzhenitsyn writes, "the howl of existentialism." For the modern individual, "the thought of death becomes unbearable. It is the extinction of the entire universe at a stroke."[12]

Today, American restlessness doesn't usually display itself as dangerous political ambition, as Hobbes feared.[13] Our self-understanding is too individualistic for us easily to connect dignity with political recognition. Instead, we find evidence of our restless pursuit of dignity in a workaholic security-consciousness among sophisticated Americans. They're laid-back or relativistic on the traditional moral issues, partly to avoid the moralism that deprives other individuals of the dignity of determining their own lives. But they are also increasingly health- and safety-conscious, and it's there that their paranoid, puritanical, and prohibitionist sides now show themselves.

Our drive to secure ourselves has, for example, caused us to be extremely moralistic about safe sex. Whatever you prefer to do is dignified as long as it's responsible, and being responsible means methodically disconnecting your sexual behavior from birth and death, from babies and fatal diseases. It's easy to imagine a complete separation of sex and procreation in the name of security, in the name of minimizing all the risk factors associated with having unprotected sex. But of course that separation will deprive our sexual behavior of the shared hopes, fears, and responsibilities that made it seem dignified in itself and the main antidote to individualistic self-obsession. The domination of eros by security-consciousness may be good for the individual's effort to continue to be, but of course he'll be more anxious than ever. Safe sex is dignified in the sense that it's a responsible choice impossible for the naturally determined animals, but it might be undignified in the sense that it's ridiculous to be that bourgeois about eros, to work too hard to prefer security over distinctively human enjoyment. Sex—like God—used to be a way we could get our minds off ourselves.[14]

Tocqueville feared that modern individuals would end up becoming so apathetic and withdrawn that they would surrender the details of their lives—their own futures—to a meddlesome, schoolmarmish administrative state.[15] But that undignified surrender of personal concern just hasn't happened. Individuals experience themselves as in many ways more on their own than ever, which is why we still increasingly connect individual dignity with personal responsibility or self-ownership. Sophisticated individuals are more aware than ever that they exist contingently in hostile environments, although their lives are in some ways more secure and certainly longer than ever. Some dignity remains in their resolute efforts to be more than accidents, and their desire not to be replaceable has intensified. That's why more of them than ever decide that it's undignified even to produce replacements—children.

## Pantheism

Arguably, the modern goal is not the achievement of real security for one's being, which is impossible, but freedom from the anxiety that accompanies our true perception of the individual's contingency. If that were so, then we should consent to anyone or anything that would deprive us of our self-consciousness. Maybe that's why there's some evidence that natural theology is making yet another comeback as a way of connecting our dignity—even our divinity—to being at home in our natural environment. The most radically modern natural theology, as Tocqueville explains, is pantheism.[16] According to the pantheist, there are two pieces of good news. First, everything is divine. Second, our individuality—what separates each of us from the other animals and our conception of God—is an illusion. Pantheism is the true theological expression of modern natural science, of, say, sociobiology. There is, our scientists say, no evidence that one species is really qualitatively distinct from another; our species has received one scientific demotion after another until nothing of our proud individuality is left. So why shouldn't we say that our struggle against nature is a senseless illusion and surrender ourselves to the natural whole that we can call god?

Certainly pantheism is at the heart of most attempts to establish a post-Christian religion in our country in our time—those of the New Agers, the neo-Gnostics, the Western Buddhists, and so forth. Tocqueville regarded pantheism as such a seductive, radically egalitarian lullaby he attempted to rally all true defenders of the true dignity of human individuality against it. The brilliant French social critic Chantal Delsol adds that the pervasiveness of pantheistic speculation today is evidence that our idea of human dignity "is now hanging by a thread."[17]

But it seems to me that the self-help in the form of self-surrender offered by pantheism is just incredible to us. I receive no solace from the fact that the matter that makes up my body continues to exist after my death as part of a tree—even a sacred tree. And it is really very, very little consolation for me to know that the genes I spread live on. I know I'm not my genes, and I also know that, even if I were, nature would soon enough disperse me into insignificance. Maybe that's why the more people become aware, through sociobiological enlightenment, that their true purpose on earth is gene-spreading, the less they end up doing it. It's surely part of our dignity that we're incapable of not resisting pantheism's seduction, incapable of not really knowing that natural theology can't account for the existence of individuals or particular persons. All of our efforts to find a post-Christian way of reinstituting a credible natural or civil theology seem doomed to fail, despite the efforts of some great philosophers and despite our human longing—one, thank God, among many—to regress to infancy or subhumanity.

## Dignity vs. Mood Control

If pantheism and other similar forms of linguistic therapy don't work, there's still the biotechnological promise to relieve us of the burden of our self-conscious freedom. Psychopharmacological mood control might free us from our anxiety and make us feel happy and safe, and it might even release reliably the serotonin that can produce feelings of dignified self-esteem without having to do anything great. Contrary to Hobbes, we might want to say that the chemical surrender of the dignified, truthful assertion of personal sovereignty is what's required to live well. Certainly the objection that we'd no longer be living in the truth is at least very questionable. If our moods are nothing more than the result of chemical reactions, as our scientists say, then who's to say which reaction is truer than another? Why shouldn't we call true whatever makes us most comfortable? Our ability reliably to produce such a mood for ourselves might be the decisive evidence for our real ability to free ourselves from our miserable natural condition.

But Hobbes would respond: The surrender of sovereignty is misguided. It would be unreasonable for me to trust anyone with unaccountable control over me. My moods, after all, are part of my capacity for self-defense, and surely I shouldn't turn them over to some expert.[18] It's bad for both my dignity and my security not to insist that I'm a free being with rights and so not an animal to be controlled through the introduction of alien chemicals into my body. Those who would compassionately assume control over others to alleviate their cruel suffering always exempt themselves from their prescribed treatment. Their compassion is always a mask for my self-destruction. Certainly the goal of every tyrant is to free subjects, allegedly for their own good, of their longing to be free. As Walker Percy reminds us, surely our right to our moods is a very fundamental one; even Hobbes takes his bearings from the moods individuals as individuals really have on their own.[19]

These concerns are worth expressing. But it's still true that the worry that our individuals can or will employ psychopharmacology to embrace happiness over worry is overblown. The truth is that free individuals want both security and self-consciousness and can't imagine themselves surrendering one aspect of themselves for the other. They certainly don't want to be deprived of the truthful awareness that allows them genuinely to be. When we think of the promise of mood control, we really believe that we can be self-conscious without being anxious. We certainly don't want to surrender our individual freedom or our personal productivity. We don't want to be so zoned out by technology-produced virtual experiences that we would lose interest in the real technology that can protect us from terrorists, asteroids, diseases, and so forth. We also want to remain alienated or moody enough to enjoy music and art, without, of course, being so moved that we try to lose ourselves in non-therapeutic drugs or even that we are habitually late for work. We want to appreciate Johnny Cash without having to suffer through actually being Johnny Cash.

If we really took mood control seriously, we would start to recover the truth that we're both more or less than free individuals, that it's as individuals that we pursue happiness, but it's as friends, lovers, family members, creatures, neighbors, and so forth that we actually are happy. If we took it seriously, we'd start to see that it's because we too readily understand ourselves as free individuals and nothing more that life seems so hard. Only such individuals could be miserable enough to think even our natural moods need to be redesigned in order to be bearable. The other animals are typically content with the moods nature has given them. Lurking behind the effort to design or engineer moods is the really bad mood. And, thank God, the perpetuation of that bad mood will be needed to fuel our pursuit of artificially good ones. We individuals just can't surrender the self that generates "the self."[20]

## From Moral Autonomy to Existentialism

Maybe our worst mood remains directed against nature as we understand it. Certainly if the evolutionists or sociobiologists or the modern scientists in general are right, there's no natural room for individual dignity. The Darwinian view is that particular animals have significance only as members of species; their behavior is oriented, by nature, toward species preservation. The future of the species doesn't depend upon my indispensable contribution; its fate is contingent on the average behavior of large numbers of anonymous people.[21] The very existence of any particular species is a meaningless accident, and my particular existence as a random member of one species among many is infinitely more accidental.

Our most extreme or whiny moral individualists—the existentialists—may say that their personal struggle for meaning in a world governed by chance and necessity is absurd, but they don't really quite believe it. For them, the dramatic personal assertion of dignity or purpose, absurd as it is in theory, produces beautiful deeds and is what makes life worth living. But for the evolutionist (including the evolutionary neuroscientist), such dramatic displays are, at this point in the development of science, somewhat inexplicable perversities that will eventually be shown to be nothing more than mechanisms for species survival. What we now think of as absurd—what we now call the behavior of the dignified human individual or person—we will eventually understand not to be absurd at all. There is, we have to admit, something Socratic (or natural-theological) about evolutionism's and neuroscience's denial of individual pretensions about one's own soul or dignified personal identity, even in their denial of "the self" that distinguishes you from me, and us from all the other animals.[22]

But sophisticated people today, even sophisticated scientists, rarely talk as if evolutionism is completely true, as if particular human beings are best understood as species fodder. They speak of human dignity, and they identify dignity with autonomy. They don't understand autonomy, of course, as the literal conquest of nature or of the limitations of our embodiment. Otherwise, nobody around right now would have dignity at all.

Our idea of autonomy comes from Kant: Human dignity comes

from neither God nor from nature, but from our personal capability to transcend natural determination through our obedience to a rational, moral law we give to ourselves.[23] We aren't contained, as Hobbes might be understood to say, by mere calculation about how to survive as biological beings in this time and place. We have the abstract and idealistic capability not to be defined by our bodily existences.[24] We have the capability to act morally, or as something other than animals with instincts, and reason can show us that our true practical standard is not merely an arbitrary assertion against impersonal necessity. The capability for moral freedom is what gives each person a unique value. It makes that person priceless. Everything exists to be used—or bought and sold at some finite cost—except us.

The idea of moral autonomy finds strength in the thought that there's no support in what we know about nature—our natures—for our freedom and dignity. The Darwinian can say that evolution accounts for everything but the irreducible freedom from natural determination of the human person. But the Kantian draws the line at evolutionism, with its view that the person's perception of his dignity or autonomy or free, rational will is merely an illusion. We are, most fundamentally, what distinguishes us from nature. We may be chimps, but we're autonomous chimps, which means we're not really chimps at all. When I give way to natural inclination—and especially to the happiness that it might make possible—I'm not being what earns me respect. To the extent that we're natural beings, we have no dignity at all.

Kant's tough and precise distinction between subhuman natural inclination and genuine free and rational obedience to a law we make for ourselves compels us to prefer intentions to results or a freedom that we can't see with our own eyes. For the Kantian, it's unreasonable to demand evidence that any particular person is free. To connect dignity with the actual practice of moral virtue produces inequality or undermines the universality required for the rational apprehension of moral autonomy. Some people act more courageously than others, and others hardly ever do. But our dignity doesn't depend on what we actually do, but on who we are as free or moral beings. We have dignity as persons deserving of respect, and not as individuals exercising their rights.

Some of our most materialistic natural scientists tend to embrace human dignity as a sort of religious dogma. That doesn't mean that they believe in the Bible, but that they find nothing reasonable about the dignity they affirm. For them, human dignity is simply an inexplicable leftover from a cosmos they can otherwise scientifically explain. Our scientists tend to exempt themselves and others like themselves, usually without good reason, from their rational or scientific account of everything that exists. They are not so much rigorous, rationalist moralists as hopeless romantics when it comes to human beings, to themselves in particular, and so they've seen no reason not to go along with the existentialists in detaching autonomy from reason defined as either the technological or the moral overcoming of our natures.[25]

## Self-Definition

Autonomy has tended to become self-definition simply. No other animal can say who he or she is, and surely what we say transforms both who we are and what we do. Self-definition allows us to waffle on whether we really make ourselves—or merely imagine ourselves—as free and singularly dignified beings. And so it allows us to waffle on whether our natural science really has room for dignity, because it certainly can make room for the imaginative qualities of the beast with speech. Self-definition leaves open the possibility, associated with the freedom of the modern individual, that whatever we can imagine we can make real, while not denying the viewpoint of natural theology that we are all governed by impersonal necessity in the end.

Self-definition straddles the line between realism and pragmatism. We can call true or real whatever makes us feel comfortable, free, and dignified. But self-definers differ from pantheists because they know their imaginative freedom has its limits: We can't imagine the self to be anything other than an end in itself. I can't define myself merely as an indistinguishable part of a greater whole, a means for someone else's ends, or as a part of some future tree.*

The Christian person or creature, the modern individual, and the

---

* I think of myself as presenting here in a simple way a somewhat confused and complicated line of thought found in the work of Richard Rorty, our most able "cultural philosopher" of recent years.

Kantian person all experience themselves as unique and irreplaceable. The self-defined self must make himself that way. Because I have to make myself out of nothing without any guidance, I can be unique without being utterly contingent only if you accord me the respect I say I deserve. I can't really be so unique that I'm not recognizable by others in my infinite dignity. So I need you to recognize my dignified uniqueness. Self-definition requires a social dimension.

This view of dignity puts a greater burden on those who must acknowledge it than the Kantian one does. According to Kant, I must respect you or treat you as an end only as a person capable of obeying the autonomous moral law. But I don't have to and even can't respect anything you do that falls short of full obedience to that law. The Kantian must distinguish between moral and immoral intentions, and Kant himself was sometimes quite judgmental or morally severe. But now we believe we must respect the intention of whatever the self-defining person chooses, even if it's affirming as one's whole identity a natural inclination, such as being gay or straight.

That means we have the duty to go further than mere indifference or non-judgmentalism. You don't accord me dignity by saying, "not that there's anything wrong with it," where "it" is whatever it is I'm doing. Your yawning, in fact, is undignified. You must respect what I do because I do it, even or especially because you wouldn't do it yourself. My dignity requires that you suspend your rational faculties and moral judgment. Otherwise, your intention might intrude upon my self-definition: I'm indignant when you employ your self-definition or life plan not to have a respectful view of mine. That indignation, of course, is merely an intensification of that felt by the individual Hobbes describes. You have to do more than merely allow me to exercise my rights for my autonomy to have its inescapably moral dimension.[26]

But the burden of autonomy defined as moral self-definition is even greater on the person who claims it. Tocqueville tells us that the characteristically modern and democratic view is that our dignity rests in our intellectual freedom. We must free our minds from the authority of parents, country, tradition, nature, God, and so forth. But that means that it's much more clear what a radically free or genuinely autonomous judgment is not than what one is. Be yourself and be unique, we're told. But the individual human mind is anxious, disoriented, and paralyzed if it has to work all by itself. The pretense of radical doubt—or pop Cartesianism—eventually leads the individual to lose confidence both in the soundness of his mind and in the personal foundation of his dignity. Modern scientific skepticism makes every particular being seem puny, impotent, and insignificant and ever more readily absorbed by forces beyond his control. Surely in a globalizing, democratizing, techno-driven world, the dignified contributions of particular individuals are harder to discern than ever.[27]

The solitude of radical freedom makes effective human thought and action impossible. That's why autonomy requires a social dimension; consciousness necessarily is knowing with others. And the genuine sharing of self-knowledge requires, Kant thought, a rational standard that we can genuinely have in common. But for the individual who looks up to no personal authority—even or especially the authority of reason as described by some moralistic philosopher—all that's left for orientation is impersonal public opinion and what the reigning experts are saying about what impersonal or objective scientific studies are showing.

The deepest question for dignity in our time is where the self-defining individual is supposed to get the point of view, the character or virtue, the genuinely inward life or conscience required to resist degrading social or scientistic conformity.[28] The self-defining individual characteristically can't lose the self in "the self" that he consciously constructs to be pleasing to or to have status in the eyes of others. But that doesn't mean it's possible for the self to resist the imperatives of "the self" without the help of nature or God or a stable tradition that embodies natural and divine wisdom. We increasingly libertarian sophisticates are so obsessed with the threat that the tyrannical moralism of others poses to our moral autonomy that we've neglected the necessarily social, natural, and personal sources of the moral resolution of the dignified "I."

Even human rights, as Delsol concludes, can't "guarantee the dignity of each human being unless they are grounded in an understanding of man that ensures his [personal] uniqueness." Her view is that a dignified democracy—one composed "of unique persons endowed with free minds and wills" depends upon the "religious partner" of "a monotheism that preaches personal eternity, one in which each irreducible being survives in his irreducibility."²⁹ The dignified person depends upon a personal eternity to survive intact in an increasingly impersonal environment.

But Delsol's conclusion is compromised, to say the least, by her modern view that there really is no personal God who grants each of us eternal life. Does human dignity really depend on each human person living beyond his biological existence? Or merely on the conscious utilitarian effort to restore a "personal theology" that does justice to human dignity in the way a natural or civil theology never could? How could that theology really survive, in our time, the modern, individualistic criticism that it leads to the undignified surrender of our real, earthly lives as particular individuals for an illusory, otherworldly one? From the radically modern view, there's nothing less dignified than the blind sacrifice of the one and only life that I will ever have.

## An American Conclusion

Our view of human dignity as human freedom from impersonal natural necessity or merely political determination may well depend on the Christian view of inner, spiritual freedom. As Bob Kraynak explains, the Christians believe that each person is radically independent of the social and political order and does not depend on external recognition from other human beings, although it may depend on my genuine recognition by the personal God who sees me as I truly am. And that inner freedom, in fact, is perfectly compatible with external servitude.³⁰ My true understanding of my freedom comes, in fact, from coming to terms with the truth about my dependence, my limitations, my inability to achieve autonomy through either technological or rational efforts. According to St. Augustine, this truthful self-understanding is impossible without faith. Otherwise, we sinful beings are blinded by unreasonable pride or fatalistic despair about our personal or individual freedom.

Does the American understanding of dignity depend upon Christian faith, or a belief in the personal God? The view expressed in our founding documents and our complex tradition is not that clear. Our understanding of human dignity draws from both the modern understanding of the free beings with rights and the Christian understanding of the dignity of the being made in the image and likeness of the personal Creator.* In our eyes, the doctrine of rights presupposes the real, infinite significance of every particular human being. For us, our dignity is guaranteed not only by the individual's own assertiveness but with some natural or divine center of personal meaning. Nature's God, for us, is also a providential and judgmental God, a personal God. That means our understanding of natural theology is not the one criticized by St. Augustine or the one that was quickly displaced by morally autonomous and "historical" claims for freedom by the modern individual.

The American view on whether we're more than natural beings, or on whether there's natural support for our personal existences, is left somewhat undetermined. That means that we waffle on whether or not we're free individuals as Locke describes them, on whether being human is all about the conquest of nature or rather about the grateful acceptance of the goods nature and God have given us. That waffling is judicious or even truthful. Even many Christians would admit that there's a lot to the Lockean criticism of Augustinian otherworldliness, if not taken too extremely. And the Americans Tocqueville describes and the American evangelicals we observe today find their dignity in both their proud individual achievement and their humble personal faith.

America is largely about the romance of the dignified citizen; all human beings, in principle, can be equal citizens of our country. The politically homeless from everywhere have found a political home here. But that's because we've regarded citizenship as more than just a convenient construction to serve free individuals. We Americans take citizenship seriously without succumbing to political theology because we can see that we're all equal citizens because we're all more than citizens. Being citizens reflects a real part, but not the deepest

---

* See the essays by Patrick Lee and Robert P. George and by Gilbert Meilaender in this volume. It can be wondered whether Lee and George's secular "natural law" argument depends on the not self-evident proposition of our creation by a personal God. And surely a shortcoming of Meilaender's argument—at least in terms of formulating American public policy—is his inability or unwillingness to connect his Christian and egalitarian view of dignity to our secular understanding of rights.

part, of human dignity.*

All human beings can, in principle, become American citizens because they are all, in another way, irreducibly homeless or alienated from political life. Human beings are free from political life because of the irreducible personal significance they all share. We regard religious freedom as for religion, for the transpolitical, personal discovery of our duties to God. Our religious liberty reflects the dignity we share as, in some sense, creatures. We seem to agree with the anti-ideological dissident Havel that each of us can be a "dignified human 'I,' responsible for ourselves," because we experience ourselves truly as "bound to something higher, and capable of sacrificing something, in the extreme cases even everything…for the sake of that which gives life meaning," to the foundation of our sense of transcendence of our merely biological existence.[31]

So there is, in our tradition, a personal criticism of the dominant modern understandings of nature and God. If human beings are naturally fitted to know and love particular persons, then their natural social instincts can't be reduced to mechanisms of species perpetuation. Our dignity, from this view, comes from the mixture of our social instincts with the self-consciousness found in members of the species that has the natural capacity for language. It comes from our ability to know and love—and to be known and loved by—other, particular persons. And, as Kass writes, "if we know where to look, we find evidence of human dignity all around us, in the valiant efforts ordinary people make to meet necessity, to combat adversity and disappointment, to provide for their children, to care for their parents, to help their neighbors, to serve their country."[32] Each of us, thank God, is given demanding responsibilities as self-conscious, loving, social, finite, and dependent beings, and so plenty of opportunity, if we think about it, to display our dignity or irreplaceable personal significance.

My personal significance doesn't depend primarily on my overcoming of an indifferent or impersonal nature or even necessarily on

---

* The American view of dignity articulated here—one that aims to reconcile the doctrine of our Declaration of Independence with the true tradition of Christian realism—is indebted, above all, to G. K. Chesterton, *What I Saw in America* (New York: Dodd and Mead, 1922). See also my *Homeless and at Home in America* (South Bend, Indiana: St. Augustine's Press, 2007), especially chapters 1-3.

my hopeful faith in a personal God. The evidence of my personal dignity comes from lovingly and sometimes heroically performing the responsibilities that I've been given by nature to those I know and love, and from living well with others in love and hope with what we can't help but know about the possibilities and limits of our true situation. My dignity depends, of course, on the natural freedom that accompanies my flawed self-consciousness, my freedom to choose to deny what I really know and not to do what I know I should. I'm given a social and natural personal destiny that I can either fulfill or betray.[33]

From this view, Augustine misled us by unrealistically minimizing the personal satisfactions that come from friendship, erotic and romantic love, family, and political life. His goal was to focus our attention on our longing for the personal God and for authentic being, but the effect of his rhetoric in the absence of that faith was to make human individuals too focused on securing for themselves their dignified independence from their natural limitations and from each other—even at the expense of the accompanying natural goods. It's just not realistic to say, as we often do today, that each human individual exists for himself. It's not even good for the species.

The truth is that our dignified personal significance is not our own creation. It depends upon natural gifts, gifts that we can misuse or distort but not destroy. Biotechnology will in some ways make us more free and more miserable. And we will continue to display our dignity even in the futile perversity of our efforts to free ourselves completely from our misery. We will continue to fail to make ourselves more or less than human, and human happiness will elude us when we're too ungrateful for—when we fail to see the good in—what we've been given, in our selves or souls. Our dignity rightly understood will continue to come from assuming gratefully the moral responsibilities we've been given as parents, children, friends, lovers, citizens, thinkers, and creatures, and in subordinating our strange and wonderful technological freedom to these natural purposes.

The bad news is that, to the extent that our dignity depends on securing our freedom from nature, we will remain undignified. The good news is that our real human dignity—even in the absence of a personal God on Whom we can depend—is more secure than we sometimes think. Thank God, we have no good reason to hope or fear that we have the power or freedom to create some posthuman or transhuman future. We're stuck with ourselves, with our souls, with being good in order to feel good.

## Notes

[1] See Chantal Delsol, *The Unlearned Lessons of the Twentieth Century*, trans. Robin Dick (Wilmington, Delaware: ISI Books, 2006), especially chapter 12.
[2] The discussion of St. Augustine here is based on his *City of God*, especially books 5-8.
[3] The account of the classical philosophic view offered here is defended by Thomas Pangle, *Political Philosophy and the God of Abraham* (Baltimore, Maryland: Johns Hopkins University Press, 2006).
[4] See John Locke, *Second Treatise of Government* (1690). Support for my view of Locke here can be found in the work of Michael P. Zuckert: *The Natural Rights Republic: Studies in the Foundation of the American Political Tradition* (Notre Dame, Indiana: University of Notre Dame Press, 1996) and *Launching Liberalism* (Lawrence, Kansas: University Press of Kansas, 2002).
[5] Tom Wolfe, "The Human Beast," the 2006 Jefferson lecture, available online at www.neh.gov/whoweare/wolfe/lecture.html.
[6] See Leon R. Kass, "The Right to Life and Human Dignity," in *Enlightening Revolutions: Essays in Honor of Ralph Lerner*, ed. Svetozar Minkov (Lanham, Maryland: Lexington Books, 2006).
[7] Ibid., p. 130.
[8] See Pierre Manent, *A World Beyond Politics*, trans. Marc A. LePain (Princeton, New Jersey: Princeton University Press, 2006).
[9] Ibid., chapters 5-7, 11.
[10] See Walker Percy, *Lost in the Cosmos: The Last Self-Help Book* (New York: Farrar, Straus & Giroux, 1983), p. 13.
[11] See the Tocquevillian/Pascalian reflections on compassionate conservatism and biology in chapter 5 of my *Stuck with Virtue: The American Individual and Our Biotechnological Future* (Wilmington, Delaware: ISI Books, 2005).
[12] Aleksandr Solzhenitsyn, *The Solzhenitsyn Reader*, ed. Edward E. Ericson, Jr. and Daniel J. Mahoney (Wilmington, Delaware: ISI Books, 2006), p. 596.
[13] Thomas Hobbes, *Leviathan*, especially chapters 11 and 18.
[14] Alexis de Tocqueville, *Democracy in America*, volume 2, part 1, chapter 5.
[15] Ibid., volume 2, part 4, chapter 6.
[16] Ibid., volume 2, part 1, chapter 7.
[17] Delsol, op. cit., p. 194.
[18] Hobbes, *Leviathan*, especially chapters 13 and 17.
[19] See Walker Percy, op. cit., pp. 73-79.
[20] Cf. my *Stuck with Virtue*, chapter 5, with the fate of Charlotte in the last chapter

of Tom Wolfe's *I Am Charlotte Simmons* (New York: Farrar, Straus & Giroux, 2003).

[21] See Mansfield, *Manliness*, pp. 59-61, 220.

[22] Cf. Tom Wolfe, "Sorry, But Your Soul Just Died," in *Hooking Up* (New York: Farrar, Straus & Giroux, 2001), with Mansfield, *Manliness*, pp. 220-224.

[23] Everything I know about Kant and human dignity and more can be found in Susan M. Shell, "Kant and Human Dignity," in *In Defense of Human Dignity: Essays for Our Times*, ed. Robert P. Kraynak and Glenn Tinder (Notre Dame, Indiana: University of Notre Dame Press, 2003), pp. 53-80; see also her essay in this volume.

[24] See Mansfield, op. cit., pp. 59-61, 220.

[25] See the work of Walker Percy here; an introduction is found in my *Postmodernism Rightly Understood* (Lanham, Maryland: Rowman & Littlefield, 1999), chapters 3 and 4, as well as in chapters 5 and 10 of my *Aliens in America* (Wilmington, Delaware: ISI Books, 2002). The best introduction to Percy's work for those with little patience for novels is his *Lost in the Cosmos*.

[26] See Manent, op. cit., pp. 191-96.

[27] See my "McWilliams and the Problem of Political Education," in *Perspectives on Political Science* 35 (Fall, 2006): 213-218. This issue of *PPS* is devoted to the work of Wilson Carey McWilliams, the most profound defender in our time of the connection between human dignity and egalitarian political community. And also see, of course, part 1 of volume 2 of Tocqueville's *Democracy in America*.

[28] This question is what animates part 1 of volume 2 of Tocqueville's *Democracy in America*. See also my *Stuck with Virtue*, especially the introduction.

[29] Delsol, op. cit., pp. 194-195.

[30] See Robert P. Kraynak, "'Made in the Image of God': The Christian View of Human Dignity and Political Order," in *In Defense of Human Dignity*, pp. 81-118, as well as the essay by Kraynak in this volume.

[31] Václav Havel, *Open Letters* (New York: Vintage Books, 1992), p. 263.

[32] Leon R. Kass, *Life, Liberty and the Defense of Dignity: The Challenge for Bioethics* (San Francisco, California: Encounter Books, 2002), p. 248.

[33] The claims in this paragraph are supported through the use of the work of Walker Percy in my *Postmodernism Rightly Understood*, chapters 3 and 4.

# 11

# Human Dignity: Exploring and Explicating the Council's Vision

## Gilbert Meilaender

Discussing the topic of murder, and replying to an "objection" (as the structure of the *Summa* calls for such replies), St. Thomas Aquinas writes, "a man who sins deviates from the rational order, and so loses his human dignity [*dignitate humana*].... To that extent, then, he lapses into the subjection of the beasts...."[1] We may contrast this with the words of Pope John Paul II in the encyclical letter *Evangelium Vitae*, released in 1995: "Not even a murderer loses his personal dignity [*dignitate*]."[2]

The seeming divergence between these two important and influential statements within the same (albeit long and extended) tradition of thought is striking. Aquinas seems to think that the murderer, by turning against what reason requires of us, becomes more beast than man—losing the dignity that characterizes human beings, the rational species. John Paul II, in a context discussing the death penalty in general and Cain's murder of Abel in particular, does not seem to think of "dignity" as something that can be lost by human beings, even when they act in ways that fall far short of the excellences that mark human nature.

The tension between these two notions of human dignity is evident, and I suspect that any time we think seriously about a range of issues in bioethics we are likely to find ourselves caught up in just this tension, looking for ways to distinguish one meaning of the term from another, or looking for other terms to mark the distinction. The work of the President's Council on Bioethics, since that work began in 2002, has made use of the concept of dignity in several different contexts (even in the title of one report, *Human Cloning and Human Dignity*), and it may be that the Council has not always clarified its use of the term as much as some would like or as it should have. Thus, arguing that "dignity is a useless concept," Ruth Macklin criticized the Council's failure to provide an analysis of the concept of dignity it used.[3] With considerably more care and precision, in remarks to the Council in its meeting on December 9, 2005—remarks that were generally appreciative of the Council's work—James Childress noted and concurred in the sense of some critics that the Council had "tended to invoke rather than really use the idea of human dignity" and had left the concept largely "unanalyzed."[4]

That is probably true, and I hope this essay will make at least a small contribution toward clarifications that are useful. Nevertheless, I suspect that some critics (among whom I do not here include Childress)—perhaps because, for whatever reasons, they operate with a reflexively jaundiced view of the Council's work—have missed some of the most important and interesting issues raised by the Council's use of the language of dignity. For there are important differences—at least differences of emphasis, and perhaps still deeper disagreements—about the meaning of dignity even among Council members whose views on substantive questions have much in common. Indeed, the most interesting disagreements are often among those whose conversations can presuppose a background of shared concern. But we will never see this or explore these important issues if we read Council documents myopically in terms of policy or politics alone.

Even if it is true that the Council has been less clear about dignity than is desirable, I suspect this is a "defect" that is inherent in discourse about the kinds of questions with which bioethics deals. So, for example, in a recent report discussing approaches that might be used to increase rates of organ donation, a committee of the Institute of Medicine of the National Academies found it necessary to resort to the language of dignity: "Most societies hold that it is degrading to human dignity to view dead bodies as property that can be bought and sold.... [B]odies are supposed to be treated with respect—with funeral rites and burial or cremation—and not simply discarded like worn out household furniture and certainly not sold by relatives (or anyone else) to the highest bidder."[5] And although an earlier chapter had interpreted the language of respect for human dignity primarily in terms of respect for autonomy, it is hard to believe that this alone could account for the sense of "degradation" which, it is said, the buying and selling of corpses would elicit in most societies.

In any case, in order to explicate and explore the idea of human dignity, I turn first to the Council's most recent report, *Taking Care: Ethical Caregiving in Our Aging Society* (September 2005).[6] Having begun with an exploration of tensions deeply buried within that report, I will then be in a position to think more generally about those tensions, well beyond the boundaries of the Council's work itself.

## Equal Dignity and Distinctions in Excellence

A distinction between two different senses in which one might speak of human dignity is emphasized in *Taking Care*. The Council speaks of this distinction in different ways. It notes, for instance, that the language of dignity might be used to mark either a "floor," a kind of respect and care beneath which our treatment of any human being should never fall—or it might be used to mark a "height" of human excellence, those qualities that distinguish some of us from others (106*f*). Similarly, it contrasts a non-comparative manner of speaking about the worthiness of human lives with various kinds of comparative assessments (whether in economic terms or in terms of nobility) of human worth (103*f*). Or yet again, it notes a difference between an "'ethic of equality' (valuing all human beings in light of their common humanity)" and an "'ethic of quality' (valuing life when it embodies certain humanly fitting characteristics or enables certain humanly satisfying experiences)" (106).

The general point is, I think, clear, and it seems right to say that, at different times and for different purposes, we are likely to speak in either of these ways. Nonetheless, trying to find a way to do justice to each of them simultaneously is no easy task. How to work out these differences in the public sphere, where equal treatment may sometimes seem to call for special attention to the needs of the vulnerable or the deprived, is among the most difficult and troubling of political issues. Of course, treating people equally need not and should not mean treating them identically, as every parent of more than one child knows.

Still, I am not persuaded that the Council's discussion is entirely successful, because it seldom does more than set the two concepts of dignity side by side. They do not interact in such a way that the meaning of one can be to some degree reshaped or transformed by the other; instead, they remain firmly fixed in separate linguistic compartments. For example, having discussed a (comparative) sense in which we might think of some human beings as manifesting greater dignity than others, the Council then turns to affirm a "*non-*comparative way of speaking about the worth of human lives" (104). Yet, attempting to affirm this non-comparative worth, it says merely: "If we value *only* the great ones, we do an injustice to the dignity of ordinary human beings" (104).

Suppose, however, that our understanding of comparative excellence were reshaped somewhat by a sense of equal human dignity. Then we might speak more as a character named Dinny does, in John Galsworthy's novel *One More River*, when reflecting on the death of old Betty Purdy:

> Death! At its quietest and least harrowing, but yet—death! The old, the universal anodyne; the common lot! In this bed where she had lain nightly for over fifty years under the low sagged ceiling, a great little old lady had passed. Of what was called "birth," of position, wealth and power, she had none. No plumbing had come her way, no learning and no fashion. She had borne children, nursed, fed and washed them, sewn, cooked and swept, eaten little, travelled not at all in her years, suffered much pain, never known the ease of superfluity; but her back had been straight, her ways straight, her eyes quiet and her manners gentle. If she were not the "great lady," who was?[7]

And suddenly what seems almost a given in the Council's

discussion—who are the great and who the ordinary human beings—may be far less obvious.

As it becomes less obvious, as the "comparative" sense of dignity begins to be transformed by the "non-comparative," as we are less sure what is the "floor" and what the "height" of human worth, we may incline to draw back a bit from some elements in the Council's discussion. For example, imagining a woman who was once a "virtuoso violinist" and is now suffering from dementia, her "treasured capacities" largely gone, the Council first affirms that she "remains a full member of the human community, equally worthy of human care." But it then expresses puzzlement about what her dignity might mean when those capacities are "fading or gone." In the case of such a virtuoso—the suggestion seems to be—dementia is especially degrading. "For all people—and perhaps most vividly for those who once stood high above the ordinary—the regression to dementia and incompetence, with all its accompanying indignities and loss of self-command, may seem dehumanizing and humiliating" (107).

This does not seem true to me. Moreover, I think there is something objectionable about this way of putting the matter. I cannot see why dementia afflicting this "virtuoso violinist" should be any more vividly dehumanizing than it would be were it to afflict, say, the woman who regularly empties the trash can in my office. Still more, I would be reluctant to call dementia in either case dehumanizing. I know of course that one might sometimes incline to the view that dementia in the case of the violinist was somehow worse than dementia in the case of the janitor, and there might be occasions when I could be inclined to suppose that dementia in either case was dehumanizing, but I would regard such inclinations as *temptations* (to be resisted as best I could).

It is when I ask myself why these inclinations should be regarded as temptations that the puzzles arise. I am reluctant to say that any living human being, even one severely disabled by dementia, has lost human dignity. Why? I am reluctant to say that some human beings—those with certain highly developed capacities—have greater dignity than others. Why?

These two puzzles are interrelated. If we assert that every human being has dignity, someone is certain to ask from us an account of what it is about human beings that gives them this equal dignity. And of almost every characteristic or property to which we might point it is likely that some human beings may lack it or lose it, or that some human beings may have it in more developed or more excellent ways (and, hence, may seem more worthy or more deserving of our respect). Each of these possibilities is buried—as temptation, in my view—in the Council's discussion summarized above. If dementia is inherently dehumanizing because it deprives human beings of the rational powers that give them their special dignity, then some living human beings may come to lack dignity entirely. If dementia is worse when it attacks the "virtuoso," diminishing qualities that were once especially highly developed, it suggests that the virtuoso and the janitor were never of equal dignity. Tackling these several aspects of our problem requires us to ask first what (if anything) about human beings is the ground of their dignity.

## Distinctions in Dignity

Discussing the morality of capital punishment, Walter Berns quotes Supreme Court Justice William Brennan's statement that "'even the vilest criminal remains a human being possessed of human dignity'"—and then disagrees emphatically:

> What sort of humanism is it that respects equally the life of Thomas Jefferson and Charles Manson, Abraham Lincoln and Adolf Eichmann, Martin Luther King and James Earl Ray? To say that these men, some great and some unspeakably vile, equally possess human dignity is to demonstrate an inability to make a moral judgment derived from or based on the idea of human dignity.[8]

We understand what Berns means, and in certain moods we are probably inclined to agree; yet, in my view, the more striking inability displayed in this passage is Berns's own inability to find a standpoint from which to see the whole truth about any and every human life. Especially when life and death are at stake, when we are forced to think about a person's life as a whole, the distinctions that we make and need to make in other contexts may lose their force.

It is obvious that, at least in certain contexts and for certain purposes, we make distinctions of merit among human beings. Academic institutions, for example, are meritocratic, and a class in which every student gets an "A"—even if welcomed for certain reasons by some students and some faculty—is understood to subvert the very nature of the undertaking. Likewise, the worlds of sport and of musical performance—to take two quite different aspects of life—are arenas in which we still strive for excellence and watch with an eye to discerning those whose performance is especially accomplished. We generally think that an eye for these distinctions and differences need not undercut our commitment to the equal dignity of human beings, and perhaps it need not. Nonetheless, impressed by the obvious importance of these distinctions for much of life, one might argue that the very notion of dignity is aristocratic rather than egalitarian.

As a starting point for examining this argument we can begin with an essay by Leon Kass, "Death with Dignity and the Sanctity of Life."⁹ Kass starts with the concept of sanctity, moving from it to dignity, but he sees the ideas as closely interrelated. What is it that makes human beings worthy of our respect? In Western culture, Kass notes, the biblical assertion that human beings have been created in God's image has often been taken as the ground of equal worth. "Human life is to be respected more than animal life, because man is more than an animal; man is said to be godlike" (241).* For Kass the ground of this special standing is the powers of "reason, freedom, judgment and moral concern" (242) that human life characteristically exhibits.

Within human life, however, those special capacities are inextricably intertwined with our bodies—with "metabolism, digestion, respiration, circulation and excretion" (244). And sometimes those bodily functions remain when reason and freedom seem to be gone.

---

* The term "godlike" does not strike me as the best choice here. For one thing, the desire to be "like God" (which, to be sure, is not quite the same as being godlike) is the description (in *Genesis* 3:5) of the primal temptation. Kass does, of course, recognize this. He writes (242): "Yet man is, at most, only godly; he is not God or a god. To be an image is also to be *different* from that of which one is an image." Given that, however, it might capture better the truth of our creation in God's image to say that human beings are neither beast nor God—but, instead, a particular kind of being made (unlike the beasts) for communion with God (on whom human life is utterly dependent).

For Kass this undermines or diminishes—he does not say "destroys"—human dignity, for it undermines human agency. Although I myself would not say that the loss of those "higher" capacities diminishes human dignity, we can understand why someone might, and we have probably all felt, at one time or another, a tug in the direction of Kass's view. More baffling to me is his suggestion that even turning to doctors for help in getting better serves to "compromise" our dignity: "being a patient rather than an agent is, humanly speaking, undignified" (245). Similarly, he writes a few pages later that "one cannot make a good end of one's life if one is buffeted about by forces beyond one's control" (248). In part, he has in mind here the ways in which caregivers and institutions may constrain and control the sick and dying, but his language seems to encompass more than just that. To think that suffering the ills which overtake us, being a patient rather than an agent, is somehow undignified seems less like an analysis of dignity than like a rebellion against the nature of human life. Were I drawn to depictions of dignity in terms of certain characteristics, I would be more inclined to say that human dignity lies in acknowledging the way in which aging and dying very often involve becoming more and more a patient (and needing to learn patience) and less and less an agent.

At any rate, dignity for Kass is an "undemocratic" idea (246). It directs us to think in terms of worthiness, honor, and nobility. "In all its meanings it is a term of distinction. Dignity is not something which, like a nose or a navel, is to be expected or found in every living human being. In principle, it is aristocratic" (246). Etymology will take us only so far, however. And these etymological observations, true though they may be if limited to a certain focus, do not successfully bring this "comparative" understanding of dignity into relation with a "non-comparative" notion of *equal* dignity. Or, perhaps I should say, to the degree that they bring them into relation, the comparative is permitted to demarcate the limits of the non-comparative. "One can, of course," Kass writes, "seek to democratize the principle [of dignity].... Yet on further examination this universal attribution of dignity to human beings pays tribute more to human potentiality, to the *possibilities* for human excellence. *Full* dignity, or dignity properly so-called, would depend on the *realization* of these possibilities" (247). This must lead in the end to some kind of distinction between *basic* and *full* humanity, with dignity accorded chiefly to the latter, to a life in which the characteristic human excellences are developed and displayed.

Such a view does, as I noted earlier, capture something almost all of us believe to be true—as is seen in the way we give grades to students or evaluate athletic and musical performances. In various areas of life, some human beings seem to move beyond the basic humanity shared with the rest of us and display excellence in ways that merit our admiration. They flourish. That is, they develop characteristic human capacities in ways that give all of us some inkling of what a human being can actually become. If we like, there is nothing to prevent us from saying that their lives display in a special way the dignity of our human nature.

Yet, there is also, at least in certain contexts, something offensive to our ears about this aristocratic way of depicting human dignity. Thus, for example, in a speech of July 17, 1858, Abraham Lincoln, while granting many human inequalities, also captured something of the problem we have with an inegalitarian concept of dignity: "I have said that I do not understand the Declaration [of Independence] to mean that all men were created equal in all respects…. [B]ut I suppose that it does mean to declare that all men are equal in some respects; they are equal in their right to 'life, liberty, and the pursuit of happiness.' Certainly the Negro is not our equal in color—perhaps not in many other respects; still, in the right to put into his mouth the bread that his own hands have earned, he is the equal of every other man, white or black."[10]

A concept of dignity that emphasizes differences of worth falls harshly on our ears because we have learned to move in the opposite direction from that which Kass takes: we have learned to let the comparative notion of dignity be transformed when brought into contact with the non-comparative and egalitarian. And we have learned this in some considerable measure because there has been a great rupture in Western culture, a rupture that gradually reshaped the classical notion of dignity (with which Kass works) by bringing it within a system of thought and practice that worshiped as God a crucified man who suffered a criminal's death on a cross. It would not be wrong to say that, though he is depicted as going to that cross willingly, he was "buffeted about by forces beyond [his] control," and he died what those of his day surely regarded as an undignified death. One would not, of course, expect these beliefs to be formative for Kass, who is Jewish; yet, I suspect that the continuing tug on him of the non-comparative understanding of human dignity is grounded both in a Jewish understanding that *every* human being has been created in the image of God and in our society's gradual development of a strong sense of human equality.

It may be that we cannot make good sense of an egalitarian and non-comparative understanding of human dignity, to which our civilization has in many ways been committed, if we abstract it entirely from the context of the religious beliefs that formed it.

That context is certainly apparent in the Declaration of Independence, upon which Lincoln relied when making his case, and it is worth articulating here. Suppose, Kierkegaard writes,

> there are two artists and one of them says, "I have traveled much and seen much in the world, but I have sought in vain to find a person worth painting. I have found no face that was the perfect image of beauty to such a degree that I could decide to sketch it; in every face I have seen one or another little defect, and therefore I seek in vain." Would this be a sign that this artist is a great artist? The other artist, however, says, "Well, I do not actually profess to be an artist; I have not traveled abroad either but stay at home with the little circle of people who are closest to me, since I have not found one single face to be so insignificant or so faulted that I still could not discern a more beautiful side and discover something transfigured in it. That is why, without claiming to be an artist, I am happy in the art I practice and find it satisfying." Would this not be a sign that he is indeed the artist, he who by bringing a certain something with him found right on the spot what the well-traveled artist did not find anywhere in the world—perhaps because he did not bring a certain something with him! Therefore the second of the two would be the artist.[11]

The truth of equal human dignity may be, as the Declaration seems to suggest, self-evident (in the sense that this truth shines by its own light and cannot be derived from other more fundamental truths), but it is not obvious. Indeed, perhaps we will see it only insofar as we "bring a certain something" with us when we look. And, for Kierkegaard, that "certain something" is very specifically the neighbor-love that Christians are enjoined to show to every human being made in God's image. I doubt, in fact, that there is any way to derive a belief in the equal worth of every human being from the ordinary distinctions in merit and excellence that we all use in some spheres of life; it is grounded, rather, not in our relation to each other but in our relation to God, from whom—to use a mathematical metaphor—we are equidistant.* "The thought of God's presence makes a person modest in relation to another person, because the presence of God makes the two essentially equal."[12]

Here, then, is our problem, from which we cannot for long continue to avert our gaze: Our society is committed to equal human dignity, and our history is in large part a long attempt to work out the meaning of that commitment. Christians and Jews have an account of persons—as equidistant from God and of equal worth before God—that grounds and makes sense of this commitment we all share. A society that rejects their account but wishes to retain the

---

* Herbert Spiegelberg has made the distinction in terms of genus and species:

"Dignity in the general sense is a matter of degree. It reflects an aristocratic picture of reality in the tradition of the 'Great Chain of Being' with higher and lower dignities. Such dignity is subject to change, to increase and decrease; it can be gained and lost. It finds its expression in such dignities as are conferred on 'dignitaries' through honors or titles, and can be expressed in dignified or undignified comportment.

"*Human* dignity is a very different matter. It implies the very denial of an aristocratic order of dignities. For it refers to the minimum dignity which belongs to every human being qua human. It does not admit of any degrees. It is equal for all humans. It cannot be gained or lost. In this respect human dignity as a species of dignity differs fundamentally from the genus."

See his "Human Dignity: A Challenge to Contemporary Philosophy," in *Human Dignity: This Century and the Next*, ed. Rubin Gotesky and Ervin Laszlo (New York: Gordon & Breach), pp. 55-56, cited in Deryck Beyleveld and Roger Brownsword, *Human Dignity in Bioethics and Biolaw* (Oxford: Oxford University Press, 2001), p. 50. I suspect, however, that in order to make sense of such a fundamental difference between genus and species we need to recount the story, to which I have alluded, of the great rupture in Western history between classical and Christian thought.

commitment faces, then, a serious crisis in the structure of its beliefs. And often, in fact, we do little more than posit an equality about which we are, otherwise, largely mute; for the truth is, as Oliver O'Donovan has assertively put it, that this belief "is, and can only be, a theological assertion."[13] We are equal to each other, whatever our distinctions in excellence of various sorts, precisely because none of us is the "maker" of another one of us. We have all received our life—equally—as a gift from the Creator.

This does not mean that equal human dignity can or will be affirmed only by religious believers. Without fully discerning the ontological ground of dignity one may have what Gabriel Marcel terms "an active and even poignant experience of the mystery inherent in the human condition."[14] We will gain insight into this mystery chiefly, Marcel thinks, when we are moved by a spirit of compassion that recognizes our shared vulnerability; hence, "dignity must be sought at the antipodes of pretension and...on the side of weakness."[15] That is to say, in our common subjection to mortality—to death, in which we must discern the meaning of a life taken whole—we may come to perceive dimly our equal dignity.

We should note, however, that relying on a sense of our shared vulnerability to ground human dignity brings with it the risk that we may come to regard relief of suffering as a moral trump card that overrides all other obligations. This has, in my view, sometimes been true of arguments put forward by Council members. Thus, for example, in a personal statement appended to the report *Alternative Sources of Human Pluripotent Stem Cells*, Janet Rowley wrote: "We talk about protecting human dignity. We should strive to help patients with serious illnesses that could potentially be treated with embryonic stem cells to live as fulfilling and dignified lives as is humanly possible."[16] Likewise, in a personal statement appended to *Reproduction and Responsibility*, Michael Gazzaniga wrote: "The Koreans have found a way to let biomedical cloning go forward with all of its spectacular promise for restoring human dignity to the seriously diseased and infirmed patients of the world while at the same time not in any way creating a social atmosphere to use such advances for baby making. What could be better?"[17] In these statements both Council members give moral priority to doing what they think necessary for achieving the dignity of a life (relatively) free of suffering. This suggests that

Leon Kass had some reason to be concerned about a concept of equal (non-comparative) dignity grounded simply in our shared vulnerability. "Modernity's preoccupation with the ways in which humans are at bottom equal in their frailty is," as he put it, "no small part of the problem."[18] To the degree this is true, we have another reason to think that our society's commitment to equal human dignity is best and most safely grounded in religious belief.

At any rate, it is not religious believers who should be ill at ease in a public square committed to the equal worth of every human being; it is those who lack the faith that animated and animates such commitment. It is not religious believers who should be mute in a public square committed to equal human dignity; it is others who find themselves mute when asked to give an account of our shared public commitment. In fact, an appreciation of the many and various distinctions in human excellence—of the sort Kass wants to press and is, in many respects, quite right to press—is safe only in a public square that can affirm the relation to the Creator which grounds our equality.

Thus, we can grant and make use of comparative notions of dignity as long as our use is shaped and transformed by our commitment to a non-comparative and equal dignity. This shaping will show itself and be important in at least two ways.[19] First, it may enable us to see what we otherwise might not were we to look only at surface differences—even *important* surface differences. It will form us as people rather like Kierkegaard's second artist, whose eye is attuned to the deeper truth that lies behind, beneath, and within the differences that distinguish us from each other.

In addition, this non-comparative concept of dignity will become relevant whenever we make what we might call "on the whole" judgments about the worth of a human life. Unable to transcend entirely our location in time and space, we never really see any life, including our own, in such a transcendent way. It presupposes, really, God's own perspective; hence, in making such judgments we think of ourselves and others in terms of the relation to God. This need not blind us to the many distinctions within everyday social life, for dissimilarity is, as Kierkegaard notes, the mark (though a confusing mark) of temporal life. "But the neighbor is eternity's mark—on every human being."[20] Since we stand equally distant from (or near to) the Eternal One, we are radically equal in those moments when our life is ju "on the whole," as only God can see it. One place, therefore, where differences in excellence or dignity can have no place, will be at "the threshold of death, when the continuance of life itself is at stake."[21] Once again, Kierkegaard sees the point: "There is not a single person in the whole world who is as surely and as easily recognized as the neighbor. You can never confuse him with anyone else, since the neighbor, to be sure, is all people.... If you save a person's life in the dark, thinking that it is your friend—but it was the neighbor—this is no mistake."[22]

We also encounter others "on the whole," (and differences in excellence become unimportant) when "they lack essential resources to participate in social communications as such."[23] It is "self-evident," as the Declaration puts it, that every human being—created by God for covenant with each other and with himself, even in the midst of the many distinctions that mark us—must have the opportunity to live within human society and participate in its common life. Thus, "the opportunity to live, and the opportunity to participate in a society, are metaphysically foundational; they correspond to our universal created nature as human beings."[24] Recognizing these two forms of "on the whole" equality need not efface our appreciation for the significance of differences among us in excellence and achievement, but it will inevitably, I suspect, democratize somewhat the judgments we make about the worth of human lives. Even within our noblest qualities and our most striking excellences, we will learn to discern "the poverty of our perfections."[25]

Here, then, is one way in which the language of dignity has played an important role in the Council's work, has perhaps been in need of some further refinement, and can, I think, be elucidated and clarified by considering the relation between human dignity in its comparative and non-comparative senses. But there is another way in which the language of dignity has entered into the Council's reports, and it also deserves attention.

## The Human Being as Neither Beast Nor God

The collection of readings titled *Being Human*, which was produced and published by the Council, contains ten chapters. Each has a very general title, under which are gathered a range of readings that seek to explore and illumine various aspects of the subject announced by the title, and the Council provides a brief introduction to each of these chapters. Chapter ten is called simply "Human Dignity." In the introduction to this chapter the tension I have been exploring above appears. Thus, for example, some of the readings collected in the chapter are said to "present supreme examples of human dignity at its finest."[26]

Significantly, however, the brief introduction to this chapter does not use the language of "excellence" only to distinguish some human beings from others. On the contrary, it refers to human dignity—the dignity of the human species taken generally—as an excellence. It recognizes, without choosing among, various kinds of reasons (some religious, some not) that one might give as the ground of this shared dignity. But human dignity itself is described as "our full humanity: not just reason or will, not just strength or beauty, but our integrated powers of body, mind, and soul."[27] This fully integrated life means living "as a man, and not as a beast."[28] It is this use of the language of dignity—to point to the specific character of human life that is lower than the gods and higher than the beasts—to which I now turn.*

Perhaps surprisingly, apart from the issues in *Taking Care* discussed above, the concept of (human) dignity is used relatively rarely in Council reports. Moreover, the Council recognizes that the concept of dignity has no explicitly recognized place in American law (in the way that concepts such as freedom, rights, and equality do).[29] I wonder, in fact, whether one reason critics have focused on the Council's use of the language of dignity may not be that their criticisms have law and policy in mind. So does the Council, of course, but it tends to put policy questions into the context of larger "anthropological" concerns.

The very first report issued by the Council (in July 2002) was

---

* This way of thinking about the Council's language of dignity was first suggested to me by Paul Weithman in a presentation made to the Council at its December 2005 meeting. Working from memory, Weithman had attributed to Kant the statement that, among the many species, man is "highest among the animals, lowest among the hosts [of heaven]." He later checked this for me and informed me that—while this captures Kant's vision of the human being as an "animal rational," the rational species that is also embodied—the phrase itself comes from Stanley Cavell.

a product. Children born of this process stand equally beside their progenitors as fellow human beings, not beneath them as made objects" (118). In other words, in distinctively human procreation the child is not simply a product of the will or choice of its progenitor. It is, instead, the internal fruition of an act of marital love. Hence, although there are different ways to produce a child, they do not all amount to *doing* the same thing; for the nature of what we do is not determined simply by what we accomplish or produce.

An anthropological vision is at work here. The human being is a particular sort of "in-between" creature. Not quite a beast. Not quite a god. Hence, to flourish as the human species, to manifest human dignity, is to live within certain limits—as creatures whose life is an integrated whole of body, mind, will, and spirit. Because we are not gods, we have to think about how we come into being and go out of being. Because we are not beasts, we can find moral meaning in the relation between the generations.

When, then, the Council speaks of "the dignity of human procreation," it has in mind the way in which the next generation of humankind comes to be not through a deliberate act of rational will (which, in godlike fashion, can be separated entirely from the sexual union of a man and a woman) but through a distinctively human relation in which reason and will are united with the body and its passions. This distinctively human form of procreation is good both for those who beget and for the child who is begotten. Procreation that is more than just an exercise in self-definition or an act of self-replication frees us from self-absorption and gives a spaciousness to the love between man and woman. And the child who is begotten, not made, becomes the natural fruition of the parental embrace, not a chosen project—a gift and a mystery, whose destiny is no one else's to determine. To speak of the "dignity" of human procreation is to use a placeholder that carries all this moral meaning—that points to a distinctively human relation between one generation and the next.

The Council may or may not be correct in the conclusions about cloning-to-produce-children and cloning-for-biomedical research that it draws on the basis of human dignity so understood, but seeing the language of dignity as a placeholder for such anthropological concerns is surely understandable and, perhaps, instructive. Nor is such an understanding by any means unique to the Council's work.

Consider, for example, a discussion of a patient's right of privacy in Tom Beauchamp's and James Childress's *Principles of Biomedical Ethics*, certainly one of the most widely read and influential works in bioethics. Childress and Beauchamp are inclined to ground a privacy right in respect for autonomy; yet, they recognize that this cannot account for all circumstances in which we would think such a right existed. "It seems intuitively correct to say that it is a violation of privacy, not merely a tasteless act of negligence, to leave a comatose person undraped on a cart in the hospital corridor. One possibility, although not one that we pursue or defend here, is to emphasize a broader conception of respect for persons that includes both respect for their autonomy *and* respect for their dignity."[31]

Such a possibility was, however, pursued—very instructively—by Paul Weithman, in his presentation to the Council at its December, 2005 meeting.[32] He noted a range of instances in which we might quite naturally have recourse to the language of dignity in order to articulate important moral concerns not easily dealt with simply in the language of rights or autonomy. So, for example, having sex in a public place may undermine human dignity even if no one's rights are violated and no one is harmed. There are conditions—such as being homeless, or being unable to feed one's children—that may seem to us to diminish human dignity, even if no one's rights have been violated. (And when, in order to express their moral concern, some people characterize such matters in terms of violations of rights, we are likely to think they have not quite gotten to the heart of the matter.) Even when rights are involved, the language of dignity may bring added moral weight. For example, we may violate someone's property rights, and we may violate someone's right not to be tortured. Why, Weithman asked, does the second seem a more weighty moral concern, so much more serious? We might well try to answer by using the language of human dignity. In addition, there are certain actions, which, even though not matters of right, call forth our respect and admiration: grace in the face of death, for example.

All of these examples seem to depend upon some image of what a truly human life ought to be, some vision of "the good life" for human beings. They are used less to distinguish those who live excellently from those who do not than to depict an ideal which we ought to seek to realize: an ideal of a life most suited to the "in-between" creatures we are.

titled *Human Cloning and Human Dignity*.[30] A reader of the report may be surprised, therefore, to discover how few actual references to dignity it makes, despite the term's prominent appearance in the title. This suggests that the term itself may be functioning primarily as a placeholder for larger understandings or background beliefs not easily articulated in shorthand ways. That possibility is reinforced when we look at the most significant instances of an appeal to human dignity within the report.

We place limits on what may be done in scientific research, the report notes, partly in order to "protect the health, safety, and dignity of the weak from possible encroachments by the strong" (17). This sort of concern indicates that the language of dignity is being associated closely with both a concern for equality and for protection against the risk of harm. Similarly, part of the point of codes of ethics governing what may be done in research is an "attempt to defend the weak against the strong and to uphold the equal dignity of all human beings" (98). This is important, but I think something more than just this is intended at a few other places in the report.

There are instances where the concern is not simply with human equality or the risk of harm but also with the kind of creature a human being is, with preserving a characteristically human life. When, for instance, the Council speaks of "the dignity of human procreation" (20), the language is serving as a placeholder for a certain vision of what it means to be human—and for our sense that the humanity of oneself or others may be wronged even when no discernible harm is suffered. The idea is this: the character of human life is degraded or diminished if we envision the relation between the generations in a way that makes some strong and others weak, in a way that makes some a "product" of the will and choice of others. This is true whether or not those who are "produced" by the will of others seem to be harmed or think themselves to have been harmed.

"The things we make are not just like ourselves; they are the products of our wills, and their point and purpose are ours to determine. But a begotten child comes into the world just as its parents once did, and is therefore their equal in dignity and humanity" (112). Or, again, "human dignity" is said to be at stake in the distinction between "making" and "begetting" because "parents beget a child who enters the world exactly as they did—as an unmade gift, not as

At one place in particular in the Council's work thus far, appeals to "dignity" understood in this way abound. That place is the third chapter ("Superior Performance") of *Beyond Therapy*.[33] Because appeals to the concept of dignity are plentiful in this chapter, it is obviously important for our topic. On the other hand, the concentration of so many appeals to dignity in a single chapter of a single report should also remind us that—in the reports of a body such as the President's Council on Bioethics—many authorial hands are at work. The use of a term may be less important than the larger understandings for which it, again, serves as a placeholder.

The principal use of the idea of dignity in this chapter is, I think, to refer to a naturally human way of being in the world. The term is often used to describe human activity—as in "the dignity of human activity" (105), or "the dignity of the activity itself" (108)—which dignity would, it is claimed, be undermined were we to use certain means to enhance performance. The dignity of the activity would be threatened, presumably, because the characteristically human form of the activity itself would be modified or subverted.

Elsewhere in the chapter, seeking to give a little more specificity to language about the dignity of human activity, the Council refers to the "dignity of embodiment" (149). This somewhat strange formulation seems to mean that the dignity we seek is to be "humanly excellent" (155), not just excellent in some other sense—not, for example, the excellence of a machine or an artifact (151). We should want to be neither mechanism (as is perhaps the beast who operates by instinct) nor master (as if we were gods). To be either of these would be to forego the dignity characteristic of human beings. I myself think that the use of a term such as "excellence" here probably confuses more than it clarifies. What this chapter on superior performance is aiming to depict might better be called "characteristically" human activity—that is, activity suited neither to a being who was all reason and will, nor to a being who was all body. This would be the activity of a complex creature composed of body, mind, will, and spirit—all operating as an integrated whole for which, though its action was "mindful" and "willful," there would be no sense of self as something separate from the body-in-motion (148). To subvert this specifically human character of our action might not harm us in obvious ways; indeed it might sometimes seem to benefit us (as in the example of enhanced athletic performance discussed by the Council). Yet, without harming us in such obvious ways, it might demean the humanity that is ours and that we ought to honor.

In my judgment, the Council is somewhat less successful in this attempt to depict (in general) a distinctively human form of activity than it was in its attempt to depict a characteristically human form of procreation. *Beyond Therapy* sees that we are divided beings for whom doer and deed are not entirely in harmony and notes that what the Greeks called *eros* was the longing for a kind of wholeness that would overcome this division within the self (149). I myself doubt that our lack of wholeness can be explained simply on its own terms, apart from any reference to the God-relation. In us, spirit and nature have quarreled. We can and do go wrong in either of two ways, and they are connected. We seek to be our own masters, as if reason and will were all that were needed for characteristically human activity (a danger the Council sees most clearly in its discussion of "the dignity of human procreation"). But also, having identified our true self with the rational will, we can come to think of the body as mere mechanism, not the body of the "animal rational" (a danger the Council underscores in its depiction of the kind of "superior performance" that does not lose the complex unity of the human being). In any case, I suspect that some of the puzzles created by the Council's use of the concept of dignity in *Beyond Therapy* are due less to the use of that concept than to an inherent difficulty: Hard as it may be to describe the ways in which we may lose the characteristic shape of human activity, it is far harder to provide an image of that activity when it is whole and undivided. To fall short in this attempt is no shame, however; it is, in fact, to be human.

What we should see by now, though, is that the Council turns to the language of dignity in order to develop some aspects of an anthropology, a vision of what the human species is and ought to be—a vision that moves well beyond the minimalistic notion that it is possible to wrong others only by harming them. We should not seek to live in disembodied ways more suited to gods than to human beings, nor should we treat our bodies as if they were things utterly open to our manipulation and not integrally involved in a characteristically human life. That is the vision for which the language of dignity serves as a placeholder. The Council may, of course, be wrong in some of the implications it draws from this vision, but the anthropological vision itself should not be beyond our understanding nor, when understood, should it seem particularly idiosyncratic.

Though not idiosyncratic, it does, however, move somewhat beyond ways in which the concept of dignity has most often been used in bioethics. Deryck Beyleveld and Roger Brownsword have distinguished three different ways in which the concept of dignity has, they believe, been used in bioethics.[34] The first they term "human dignity as empowerment." The central idea here is that one's dignity is violated if one's autonomy is not respected, and this concept leads quite naturally to an emphasis upon informed consent (11). Why exactly human beings should be thought to have such dignity is not clear, however. Beyleveld and Brownsword note that, if we cannot offer some ground that supports the attribution of dignity, the notion that all human beings possess such dignity will rest "entirely on contingent acceptance—it depends on humans having the right attitude" (22). And, as I noted earlier, insofar as we set aside our inherited religious grounding for human dignity while wishing to retain the commitment, we face a deep structural problem in our beliefs. Assertions that lack grounding often begin to sound a bit shrill.

The second concept of dignity Beyleveld and Brownsword call "human dignity as constraint"—that is, constraint on individual choices. This concept stands in clear tension with the first, for this sort of appeal to dignity may be used to control (or prohibit) activity to which one freely consents and which seems to harm no one else. As an example of the clash between these two concepts, they use a dwarf-throwing case from France, in which the police were authorized to stop the attraction of dwarf-throwing in clubs.

> The legality of the bans was challenged by, among others, one of the dwarfs…, who argued that he freely participated in the activity, that the work brought him a monthly wage (as well as allowing him to move in professional circles), and that, if dwarf-throwing was banned, he would find himself unemployed again. To this, the Conseil d'État responded that the dwarf compromised his own dignity by allowing himself to be used as a projectile, as a mere thing, and that no such concession should be allowed (26).

A third concept, somewhat different from the first two, is that of "dignified conduct." Whereas the first two concepts, however different from each other, might be described as notions of an intrinsic dignity, this third concept will make place for higher and lower ranks of dignity. The issues it raises I have dealt with earlier in discussing the tension between equal human dignity and distinctions in dignity.

Of these three concepts, it is the second—human dignity as constraint—that most closely approximates the position I have been developing, in which "dignity" functions as a placeholder for a richer, more developed anthropology of human nature and activity. Nevertheless, Beyleveld and Brownsword's notion of "dignity as constraint" does not fully capture the texture of the Council's vision. For one thing, it is an almost entirely negative notion, setting limits on otherwise autonomous action. As such, it lacks the positive (and, we must admit, very ambitious) attempt the Council makes to depict more fully the distinctively human form of certain activities—and it lacks the underlying metaphysic, the vision of the human being as a certain sort of creature.

In addition, for Beyleveld and Brownsword "dignity as constraint" articulates simply "a preferred version of the good life" (36). That is insufficient, in their view, because "modern societies are often pluralistic societies" (45), some of whose members may not, in fact, be committed to the good life so understood. This will seem like an insuperable problem however, only if our attention is focused almost entirely on policy questions, and if we assume, mistakenly, that there are ways of reaching consensus on such policy questions that involve no larger commitments about what it means to be human.

But there are not. To take just one example relevant to the Council's treatment of "the dignity of human procreation": An approach unlike the Council's, which (emphasizing the mastery of will and choice) disaggregated reproduction into its several parts and then combined them in new and different ways (with, for example, donor gametes or a surrogate womb), would hardly be free of metaphysical baggage. Rather, as Paul Ramsey once noted, it would simply embrace a new myth of creation, according to which human beings are created with two separate capacities—the body to express the unity of the partners through sexual relations, and the power to produce children through "a cool, deliberate act of man's rational will."[35] To their credit, Beyleveld and Brownsword recognize this at least in part. They note that the concept of "human dignity as empowerment" for autonomous choice has great difficulty offering a ground or reason why we should think human beings possess dignity in that sense. Indeed, it also begins to look like little more than another "preferred version of the good life," and certainly the concept of rights or respect for persons—even if it has a history within our law—is no less disputed or metaphysically thorny than is the concept of dignity.[36]

Here we stand on the border of another and equally difficult set of questions, having to do with the place of rich and developed conceptions of human nature within public argument and debate, but that is a matter for another time. It is for now sufficient to see that the President's Council on Bioethics, though it has used the concept of human dignity only infrequently, has used it to address questions that bioethics cannot avoid. In a society such as ours, committed as we are to human equality, we cannot avoid worrying about distinctions in dignity, and we cannot forever avert our gaze from the question of what grounds our commitment. And in any society, but certainly in one with our history, we must think carefully about what sort of creature—highest among the animals because rational and made for union with God, lowest among the hosts because embodied—the human being is, and how best to live in ways befitting such a creature.

## Notes

[1] *Summa Theologiae*, IIaIIae, q. 64, a. 2, ad. 3. We should not imagine that this idea is a peculiarity of Aquinas. Thus, for example, in his *Second Treatise* (1690), John Locke writes (paragraph 11) that a murderer may be killed in order "*to secure* Men from the attempts of a Criminal, who having renounced Reason, the common Rule and Measure, God hath given to Mankind, hath by the unjust Violence and Slaughter he hath committed upon one, declared War against all Mankind, and therefore may be destroyed as a *Lyon* or a *Tyger*, one of those wild Savage Beasts, with whom Men can have no Society nor Security."

[2] John Paul II, *The Gospel of Life* (Boston: Pauline, 1995), par. 9. In a rather free translation of the Latin, the English version has "personal dignity" for the Latin *dignitate*.

[3] Ruth Macklin, "Dignity is a Useless Concept," *BMJ* 327 (2003): 1419-1420.

[4] See Childress's remarks in the transcript at www.bioethics.gov/transcripts/dec05/session5.html. See also James F. Childress, "Epilogue: Looking Back to Look Forward," in *Belmont Revisited: Ethical Principles for Research with Human Subjects*, ed. James F. Childress, Eric M. Meslin, and Harold T. Shapiro (Washington, D.C.: Georgetown University Press, 2005), p. 246: "[T]he principle of human dignity is central...[in the Council's report, *Human Cloning and Human Dignity*], and the concept of dehumanization is parasitic on that principle. However, while referred to approximately fifteen times in the report, human dignity is nowhere clearly spelled out. Hence, readers cannot easily determine whether, how, and why human reproductive cloning constitutes dehumanization."

[5] *Organ Donation: Opportunities for Action*, ed. James F. Childress and Catharyn T. Liverman (Washington, D.C.: The National Academies Press, 2006), p. 233.

[6] References will be given by page number in parentheses within the text.

[7] John Galsworthy, *One More River* (New York: Charles Scribner's Sons, 1961 [1933]), p. 104.

[8] Walter Berns, *For Capital Punishment* (Lanham, Maryland: University Press of America, 1991), p. 163.

[9] Leon R. Kass, *Life, Liberty and the Defense of Dignity: The Challenge for Bioethics* (San Francisco, California: Encounter Books, 2002), pp. 231-256. References will be given by page number in parentheses within the text.

[10] *The Life and Writings of Abraham Lincoln*, ed. Philip Van Doren Stern (New York: The Modern Library, 1940), pp. 455-456.

[11] Søren Kierkegaard, *Works of Love* (Princeton, New Jersey: Princeton University Press, 1995 [1847]), p. 158.

[12] Ibid., p. 342.

[13] Oliver O'Donovan, *The Ways of Judgment* (Grand Rapids, Michigan: Eerdmans, 2005), p. 40.

[14] Gabriel Marcel, *The Existential Background of Human Dignity* (Cambridge, Massachusetts: Harvard University Press, 1963), p. 134.

[15] Ibid., p. 134.

16 The President's Council on Bioethics, *Alternative Sources of Human Pluripotent Stem Cells: A White Paper* (Washington, D.C.: Government Printing Office, 2005), p. 90.

17 The President's Council on Bioethics, *Reproduction and Responsibility: The Regulation of New Biotechnologies* (Washington, D.C.: Government Printing Office, 2004), p. 239. Gazzaniga wrote this in 2004. Perhaps, given what we have since learned about Korean "advances" in cloning-for-biomedical-research, he would wish to modify it somewhat.

18 Leon R. Kass, "Human Frailty and Human Dignity," *The New Atlantis* 7 (Fall 2004/Winter 2005), p. 116.

19 In what follows immediately, I am relying in considerable measure on O'Donovan, op. cit., pp. 42-49.

20 Kierkegaard, op. cit., p. 89.

21 O'Donovan, op. cit., p. 44.

22 Kierkegaard, op. cit., pp. 51-52.

23 O'Donovan, op. cit., p. 45.

24 Ibid., p. 48.

25 A wonderful phrase, which I owe to Russell Hittinger. See also *Luke* 17:7-10.

26 *Being Human: Core Readings in the Humanities* (New York: Norton, 2004), p. 568; this is a republication of *Being Human: Readings from the President's Council on Bioethics* (Washington, D.C.: Government Printing Office, 2004).

27 Ibid., p. 567.

28 Ibid., p. 568.

29 *Reproduction and Responsibility*, p. 11.

30 The President's Council on Bioethics, *Human Cloning and Human Dignity* (New York: Public Affairs, 2002). References will be given by page number in parentheses within the text.

31 Tom L. Beauchamp and James F. Childress, *Principles of Biomedical Ethics*, 4th ed. (New York: Oxford University Press, 1994), p. 411.

32 See www.bioethics.gov/transcripts/dec05/session5.html.

33 The President's Council on Bioethics, *Beyond Therapy: Biotechnology and the Pursuit of Happiness* (Washington, D.C.: Government Printing Office, 2003). References will be given by page number in parentheses within the text.

34 Deryck Beyleveld and Roger Brownsword, *Human Dignity in Bioethics and Biolaw* (Oxford: Oxford University Press, December 2001). References will be given by page number in parentheses within the text.

35 Paul Ramsey, *Fabricated Man: The Ethics of Genetic Control* (New Haven, Connecticut: Yale University Press, 1970), p. 36.

36 A point that Ruth Macklin (see note 3 above), despite her call for greater precision in the use and analysis of concepts, fails to see.

# Commentary on Meilaender and Dennett

## Peter Augustine Lawler

These comments began as a comparison I gave at the February 2007 meeting of the President's Council of the essays in the volume by Gilbert Meilaender and Daniel Dennett. My aim is to highlight some obvious differences and unexpected similarities between their two egalitarian views of dignity. I distinguish both of them from the more complex or ambivalent view of the relationship between dignity and equality given by Leon Kass, and I comment on Diana Schaub's provocative suggestion that Americans should distinguish clearly between equal rights and unequal dignity. My overall intention is to call attention to the significance of this volume: In this technological and biotechnological age we have more reason than ever to be concerned about human dignity, but we're stuck with some pretty basic disagreements over what dignity is.

From one view, Meilaender's and Dennett's essays defend two extreme and incompatible positions. Dennett prides himself on being a rather extreme or dogmatic atheist. And Meilaender, at least in his defense of the equal dignity of us all, is a rather extreme theist—that is, an Augustinian. In both cases we're reminded that extremism in defense of dignity is surely no vice, and we can add that both men, for the most part, lack the self-righteousness that often accompanies extreme defenses of dignity. Each man portrays himself, with good reason, as a nice-guy extremist.

And their extreme positions are far from completely incompatible. Meilaender and Dennett agree, for example, that dignity is not a useless concept. They also agree that dignity has to be saved from the inhuman reductionism of modern science, or at least from pervasive misunderstandings of what modern science actually teaches. They even seem to agree that our understanding of dignity—or at least the inherited understanding of dignity that has distinguished and ennobled our tradition—is Christian.

Meilaender claims that we are right to believe in the dignity of each unique and irreplaceable human person and the only sensible explanation for our faith in that observed phenomenon is the Christian one; we were all given infinite significance by a personal Creator. Our belief in the equal dignity of all human beings is an indispensable part of our Christian inheritance. And our attempts to find a foundation for that belief without Christianity become increasingly shrill as they become more obviously futile.

Dennett agrees, with scientific condescension, that all our claims for the reality of human dignity have been Christian. He adds that all the Christian claims about the soul or some immaterial dimension of personal existence have been refuted by modern science. For Dennett, the belief in the soul or in dignity has the same status as belief in mermaids. It's no more silly to believe in some half-woman/half-fish that nobody has ever really seen than it is to believe in a half-soul/half-body that nobody has ever really seen. Everything that we do, we now know, has a material explanation. In the spirit of Dennett's analysis, we might add two observations: Not so long ago, very smart and astute people believed in souls, while mermaid-believers have always been rather silly. And in the near future, biotechnology might allow us to combine the materials of a woman and a fish to create something like a mermaid. But we never will be able to create a soul, to free ourselves from our essentially material being.

Dennett does claim to see with his own eyes—and this is very important—that our need to believe in equal, personal dignity is real. It is an observable characteristic of the type of being human beings alone are. We are the social animals who conceive of projects to live good, purposeful lives, although there is no scientific foundation for human conceptions of either virtue or purpose. So we can't get by without believing in some useful illusions—such as free will, love, and dignity. And we can't help but adhere to those beliefs in the face of what we really know about our accidental, evolutionary, and wholly material existences.

Dennett's ingenious solution to the problem of the incompatibility between scientific truth and dignified belief is to say, quite candidly, that we're hardwired to believe. And our allegiance to our belief in equal human dignity can be supported by the good life it makes possible for us. That our belief makes possible our flourishing can be enough to sustain it; we can stop obsessing about whether it's actually true by just accepting the fact that it's not. All we need to know is that when we do believe we're better off as social animals.

So the big difference between Dennett and Meilaender is not over utility, but truth. For Meilaender, each of us is a unique and irreplaceable being, hence not merely species fodder. And he would deny, of course, that it's either possible or useful to stop caring about whether our dignified beliefs are actually true. Our belief in our dignity corresponds to the mystery we can actually observe about members of our species—human persons—alone.

That mystery has nothing to do with the separate existence of the soul from the body. For Meilaender, almost nothing is more deceptive than thinking of ourselves as somehow detached from our bodies, as "souls" or "spirits" or "autonomous agents" somehow looking down on our bodies from some undisclosed location. He agrees with Dennett that we can't separate ourselves from our embodiment, and so, from his view, Dennett presents at best a crude and fundamentally misleading caricature of what Christians actually believe.

For Meilaender, the mystery of human life is that we are the only beings, as far as we know, who are given the dignified responsibility of living well or badly with what we really know and who we really love, who are conscious of both our limitations and our purposes, of our biological mortality and our transcendence. Our awareness of this mystery in no way depends on knowledge of a separable soul, knowledge we simply don't have. But we also know, when we don't divert ourselves from ourselves, that we have no fully adequate scientific explanation for the mystery of being and human being. And it makes perfectly good sense that our dignified experience of a mysterious but nonetheless real personal responsibility was given to us by a personal, loving God Who eludes our comprehension and control.

For Dennett, nothing human or natural or material is mysterious. Everything can or will be comprehended by science and scientists. That's good because it means we can understand scientifically why we have attributed dignity to ourselves. Insofar as we believe our dignity is mysterious, we can't consciously and rationally employ it for the purpose of our social flourishing. So modern science, properly understood, can make our dignity more effective. Dennett, of course, has the merit of joining Meilaender in criticism of those who connect our dignity with our autonomy, with our freedom from natural limitations for laws or choices we impose on ourselves. For him, dignity also, in a way, has its roots in our truthfully confronting our natural limitations. Our fictional dignity properly understood depends on our awareness of our real material situation. We are tempted to tell Dennett that what he really means is that we have dignity as the beings who can consciously shape our lives around a fictional concept of dignity. He would respond: That's not really dignity, because, in truth, we're not really choosing freely but just facing up to necessity.

These two extremists also share an egalitarian view of dignity, and that separates them from members of the President's Council—such as Leon Kass and Diana Schaub—who tend to think that dignity is fundamentally aristocratic, a display of one's distinctive personal excellence. Meilaender and Dennett deny that my dignity is dependent on the excellence or virtue that I display in a particular social context. That's easy for Dennett to do: his view is that there's nothing I can do that would really make me dignified. Meilaender's view is that nothing that I can do can really make me undignified.

We can wonder, as Kass and Schaub do, how successful the two extremists are in disconnecting dignity from real human achievement in thought and action. Meilaender criticizes Kass for saying that because patients lack agency they lack the capacity to be dignified. To support his case, he gives the example of the dignified patient who acts with patience in light of the truth about his dependent human condition. He explains how patients can even be more truthful or more dignified than manly or magnanimous men who take pleasure in forgetting about the truth about their embodied, social, and natural dependence and limitations. The patient he describes doesn't disconnect dignity from gratitude and so is more dignified than those who engage in that self-deception.

Kass responds that Meilaender's dignified patient depends upon his capacity to engage in action and thought appropriate to his human situation. That patient is not really pure patient. He's partly a patient and partly not; a pure patient—someone, say, in the last stages of Alzheimer's—would be perfectly passive and so incapable of displaying dignified virtue. Dennett claims it's enough to say that we will have better lives if we regard pure patients as having equal dignity. But maybe the truth isn't self-evident. And Kass is never that clear about why we must accord pure patients dignity. Meilaender's faith gives him confidence enough that every human life has equally irreplaceable significance, and so he never has to engage in deliberation about the dignity of any particular human patient.

So far the evidence is that, not only do most Americans share Meilaender's faith, but the results are disastrous when we make public policy based on skepticism about its truth. The monstrous tyrannies of the 20th century were all based on the premise that some human beings exist for others—one race is expendable for another's benefit, or today's individuals can be sacrificed indiscriminately for the perfect society of the future. And surely we all agree that an undignified temptation of biotechnology is the engineering or manufacturing of human beings for the benefit of others—as, for example, sources of spare parts, or as material for medical research. The undoubted moral premise of our individualism is that no particular human being exists merely for others; so our law depends on the thought that each of us is a dignified end, not a dispensable means.

Dennett's utility argument actually points to the conclusion that our humane belief in dignity is useful only if we have faith, with Meilaender, that it's really true. An urgent question before us is to what extent that faith is reasonable apart from real belief in the personal God of the Bible. Another is to what extent Kass, Meilaender, and Dennett finally share the same answer to that question. Surely only Dennett is sanguine about the reasonableness of belief that is not really true.

Another point of agreement between Dennett and Meilaender worth emphasizing is that they both defend human dignity as a way of fending off human degradation. They both write to preserve the qualities that distinguish human beings from their assault by modern science and potentially by biotechnology. Even Dennett seems to write to preserve the real existence of beings capable of believing and acting in a dignified way from biotechnology that would, say, suppress those parts of the brain that make dignity indispensable.

Both of our extremists are open to the criticism that, when formulating public policy, Americans have always thought in terms of protecting rights, not dignity. Because we can speak so clearly and certainly of rights, why should we employ a term as murky—as controversial and as self-righteous—as dignity? There are actually good reasons to think of dignity as at least politically useless. When Leon Kass wrote of "Life, Liberty, and the Defense of Dignity," it can be argued, he was imposing upon our country a needlessly innovative and contentious idea. According to Diana Schaub, our political community is sufficiently formed by our concern with equal rights, and dignity—which is necessarily unequal—should remain a private or personal goal.

Our need to speak of dignity, I think, comes from reflection on our experiences of the 20th and 21st centuries. What the ideology-driven, totalitarian regimes of the 20th century did to human beings was a lot worse than merely violating rights. The Nazis and the Communists were at war against the very existence of beings capable of experiencing the dignity of human individuality, of (as the dissidents Solzhenitsyn, John Paul II and Havel wrote) living responsibly in light of the truth. It's in the courageous and truthful thought and action of these dissidents that we find evidence of dignity that is trivialized by the view that they were merely exercising their rights. And in the 21st century, as Kass has shown, biotechnology could actually provide us with ways of changing our nature in undignified ways that would promise to maximize our comfort, security, and happiness. Our spirit of resistance to such changes in our nature surely will be insufficiently animated by the ambiguous phrase, "natural rights."

I have to add that it may show a lack of faith—or it may just be unrealistic—to believe that we are capable of making ourselves anything other than beings with dignity. Both totalitarian and biotechnological efforts to eradicate those aspects of our nature that make us dignified beings—that make us stuck with virtue to live well with what we can't help but know—are, as far as I can tell, doomed to fail.

# Commentary on Meilaender and Lawler

## Diana Schaub

In his very fine essay, Gilbert Meilaender argues that Christianity has transformed the Greek emphasis on comparative dignity by bringing it into contact with egalitarian dignity. Christianity, he says, marks "a great rupture in Western culture." He further argues that this Christian egalitarianism is the inspiration behind the American assertion of man's equality in the Declaration of Independence. He suggests that one needs belief in the fatherhood of God for the brotherhood of men to be seen as self-evident. He worries that, with the decline in religious belief—and the unwillingness to acknowledge the connection between religion and politics—we are increasingly in a situation where our commitment to equal human dignity is ungrounded and, hence, unsustainable.

Meilaender wants us back on firm ground and, in particular, he argues that there are two places where differences in excellence or dignity must not matter: the first is at "the threshold of death, when the continuance of life itself is at stake," and the other is "the opportunity to live within human society and participate in its common life."

While Meilaender makes plain his discomfort with the aristocratic ancient Greek take on dignity (even calling it "a temptation" that ought to be resisted), there were moments in which he seemed more of a Hellenizer than he admits. Perhaps the distance between Meilaender and Kass is not as great as either believes.

Let me cite a couple of instances. Early in the paper, Meilaender presents us with a character from a Galsworthy novel. He offers old Betty Purdy as an individual who confounds our aristocratic presumptions about greatness and dignity. The passage he cites does indeed show the falsity of status and wealth as markers of human dignity, but it does not at all argue for equal human dignity. The greatness of this little old lady came from the moral virtues she displayed in the midst of the ordinariness of her life. Her greatness depended on her comparative excellence, not her equal human dignity. We are told of the meagerness of her material existence and her limited range of action, "but her back had been straight, her ways straight, her eyes quiet and her manners gentle." I take it we are to admire her fortitude and her probity and her kindness. Those are not qualities equally possessed. If the woman had instead lived in Buckingham Palace with the world as her stage, real greatness would still have depended on her moral virtues. That is one of the points made by the wonderful movie *The Queen*, starring Helen Mirren[1]. Of the queen also it could be said that "her back had been straight, her ways straight, her eyes quiet and her manners gentle."

I suppose one might argue that the disposition to see moral excellence in humble places owes something to Christianity. However, one can find even in Homer admiration not only for the fierce-hearted, but also the patient-hearted.

It is particularly over the status of the patient that Professors Meilaender and Kass conflict. Meilaender quotes Kass as saying "being a patient rather than an agent is, humanly speaking, undignified." Meilaender dissents and counters that "human dignity lies in acknowledging the way in which aging and dying very often involve becoming more and more a patient (and needing to learn patience) and less and less an agent." However, what Meilaender describes—namely, "acknowledging" aging and "learning" patience—are the actions of an agent in the face of suffering. Patience is a virtue, and a difficult one for most of us. A human being displaying patience suffers in a way very different from an animal, despite the fact that an animal might seem just as stoic and uncomplaining. A patient sufferer displays a dignity and excellence that a passive and uncomprehending animal does not.*

Although Meilaender reiterates that he finds "something offensive" about the aristocratic view of human dignity, it seems to me that he himself regularly recurs to a version of it and that he can't help but do so. After all, in Christianity, the message to respect basic humanity came from the fullest and purest humanity. The bearer of the message was not just a godly man, but God become man. We are to imitate His perfection. Christian virtues may be different from classical virtues, but the standard is if anything higher.

Meilaender appeals to Lincoln for evidence of what he calls "the problem we have with an inegalitarian concept of dignity." I too accept Lincoln as an authority. However, I don't find Lincoln at all offended by the aristocratic view. In fact, Lincoln always starts his explications of the meaning of the Declaration by acknowledging the fact of human inequality. Men are not equal in all sorts of features and capacities, and Lincoln lists many of them. For Lincoln, admitting the existence of various politically and socially significant inequalities should not in any way imperil the real truth of the Declaration, namely that men are equal in their natural rights to life and liberty. Lincoln speaks of equal rights, not equal dignity. I suspect that we may have gone awry when we confounded the language of dignity with that of equality. Dignity was not a word either the Founders or Lincoln employed much, and when they did it was in a frankly meritocratic sense.

Moreover, in the passage Meilaender cites it is worth noting that Lincoln illustrates the equality of rights by saying that human beings are equal in their right to eat "the bread that...[their] own hands have earned." Even this equal right hinges on earning. Labor is the title to property, and men will labor unequally. Lincoln does not here tell us what those who are unable to labor are entitled to. I don't

---

* In fairness, however, to the other animals, I would just note that Homer ascribes virtues to them as well. Penelope is not the only paragon of patience in the *Odyssey*. When Odysseus finds his great-hearted dog Argos on a dung heap, covered in ticks, awaiting his return, he sheds tears for his faithful companion. (See Homer, *Odyssey* 17.300*ff*.) Though Penelope too suffers from an infestation of the human equivalent of dog ticks (the suitors), her wit is a resource that Argos does not have. Perhaps that is why Odysseus is able to suppress his tears for the long-suffering Penelope.

mean to suggest that Lincoln would have denied sustenance to the young or the elderly or the sick. Lincoln was attacking the injustice of slave labor, and his arguments were marshaled accordingly. I have no doubt that Lincoln would defend the right to life as vigorously as he defended the right to liberty. We have evidence of his capacious humanity in the closing lines of the Second Inaugural when he calls on Americans "to care for him who shall have borne the battle, and for his widow, and his orphan."

The example of Lincoln leads me to think that we have a model for how to combine and celebrate both the respects in which human beings are equal and the respects in which they are unequal. One need not imperil the other. Indeed, the life of Lincoln—a superior man who devoted and sacrificed his life to the teaching of equality—reminds us that we can't have one without the other. We shouldn't lose sight of the success of the American Founders, among whom I include Lincoln, in combining the egalitarian and the inegalitarian. They didn't seem to struggle with it as we do. They were a happy amalgam: Greco-Roman, Judeo-Christian Lockeans. Whether this synthesis coheres in theory or not, perhaps we need to take it more seriously as a basis for sound policy guidance

Meilaender asserts that there are two places where judgments of individual worth should not be given any scope: at the threshold of death and participation in human society. Meilaender seems to say these are absolutes. He quotes Kierkegaard approvingly: "If you save a person's life in the dark, thinking that it is a friend—but it was the neighbor—this is no mistake." I can imagine scenarios in which it might have been a very big mistake: what if your neighbor also happened to be your enemy and you happened to have been on a nighttime reconnaissance mission? Kierkegaard's statement is radically apolitical; it abstracts entirely from the distinction between friend and foe. Does the political fact that some neighbors are friends and allies while others are deadly and inveterate foes require that individuals in authority be entrusted with the power of life and death over other individuals? Or are the claims of "the neighbor" indeed absolute? If human judgments have no place at the threshold of death does that require not only opposition to the death penalty but thoroughgoing pacifism as well?

This question points back to the striking contrast between St.

Thomas Aquinas and Pope John Paul II with which Meilaender begins his essay and which is worth repeating. For Aquinas, a murderer "loses his human dignity," "lapses into the subjection of the beasts," and presumably can be treated accordingly, in order to defend the life and dignity of other men and society in general. For Pope John Paul II, the human dignity of the murderer remains intact. Although I'm no expert on the evolution of Vatican teaching, I suspect that the embrace of the apolitical language of inherent and immutable dignity is connected to the Church's newfound ambivalence about capital punishment. While the Catholic Church has not officially denied the theoretical legitimacy of capital punishment or overturned its just war doctrine, the trend is toward non-judgmentalism and the unilateral disarmament of the decent.

I have similar reservations about the assertion that all human beings "must have the opportunity to live within human society and participate in its common life." Does this mean that we are not allowed to deprive others of liberty and social interaction through imprisonment, including solitary confinement? If incarceration is permitted, then we are making judgments about an individual's viciousness and exclusion from society.

In both these cases, it seems to me that the language of equal rights is preferable to the language of equal dignity. Rights are inalienable, but they also imply reciprocity and responsibility. Those who violate the rights of others have rendered some of their own rights forfeit. A rights-based approach protects the innocent and weak, about whom Meilaender and all of us are concerned, but does not require us to abandon human judgments about virtue and vice.

As to Meilaender's claim that our nation's founding doctrine is grounded in Christianity, it is true that the Declaration refers to men as "created" equal and endowed by their "Creator" with certain inalienable rights. It is also true that Jefferson shared Meilaender's worry that, once religious belief falters, the commitment to equality will be hard to sustain. Here's how Jefferson put it:

> And can the liberties of a nation be thought secure when we have removed their only firm basis, a conviction in the minds of the people that these liberties are of the gift of God? That they are not to be violated but with his wrath?[2]

Having granted that much, I would point out that the Declaration refers to the "Laws of Nature and Nature's God." I suspect that Nature's God is not quite the same as the Biblical God. Meilaender says that the truth of human equality is a "theological assertion," but how strong a theology is required? In other writings, Jefferson argued that it is not religion, but rather reason and science that will reveal the truth of the Declaration. In a letter written just days before his death, Jefferson said that

> All eyes are opened, or opening, to the rights of men. The general spread of the light of science has already laid open to every view the palpable truth that the mass of mankind has not been born with saddles on their backs, nor a favored few booted and spurred, ready to ride them legitimately, by the grace of God.[3]

As we know, even if equal rights are self-evident, they are not self-establishing. The paradox of rights is that you have to hazard your life and liberty in order to secure your right to life and liberty. The vindication of the essential dignity of humanity depends upon the actions of individuals who do amazing things like "mutually pledge to each other our lives, our fortunes, and our sacred honor." As Frederick Douglass never tired of telling his enslaved brothers:

Hereditary bondmen, know ye not,
Who would be free, themselves must strike the blow.[4]

This was a heartening message for both blacks and women, who had the wherewithal to strike the blow and secure the dignified treatment to which they were by nature entitled.

It may not be such a cheering message for the young or the drastically impaired—although perhaps the answer that Locke gives about the young is sufficient. He says: "*Children*, I confess are not born in this full state of *Equality*, though they are born to it."[5] Consequently, our handling of them must always be aware of their directedness towards rational liberty. Children are rights-bearers too. Accordingly, the power of parents and guardians is limited; Locke insists it does not extend to life and death. Immature human beings (embryos included) have, by nature, the same bodily immunity as adults. There is a fundamental human right not to have one's body captured or controlled by others for their ends and purposes.

In the case of the weak and immature, respect for this basic right to life will continue to depend on the deference of the strong. In his speeches, Lincoln deployed his relentless logic to get those who had the upper hand to realize the momentary and fragile character of their strength. He stressed that the only guarantee of one's own rights lies in the recognition of the rights of others. "As I would not be a *slave*, so I would not be a *master*."[6] And again, "In *giving* freedom to the *slave*, we *assure* freedom to the *free*—honorable alike in what we give, and what we preserve."[7] This is a version of neighbor love and brotherhood that is reasonable and republican in character. It doesn't deny the fatherhood of God, but it doesn't draw attention to it either.

At the risk of impiety, I will suggest that brothers can get along pretty well when the father, whether human or divine, remains in the background. After all, the first story of brothers in the Bible is a story of fratricide in response to God's favoring the gift of one brother over the other. I'm not so certain that it helps our sense of human equality to view matters under the aspect of eternity. As I read the Bible, some of us will be eternally damned and others saved. We are not equidistant from God, either here on earth or later. I'm quite certain that Professor Meilaender is "nearer my God to thee" than I am, but I think that we can still be equal citizens, mutually acknowledging our individual rights and brotherly responsibilities.

\*

Though one might legitimately doubt the adequacy of rights language—particularly in light of the corruption of that language and its contemporary links to notions of radical autonomy—it nonetheless seems to me still the best way to approach the bioethical issues that arise at both the beginning of life and the end of life. When life is at its simplest, it is the right to life that should guide our reflections. I am not arguing for a return exclusively to rights language, since I agree that it does not reach to all bioethics questions, particularly those that involve the highest human possibilities. So, for instance, in the *Beyond Therapy* report, the Council rightly (and profoundly) spoke about human flourishing—in other words, not just about the right to the pursuit of happiness, but about the nature of happiness itself. It investigated the character of mature and meaningful human action and how certain biotech developments might impair, cheapen, or debase such activities. The report was a defense of human dignity and, as such, a demonstration or enactment of dignity. But, even here, the language of dignity is inseparable from the language of rights. We ask the question "what is happiness?" so that the answer might guide our pursuit of it and so that we might better understand how to secure the right to the pursuit of it.

Peter Lawler argues, both in his essay in this volume and, more extensively, in the Council session devoted to this volume,[8] that the language of rights was insufficient to either describe or confront the horrors of fascism and communism (and that it may be similarly inadequate today to the extent that biotechnology could be perverted so as to "be at war with the very aspects of our nature that allow us to be dignified beings"). Lawler remarks that dissidents like Solzhenitsyn, Havel, and Pope John Paul II "were big on bringing back the word 'dignity' because the word 'rights' just wasn't enough." I'm not so sure. Perhaps they appealed to "dignity" because they didn't come from a rights-based tradition and weren't aware of its range and rhetorical power. Certainly, Churchill was eloquent in condemnation of modern totalitarianism and adamant in resistance without recourse to the word "dignity." In his "War Speech" in the House of Commons, Churchill explained the war against the "pestilence of Nazi tyranny" as "a war, viewed in its inherent quality, to establish, on impregnable rocks, the rights of the individual, and it is a war to establish and revive the stature of man."[9] For Churchill, that "stature" (which might be construed as a synonym for dignity—of the "aristocratic" variety) is inseparable from the assertion and protection of individual rights. The human heights of a few are achieved on the firm ground of the rights of all. Similarly, in response to the Soviet menace in his "Iron Curtain" address, Churchill declared:

> We must never cease to proclaim in fearless tones the great principles of freedom and the rights of man which are the joint inheritance of the English-speaking world and which

through Magna Carta, the Bill of Rights, the Habeas Corpus, trial by jury, and the English common law find their most famous expression in the American Declaration of Independence.[10]

Churchill, of course, was viewing these regimes from the outside. One might argue that those whom Lawler calls "the great dissident opponents" experienced a deeper truth, namely that Hitler and Stalin weren't just violating rights but "were at war against the being capable of experiencing dignity." If so, the ideologues were notably unsuccessful, since they brought some, at least, of their victims not to the depths of dehumanization but to the depths of wisdom and humane insight. The American experience, also, offers examples of individuals who felt the full effects of soul-destroying tyranny and yet emerged fortified in spirit. Frederick Douglass is one of the great dissidents. Like the Founders and Lincoln, Douglass very rarely employed the word "dignity." I suspect that Frederick Douglass would have had the language to denounce fascism and communism just as he had the language to denounce the slaveocracy, with nary a mention of dignity. As Lawler also notes, these monstrous offenses—which "can't be described as mere violations of rights"—were perpetrated by ideologists who denied the existence of individual rights. Violations of rights are never "mere." It may be that the surest route to attain and sustain human dignity is through the defense of human rights. While Douglass didn't speak of dignity, his every action displayed and demonstrated it.

Our contemporary tendency to bandy the word about is an ominous sign that we no longer agree about its content. Because we no longer share what Meilaender calls a "vision of what it means to be human," perhaps we are obliged to be more explicit than in the past about the conditions and limits of human dignity. As Meilaender details so well in the final section of his paper, the Council has done valuable work in articulating an anthropological vision (as opposed to a transhumanist vision), in its discussions both of characteristically human procreation and of superior human performance (athletic and other). I don't know whether an anthropology is necessary to being human, but if a science of man can help either to keep us men or make us good men I'm all for it.

## Notes

[1] *The Queen,* directed by Stephen Frears, Miramax Films, Pathé Productions, and Granada, 2006.
[2] Thomas Jefferson, *Notes on the State of Virginia,* Query XVIII, "Manners," in *The Portable Thomas Jefferson,* ed. Merrill D. Peterson (New York: Viking Penguin, 1975), p. 215.
[3] Thomas Jefferson, "To Roger C. Weightman," June 24, 1826, in *The Portable Thomas Jefferson,* p. 585.
[4] See, for example, Frederick Douglass, *My Bondage and My Freedom* (New York: Penguin, 2003 [1855]), chapter 17, "The Last Flogging." Douglass is quoting Lord Byron, *Childe Harold's Pilgrimage* (1812-1818), Canto 2, Stanza 76.
[5] John Locke, *The Second Treatise of Government,* in *Two Treatises of Government,* ed. Peter Laslett (Cambridge: Cambridge University Press, 1994), chapter VI, "Of Paternal Power," paragraph 55, p. 304.
[6] Abraham Lincoln, "My Idea of Democracy," in *The Political Thought of Abraham Lincoln,* ed. Richard N. Current (New York: Macmillan, 1967), p. 327.
[7] Abraham Lincoln, "Second Annual Message to Congress, 1862" in *The Political Thought of Abraham Lincoln,* p. 234.
[8] See the transcript of the Council's discussion on Friday, February 6, 2007, online at www.bioethics.gov/transcripts/feb07/session6.html.
[9] Winston S. Churchill, "War Speech," September 3, 1939, House of Commons, in *Winston S. Churchill: His Complete Speeches 1897-1963,* ed. Robert Rhodes James (New York: Chelsea House, 1974) vol. 6; available online at www.winstonchurchill.org/i4a/pages/index.cfm?pageid=878.
[10] Winston S. Churchill, "Sinews of Peace," March 5, 1946, Fulton, Missouri, in *Winston S. Churchill: His Complete Speeches 1897-1963,* vol. 7; available online at www.winstonchurchill.org/i4a/pages/index.cfm?pageid=429.

# Part IV.
# The Sources and Meaning of Dignity

# 12

# Defending Human Dignity

## Leon R. Kass

*It is difficult to define what human dignity is. It is not an organ to be discovered in our body, it is not an empirical notion, but without it we would be unable to answer the simple question: what is wrong with slavery?*—Leszek Kolakowski[1]

In American discussions of bioethical matters, human dignity, where it is not neglected altogether, is a problematic notion. There are disagreements about its importance relative to other human goods, such as freedom or justice. There are differences of opinion about exactly what it means and what it rests on, a difficulty painfully evident when appeals to "human dignity" are invoked on opposite sides of an ethical debate, for example, about whether permitting assisted suicide for patients suffering from degrading illnesses would serve or violate their human dignity. There are also disagreements about the extent to which considerations of human dignity should count in determining public policy.

We friends of human dignity must acknowledge these difficulties, both for practice and for thought. In contrast to continental Europe and even Canada, human dignity has not been a powerful idea in American public discourse, devoted as we are instead to the language of rights and the pursuit of equality. Among us, the very idea of "dignity" smacks too much of aristocracy for egalitarians and too much of religion for secularists and libertarians. Moreover, it seems to be too private and vague a matter to be the basis for legislation or public policy.

Yet, that said, we Americans actually care a great deal about human dignity, even if the term comes not easily to our lips. In times past, our successful battles against slavery, sweatshops, and segregation, although fought in the name of civil rights, were at bottom campaigns for human dignity—for treating human beings as they deserve to be treated, *solely because of their humanity.* Likewise, our taboos against incest, bestiality, and cannibalism, as well as our condemnations of prostitution, drug addiction, and self-mutilation—having little to do with defending liberty and equality—all seek to defend human dignity against (voluntary) acts of *self*-degradation. Today, human dignity is of paramount importance especially in matters bioethical. As we become more and more immersed in a world of biotechnology, we increasingly sense that we neglect human dignity at our peril, especially in light of gathering powers to intervene in human bodies and minds in ways that will affect our very humanity, likely threatening things that everyone, whatever their view of human dignity, holds dear. Truth to tell, it is beneath our human dignity to be indifferent to it.

As part of its effort to develop and promote a "richer" bioethics, the President's Council on Bioethics, in its previously published works, has paid considerable attention to various aspects of human dignity that are at risk in our biotechnological age: the dignity of human procreation, threatened by cloning-to-produce-children and other projected forms of "manufacture"; the dignity of nascent human life, threatened by treating embryonic human beings as mere raw material for exploitation and use in research and commerce; the dignity of the human difference, threatened by research that would produce man-animal or man-machine hybrids; the dignity of bodily integrity, threatened by trafficking in human body parts; the dignity of psychic integrity, threatened by chemical interventions that would erase memories, create factitious moods, and transform personal identity; the dignity of human self-command, threatened by methods of behavior modification that bypass human agency; the dignity of human activity and human excellence, threatened by reliance on performance-enhancing or performance-transforming drugs; the dignity of living deliberately and self-consciously, mindful of the human life cycle and our finitude, threatened by efforts to deny or eliminate aging and to conquer mortality; the dignity of dying well (or of living well while dying), threatened by excessive medical intervention at the end of life; and the dignity of human being as such, threatened by the prospect of euthanasia and other "technical solutions" for the miseries that often accompany the human condition.[2] Beyond these practical issues, the Council has also tried to call attention to the dignity of proper human self-understanding, threatened by shallow "scientistic" thinking about human phenomena—for example, views of human life that see organisms as mere means for the replication of their genes, the human body as a lifeless machine, or human love and moral choice as mere neurochemical events.[3] In my own personal writings on biology and human affairs, spanning over thirty-five years, I have dealt with many of the same aspects of human dignity and the dangers they face from the new biology, both to our practice and to our thought.[4]

Yet neither the Council nor I have tried to articulate a full theoretical account of human dignity; neither have we tried to reconcile some of the competing views that are held by the various members, all bidding fair to gain our assent. This essay is offered as a contribution toward the development of such a conceptual account. Specifically, it aims to do three things: to defend a robust role in bioethics for the idea of human dignity; to make clearer what human dignity is and what it rests on; and to try to show the relationship between two equally important but sometimes competing ideas of human dignity: the *basic* dignity of human *being* and the *full* dignity of being (actively) *human*, of human *flourishing*.\*

---

\* Application to specific bioethical topics and debates of any conceptual clarifications found in this essay must await subsequent exploration. The purpose of this paper is entirely philosophical; and it intends no immediate or direct implications for public policy in any substantive field of bioethics.

## Why Bioethics Must Care About Human Dignity: Old and New Concerns

Attention to human dignity is important in nearly all arenas of bioethical concern: clinical medicine; research using human subjects; uses of novel biotechnologies "beyond therapy" (especially for so-called "enhancement" purposes); and "transhumanist" activities aimed at altering and transcending human nature. But because the central ethical concerns in these domains differ, *each realm of bioethics gives special salience to a different aspect of human dignity.*

In clinical medicine, a primary ethical focus is on the need to respect the equal worth and dignity of each patient at every stage of his or her life—regardless of race, class or gender, condition of body and mind, severity of illness, nearness to death, or ability to pay for services rendered. Defenders of human dignity rightly insist that every patient deserves—from every physician, nurse, or hospital—equal respect in speech and deed and equal consideration regarding the selection of appropriate treatment. Moreover, they also rightly insist that no life is to be deemed worthier than another and that under no circumstances should we look upon a fellow human being as if he or she has a "life unworthy of life" and deserves to be made dead. The ground of these opinions, and of the respect for human dignity they betoken, lies not in the patient's autonomy or any other of his personal qualities or excellences, but rather in the patient's very being and vitality. Doctors should always respect the life the patient has, all the more because he has entrusted it to their care in the belief that they will indeed respect it to the very last.

Regarding research with human subjects, the major ethical issues concern not only safeguarding the subject's life and health but also respecting the subject's humanity, even as he is being treated as an experimental animal. Concern for human dignity focuses on enlisting the human subject as a knowing and willing co-partner in the research enterprise. Soliciting voluntary informed consent pays tribute to the humanity of the human subject, even as that humanity will be largely overlooked in the research protocol. Bioethicists usually believe that respecting human dignity here means respecting autonomy—the freedom of the subject's will—and so it does; more to it. It involves respecting also the subject's courage in accepting risks and discomforts, his philanthropic desire to contribute to a worthy cause, and his generosity of time and trouble in embracing activities from which he will receive no direct benefit.

In these domains of clinical medicine and research involving human subjects, appeals to human dignity, while tacitly employing an ideal of proper treatment and respect, function explicitly and mainly as bulwarks against abuse: patients should not be reduced to "thing-hood" or treated as mere bodies; research subjects should not be utilized as mere means or treated only as experimental animals. This "negative" function of the concept of human dignity in these domains makes perfect sense, inasmuch as it is intended—and needed—to restrain the strong in their dealings with the weak. It makes even more sense once we remember the origins of modern biomedical ethics: a concern for human dignity hovers over all of modern biomedical ethics owing to the world's horror at the Nazi atrocities, atrocities in which German scientists and German doctors were deeply implicated. They more than lent a hand with eugenic sterilization, barbaric human experimentation, and mass extermination of the "unfit"—all undertaken, mind you, in order to produce "a more perfect human." The rise to prominence of the idea of "human dignity" in post-World-War-II Europe, expressed in the laws of many nations and especially in the United Nations' *Universal Declaration of Human Rights*, was surely intended to ensure that no human beings should ever again be so abused, degraded, and dehumanized—and, of course, annihilated.

But a more robust notion of human dignity is needed when we turn from these traditional domains of medical ethics to the moral challenges raised by new biotechnological powers and the novel purposes to which they are being put, and when we turn from concerns with abuse of power that the strong inflict upon the weak to concerns with ethically dubious uses of powers that the strong—indeed, most of us—will choose to exercise for and on ourselves. Our desires for a better life do not end with health, and the uses of biotechnology are not limited to therapy. Its powers to alter the workings of body and mind are attractive not only to the sick and suffering, but to everyone who desires to look younger, perform better, feel happier, or become more "perfect."

We have already entered the age of biotechnical enhancement:

growth hormone to make children taller; pre-implantation genetic screening to facilitate eugenic choice (now to rule out defects, soon to rule in assets); Ritalin and other stimulants to control behavior or boost performance on exams; Prozac and other drugs to brighten moods and alter temperaments—not to mention Botox, Viagra, and anabolic steroids. Looking ahead, other invitations are already visible on the horizon: Drugs to erase painful or shameful memories or to simulate falling in love. Genes to increase the size and strength of muscles. Nano-mechanical implants to enhance sensation or motor skills. Techniques to slow biological aging and increase the maximum human lifespan. Thanks to these and other innovations, venerable human desires—for better children, superior performance, ageless bodies, and happy souls—may increasingly be satisfied with the aid of biotechnology. A new field of "transhumanist" science is rallying thought and research for wholesale redesign of human nature, employing genetic and neurological engineering and man-machine hybrids, en route to what has been blithely called a "posthuman future."

Neither the familiar principles of contemporary bioethics—respect for persons, beneficence (or "non-maleficence"), and justice—nor our habitual concerns for safety, efficacy, autonomy, and equal access will enable us to assess the true promise and peril of the biotechnology revolution. Our hopes for self-improvement and our disquiet about a "posthuman" future are much more profound. At stake are the kind of human being and the sort of society we will be creating in the coming age of biotechnology. At stake are the dignity of the human being—including the dignity or worth of human activity, human relationships, and human society—and the nature of human flourishing.

To be sure, the biotechnological revolution may, as the optimists believe, serve to enhance human dignity. It may enable more and more people to realize the American dream of liberty, prosperity, and justice for all. It may enable many more human beings—biologically better-equipped, aided by performance-enhancers, liberated from the constraints of nature and fortune—to live lives of achievement, contentment, and high self-esteem, come what may.

But there are reasons to wonder whether life will really be better if we turn to biotechnology to fulfill our deepest human desires. There is an old expression: to a man armed with a hammer, everything looks like a nail. To a society armed with biotechnology, the activities of human life may come to be seen in purely technical terms, and more amenable to improvement than they really are. We may get more easily what we asked for only to realize it is vastly less than what we really wanted. Worse, we may get exactly what we ask for and *fail* to recognize what it cost us *in coin of our humanity*.

We might get better children, but only by turning procreation into manufacture or by altering their brains to gain them an edge over their peers. We might perform better in the activities of life, but only by becoming mere creatures of our chemists or by turning ourselves into bionic tools designed to win and achieve in inhuman ways. We might get longer lives, but only at the cost of living carelessly with diminished aspiration for living well or becoming people so obsessed with our own longevity that we care little about the next generations. We might get to be "happy," but only by means of a drug that gives us happy feelings without the real loves, attachments, and achievements that are essential for true human flourishing. As Aldous Huxley prophetically warned us, in his dystopian novel *Brave New World*, the unbridled yet well-meaning pursuit of the mastery of human nature and human troubles through technology can issue in a world peopled by creatures of human shape but of shrunken humanity—engaged in trivial pursuits; lacking science, art, religion, and self-government; missing love, friendship, or any true human attachments; and getting their jollies from high-tech amusements and a bottle of soma.

This is not the place to argue whether we have more to fear than to hope from biotechnological enhancement or the pursuit of a posthuman future. I happen to share Huxley's worries, and I surely see no reason to adopt the optimism of the transhumanists—especially because they cannot provide a plausible picture of "the new posthuman being," and, worse, can offer no standards for judging whether their new "creature" will be *better* than *Homo sapiens*. But for present purposes, my point is simply this: we cannot evaluate *any* proposed enhancements or alterations of our humanity unless we have some idea of human dignity, some notion of what is estimable and worthy and excellent about being human. In order to know whether change is progress rather than degradation, we need a standard of the *un*degraded and the admirable. We need to understand the natu and worth of human flourishing in order to recognize both the true promise of self-improvement and the hazards of self-degradation; we need to understand the nature and worth of human agency and human activity in order to recognize both enhancement and corruption of our ways of encountering the world and one another; we need to understand the nature and worth of human aspiration and human fulfillment in order to assess not only the means but also the ends that we will be pursuing in the coming age of biotechnology, both for ourselves as individuals and for our society. We need, in short, wisdom about human dignity and what sustains and enhances it— and what destroys it.

Concerns for human dignity in bioethical matters take mainly two forms: concerns for the dignity of life around the edges (the "life and death" issues) and concerns for the dignity of life in its fullness and flourishing (the "good life" and "dehumanization" issues; the "Brave New World" issues). In the former case are questions regarding what we owe to nascent life (including fetal and embryonic life, *in vivo* and *in vitro*) that has yet to attain full development of human powers, and what we owe to fading or dying human life, life not only past its prime but, in many cases, life with the most human of our powers dwindling to near-nothingness. Especially poignant are those cases in which—often thanks to previous medical successes, and the ease of combating potentially lethal infections—individuals are sustained, often for years, in greatly degraded conditions, incapable of living dignifiedly while dying or having a timely end to their life. In the latter case are questions regarding what makes for true human flourishing and how to keep human life human, in the face of the soul-flattening and dehumanizing dangers of a Brave New World. Especially difficult here will be discerning which proposed enhancements of body or mind actually conduce to human dignity and to living well and which do not—and which, tragically, at once improve and degrade.

Depending on which of the two dangers most trouble us, defenders of human dignity will emphasize either the basic dignity of human life or the full dignity of being (flourishingly) *human*.\* If one

---

\* and meaning of the names given here will be made clearer in
hree of this paper. Another set of terms I considered using were
nd "human *dignity*," the former to stress the horizontal dimen-

believes that the greatest threat we face comes in the form of death and destruction—say, in the practices of euthanasia and assisted suicide, embryo research, or even just denial of treatment to the less than fully fit—then one will be primarily concerned to uphold the equal dignity of every still-living human being, regardless of condition. If, conversely, one thinks that the greatest threat we face comes *not* from killing the creature made in God's image but either from trying to redesign him after our own fantasies or from *self*-abasement owing to shrunken views of human well-being (à la Nietzsche's "last man"), then one will be primarily concerned to uphold the full dignity of human excellence and rich human flourishing.

The two aspects of human dignity do not always have the same defenders, especially when concerns for equality and life seem to be at odds with concerns for excellence and living well. Indeed, defenders of one aspect of dignity sometimes ignore the claims made on behalf of the other. Certain pro-lifers appear to care little whether babies are cloned or even "born" in bottles, so long as no embryo dies in the process; and others insist that life must be sustained come what may, even if it means being complicit in prolonging the degradation and misery of loved ones. Conversely, certain advocates of so-called "death with dignity" appear to care little whether the weak and the unwanted will be deemed unworthy of life and swept off the stage, so long as *they* get to exercise control over how *their own* life ends; and patrons of excellence through biotechnological enhancement often have little patience with the need to care, here and now, for those whose days of excellence are long gone. Meanwhile, those who dream of posthuman supermen appear to care not a fig either for the dignity of human being or for the dignity of being human, since they esteem not at all the dignity of us ordinary mortals, never mind those of us who are even less than merely ordinary.

Yet there is no reason why friends of human dignity cannot be—and, indeed, should not be—defenders of *all* aspects of human dignity, both the dignity of "the low" and the dignity of "the high." Yes, there will be times when there will be tensions between them,

---

sion of universal "human-all-too-human"-ness, carried by the term "human," the latter to stress the vertical dimension of excellence or worthiness, carried by the term "dignity." Once again, the discussion below should clarify matters beyond such attempts at finding the right shorthand phrases.

demanding prudent and loving attention lest we make major mistakes. Yes, each aspect if emphasized single-mindedly may appear to threaten the other: concern for the dignity of human flourishing may appear to look down invidiously on the less than excellent; concern for the dignity of ("mere") human aliveness may appear willing to level all higher human possibilities. But precisely to avoid the dangers of myopic single-mindedness, we can, and must, defend both the dignity of human *being* and the dignity of being *human*. In fact, as I will suggest at the end, when properly understood, the two notions are much more intertwined than they are opposed. But first, we need to look at each more closely, beginning with the dignity of being human—the dignity of human flourishing, the dignity of living well.

## Full Human Dignity: The Dignity of Being Human

Discussions of human dignity are, alas, not generally known for their concreteness. The term itself is abstract and highly ambiguous,* as are many of the notions—for example, "human worth" or "high moral standing"—we invoke when trying to explain what we mean by "dignity." Yet despite these difficulties, we can in fact readily recognize dignity, both when we see it shining and when we see it extinguished. Here are some vivid examples, one positive and one negative.

Among the many moving songs from the American Civil War, one in particular always gives me gooseflesh: the "First Arkansas Marching Song," written for and sung by a regiment made up entirely of ex-slaves fighting on the side of the Union:[†]

> Oh we're the bully soldiers of the "First of Arkansas,"
> We are fighting for the Union, we are fighting for the law;
> We can hit a Rebel further than a white man ever saw,
> As we go marching on.

---

* For a most valuable explication of the most prominent understandings of human dignity, see the essay by Adam Schulman in this volume.
† Sung to the tune of "John Brown's Body." There are seven verses, of which I use the first, third, and last. A full text can be found online at www.civilwarpoetry.org/union/songs/arkansas.html.

(Chorus: Glory, glory, hallelujah, etc.)

We are done with hoeing cotton, we are done with hoeing corn,
We are colored Yankee soldiers, now, as sure as you are born;
When the masters hear us yelling, they will think it's Gabriel's horn,
As we go marching on.

Then fall in, colored brethren, you'd better do it soon,
Can't you hear the drums a-beating the Yankee Doodle tune;
We are with you now this morning, we'll be far away at noon,
As we go marching on.

Debased ex-slaves, only recently hoeing cotton and corn for their masters, transform themselves into brave soldiers "fighting for the Union…fighting for the law." Although formally emancipated by Lincoln's proclamation months earlier, they were truly lifted up from slavery not by another's largesse but by their own power and choice. They celebrate here their new estate, singing out their newly found dignity and beckoning others to join the cause. Our heart is stirred by this simple display of noble humanity, especially because it actively reverses their previous degradation and because it fully refutes the dehumanizing conclusions some had drawn from their prior servitude and submissiveness, namely, that anyone who accepts a life in slavery must have a slavish soul. I am particularly moved by the ex-slaves' dedication to a cause higher than their own advantage. And my imagination thrills to the picture of their marching through Southern towns and past slave-holding plantations, summoning their brethren to affirm their own dignity by putting their lives also in the service of freedom and Union.

Opposite to this example of dignity triumphing over degradation is the self-inflicted dehumanization of Herr Professor Immanuel Rath in the classic German movie, *The Blue Angel* (1930).[5] A strict, upright, gymnasium English teacher, Professor Rath goes to the local night club to reprimand his wayward students who have been attracted there by the siren singer, Lola Lola, and to scold her for corrupting the young. But on entering into her presence, Rath is smitten by Lola's charms, and he returns the next night filled with desires of his own. When he gallantly "defends her honor" against a brutish sea captain seeking sexual favors, Lola, touched by his chivalry on her behalf, invites him to spend the night. Exposed in school the next morning by his students, the honorable professor declares his intention to marry Lola Lola, for which decision he is promptly dismissed from his position. After laughing uncontrollably at his proposal, Lola Lola unaccountably accepts him; yet at the wedding feast, in front of all the guests, Rath is made to cock-a-doodle-do like a rooster in love. The married professor now joins the traveling show, first as Lola's servant, later as a performing clown. Eventually, when the traveling entertainers return to his hometown, Professor Rath is made co-star of the vaudeville show. With her latest lover at her side, Lola forces Rath to play a (cuckolded) crowing rooster while eggs are cracked upon his skull before a full house of roaring spectators, including his former students and neighbors. It is a scene of human abasement that is unbearable to watch.

What human goods and evils are at issue in these two vignettes? Not liberty or equality or health or safety or justice, but primarily the gain or loss of worthy humanity—in short, the display or the liquidation of human dignity. In the first case, degraded human beings knowingly assert their humanity and their manhood, committing their lives to the cause of freedom, union, and law; anyone who is not humanly stunted admires and applauds their nobility, their courage, and their devotion to a righteous purpose higher than themselves. In the second case, an upright and proper man of learning loses, first, his wits and his profession to his infatuation and, finally, every shred of dignified humanity, as he shrinks to impersonate an inarticulate barnyard animal; anyone who is not humanly stunted shudders at his utter degradation, notwithstanding the fact that he brought it on himself.

With these examples of dignity and its degradation before us, let me try to specify what I think we should mean by the "dignity of being human." On anyone's account, the idea of "dignity" conveys a special standing for the beings that possess or display it. Both historically and linguistically, "dignity" has always conveyed something elevated, something deserving of respect. The central notion, etymologically, both in English and in its Latin root (*dignitas*),* is that of

---

* Additional linguistic evidence may enrich our inquiry. *Dignitas* means (1) a being worthy, worthiness, merit, desert, (2) dignity, greatness, grandeur, authority, rank,

worthiness, elevation, honor, nobility, height—in short, of excellence or virtue. In all its meanings it is a term of distinction; dignity was not something that, like a nose or a navel, was to be expected or found in every living human being. *Dignitas* was, in principle, "aristocratic," less in the sense of social class, more in the sense of human excellence (*aristos*, from the Greek, means "best"). Even in democratic times, as the soldiers of the First of Arkansas make clear, "dignity" still conveys the presence and active display of what is humanly best.

Before attempting further specification of dignity's substance, let me address a couple of objections that I anticipate even to what little I have already said. Some people complain that all notions of dignity are merely social constructs, projections of the prejudices of (aristocratic) societies and conferred or attributed from the outside—as are honor and office. In the same spirit, others object that notions of dignity that appeal to excellence necessarily deny human dignity to many or most people, because they are essentially *comparative*. But if carefully examined, these complaints are not justified. Yes, societies accord honor to human excellence—and, yes, different societies esteem different virtues differently—but in many (if not most) cases the virtues esteemed are truly marks of superior humanity: the fireman who rushes into a burning building to save a child or the soldier who falls on a grenade to save his buddies is deserving of our admiration, and he will win it in many if not all societies. Mother Theresa and the Dalai Lama justly earn nearly universal applause; Saddam Hussein

---

and (3) (of inanimate things) worth, value, excellence. The noun is cognate with the adjective *dignus* (from Greek and Sanskrit roots *DEIK* and *DIC*, meaning "to bring to light," "to show," "to point out"), literally, "pointed out" or "shown," and hence, "worthy" or "deserving" (of persons), and "suitable," "fitting," "becoming," or "proper" (of things). "Dignity," in the *Oxford English Dictionary*, is said to have eight meanings, the four relevant ones I reproduce here: (1) The quality of being worthy or honourable; worthiness, worth, nobleness, excellence (for instance, "The real dignity of a man lies not in what he has, but in what he is," or "The dignity of this act was worth the audience of kings"); (2) Honourable or high estate, position, or estimation; honour, degrees of estimation, rank (for instance, "Stones, though in dignitie of nature inferior to plants," or "Clay and clay differs in dignity, whose dust is both alike"); (3) An honourable office, rank, or title; a high official or titular position (for instance, "He…distributed the civil and military dignities among his favorites and followers"); (4) Nobility or befitting elevation of aspect, manner, or style; becoming or fit stateliness, gravity (for instance, "A dignity of dress adorns the Great").

and Pol Pot justly earn nearly universal condemnation. The dignity of the First of Arkansas is displayed from within, not conferred from without; the dehumanization of Immanuel Rath is self-evident and intrinsic, not stipulated or attributed.

Although we often do contrast the virtue of one person with the vice of another—as I have just done—such judgments of excellence and its opposite are, in fact, only *accidentally* comparative. When we recognize the superior dignity of Mother Theresa we do so not by comparing her against Saddam Hussein or even against merely moderately virtuous human beings. We judge not that she is better than others (as we do in competitive sports)—though, in fact, it happens that she is—but rather that she measures up to and even exceeds a high standard of excellent character and dignified conduct. We are not comparing individuals against each other; we are measuring them against a standard of goodness. Proof: courageous or generous deeds would still be courageous or generous deeds—equally dignified and equally honorable—even if *everyone* practiced them regularly. Thus, the seemingly inegalitarian nature of dignity grounded in excellence of character is not *in its essence* undemocratic, even if ethical virtue is not, in fact, displayed equally by everyone. Indeed, the fact that most of us esteem and honor conduct better than our own is strong evidence that we do not feel ourselves diminished by it. On the contrary, just as taste honors those who *appreciate* genius almost as much as it honors those who *display* genius, so the appreciation of exemplary human dignity honors also the dignity of those who can recognize and esteem it. Excellence is only accidentally invidious; and the need to make discriminating judgments is no reason to shy away from caring for dignity.

The trouble with dignity is not that dignity is conventional rather than natural, ascribed or attributed rather than intrinsic, or that it involves making discriminations of worthiness that, alas, find some people lacking. The serious difficulty in speaking about dignity is entirely substantive: *Which* intrinsic excellences or "elevations" are at the heart of human dignity and give their bearers special worth and standing? Let me review some candidates, beginning with the dignity of heroes.

Although they did not have the term, dignity as honor linked to excellence or virtue would certainly be the view of the ancient Greeks.

In the world of the poets, the true or full human being, the hero who drew honor and prizes as his dignity, displayed his worthiness in noble and glorious deeds. Supreme was the virtue of courage: the willingness to face death in battle, armed only with your own prowess, going forth against an equally worthy opponent—think Achilles against Hector—who, like you, sought a victory not only over his adversary but, as it were, over death itself. This heroic dignity, esteemed because it does not hide from the affront of our mortality but goes forward to meet it face to face, is poles apart from our bourgeois fear of death and love of medicine, though, paradoxically, it honors the human body as a thing of beauty to a degree unsurpassed in human history. Heroic excellence, following the Socratic turn, was later supplanted in Greek philosophy by the virtue of wisdom; the new hero is not the glorious warrior but the man singularly devoted to wisdom, living close to death not on the field of battle but by a single-minded quest for knowledge eternal.

Yet attractive though these candidates are (we can still read about Achilles and Socrates with admiration), the Greek exemplars are of little practical use in democratic times and, especially, in bioethical matters. True enough, courage and wisdom still contribute to dignity, and they are admirable beyond the confines of war or philosophical pursuit. For example, part of what we mean by "dignified dying" is seen in the courage with which death is faced and in the degree to which the dying person knows the score and does not shrink from the grim truth. Nevertheless, the dehumanization evident in Huxley's *Brave New World* is not primarily that it lacks glorious warriors or outstanding philosophers (or artists or scientists or statesmen)—though the fact that they are not appreciated in such a world is telling. The basic problem is the absence of kinds of human dignity more abundantly found and universally shared.

In Western philosophy the most high-minded attempt to supply a teaching of universal human dignity belongs to Kant, with his doctrine of respect for *persons*. Persons, *all* persons or rational beings (human or not), deserve respect not because of some realized excellence of achievement but because of a universally shared participation in morality and the ability to live under the moral law. However we may finally judge it, there is something highly dignified in Kant's effort to find a place for human freedom and dignity in the face of the

Newtonian world view that captures even the human being, omitting only the rational will. And there is something austerely dignified in the Kantian refusal to confuse reason with rationalization, duty with inclination, and the right and the good with happiness (pleasure). Whatever persists of a non-utilitarian ethic in contemporary academic bioethics descends largely from this principled moralistic view.* Never mind that, for most people, human "autonomy" no longer means living under the universalizable law that self-legislating reason prescribes for itself, but has come to mean "choosing for yourself, whatever you choose," or even "asserting yourself authentically, reason be damned." Lurking even in this debased view of the "autonomous person" is an idea of the human being as something more than a bundle of impulses seeking release and a bag of itches seeking scratching. "Personhood," understood as genuine moral agency, may indeed be threatened by powers to fiddle around with human appetites through psychoactive drugs or computer chips implanted in brains. We are not wrong to seek to protect it.

Yet Kant's respect for persons is largely formal, abstracting from how persons actually *exercise* their freedom of will. If, as he suggests, universal human dignity is grounded in the moral life, in that everyone faces and makes moral choices and is capable of living under the moral law, greater dignity would seem to attach to having a *good* moral life, that is, on choosing *well* and on choosing *rightly*. Is there not more dignity in the courageous than in the cowardly, in the moderate than in the self-indulgent, in the righteous than in the wicked, in the honest man than in the liar?† Should we not distinguish between the basic dignity of *having* freedom and the greater dignity of *using it well?*

But there is a deeper difficulty with the Kantian dignity of "personhood." It is finally inadequate for our purposes, not because it is

---

* The respect for persons so widely celebrated in the canons of ethics governing human experimentation is in fact a descendant of Kant's principle of human autonomy and the need to protect the weak against the powerful.

† This is not to say that one should treat other people, including those who live immorally and eschew dignity, as if they lacked it. To the contrary, it may be salutary to treat people on the basis of their capacities to live humanly and with dignity, despite even great fallings short or even willful self-degradation. Yet this would require that we expect and demand of people that they behave worthily and that we hold them responsible for their own conduct.

undemocratic or too demanding, but because it is, in an important respect, inhuman. Precisely because it dualistically sets up the concept of "personhood" in opposition to nature and the body, it fails to do justice to the concrete reality of our embodied lives, lives of begetting and belonging no less than of willing and thinking. Precisely because it is universalistically rational, it denies the importance of life's concrete particularity, lived always locally, corporeally, and in a unique trajectory from zygote in the womb to body in the coffin. Precisely because "personhood" is distinct from our lives as embodied, rooted, connected, and aspiring beings, the dignity of rational choice pays no respect at all to the dignity we have through our loves and longings—central aspects of human life understood as a grown-togetherness of body and soul. Not all of human dignity consists in reason or freedom.

It is, I note in passing, easy to see why the notion of "personal dignity" is of limited value in the realm of bioethics. Although the bioethics of personhood is very good at defending those aspects of human dignity tied to respect for autonomy against violations of human will, including failures to gain informed consent and excessive paternalistic behavior by experts and physicians, this moral teaching has very little to offer in the battle against the dehumanizing hazards of a Brave New World. For it is, in fact, perfectly comfortable with embryo farming, surrogate motherhood, cloning, the sale of organs, performance-enhancing drugs, doctoring of memory, chemical happiness, man-machine hybrids, and even extra-corporeal gestation—Why?—because these peculiar treatments of the body or uses of our embodiments are no harm to that homunculus of personhood that resides somewhere happily in a morally disembodied place. *Pace* Kant, the answer for the threat to human dignity arising from sacrificing the humanly high to the humanly urgent, the soul to the body, is not a teaching of human dignity that severs mind from body, that ignores the urgent, or that denies dignity to human bodily life as lived. The defense of what is humanly high requires an equal defense of what is seemingly "low."

The account of human dignity we badly need in bioethics goes beyond the said dignity of "persons" to embrace the worthiness of embodied human life, and therewith of our natural desires and passions, our natural origins and attachments, our sentiments and repugnances, our loves and longings. What we need is a defense of the dignity of what Tolstoy called "real life," life as ordinarily lived, everyday life in its concreteness. Our theories about human dignity need to catch up with its widespread, not to say ubiquitous, existence.

As we learn from everyday life, the dignity of being human is perfectly at home in ordinary life, and I would add, in democratic times. Courage, moderation, generosity, righteousness, and the other human virtues are not solely confined to the few. Many of us strive for them, with partial success, and still more of us do ourselves honor when we recognize and admire those people nobler and finer than ourselves. We frequently give our wayward neighbors the benefit of the doubt, and we strongly believe in the possibility of a second chance. No one ever knows for sure when a person hitherto seemingly weak of character will rise to the occasion, actualizing an ever-present potential for worthy conduct. No one knows when, as in the case of the ex-slaves of the First of Arkansas, human dignity will summon itself and shine forth brightly. With suitable models, proper rearing, and adequate encouragement—or even just the fitting occasion—many of us can be and act more in accord with our higher natures.

In truth, if we know how to look we find evidence of human dignity all around us, in the valiant efforts ordinary people make to meet necessity, to combat adversity and disappointment, to provide for their children, to care for their parents, to help their neighbors, to serve their country. Life provides numerous hard occasions that call for endurance and equanimity, generosity and kindness, courage and self-command. Adversity sometimes brings out the best in a man, and often shows best what he is made of. As the example of Tolstoy's Ivan Illich shows, even confronting our own death provides an opportunity for the exercise of admirable humanity, for the small and great alike.

Beyond the dignity of virtue and the dignity of endurance, there is also the simple but deep dignity of human activity—sewing a dress, throwing a pot, building a fire, cooking a meal, dressing a wound, singing a song, or offering a blessing made in gratitude. There is the simple but deep dignity of intimate human relations—bathing a child, receiving a guest, embracing a friend, kissing one's bride, consoling the bereaved, dancing a dance, or raising a glass in gladness. And there is the simple but deep dignity of certain ennobling human passions—hope, wonder, trust, love, sympathy, gratitude, awe, and reverence for the divine. No account of the dignity of being human is worth its salt without them. And no technologically driven world of the future that fails to safeguard the dignity of everyday life deserves our assent.

## Basic Human Dignity: The Dignity of Human Being

The humanity that shines forth in human beings, whether in the great or in the small, is always something that arouses our admiration and our respect. Even when universalized, it retains the character of excellence or worthiness. Yet there are partisans of human dignity who will have none of these judgments of excellence or worth. Even when they gladly acknowledge the difference between virtue and vice, they are loath to say that one person lives a life more worthy than another. They insist that human dignity, rightly understood, is something all human beings—the base as well as the noble, the wicked as well as the righteous—enjoy *equally*, simply by virtue of their human *being*.* Why do they do so, and what can we make of this claim?

To begin with, they assert the equal dignity of every human being for certain express purposes, limited ones to be sure, but crucial for any decent society: to prevent the display of contempt, and especially *"capital"* contempt with lethal consequences, for those who do not "measure up." They seek to insure a solid level of human worth that no one can deny to any fellow human being; they wish to lean against the widespread tendency to treat the foreigner and the enemy, the misfit and the deviant, or the demented and the disabled as less human or less worthy than oneself—and especially as unworthy of basic respect and continued existence. And, following the unspeakable horrors perpetrated in the 20th century, they wish at the very least to provide a moral barrier against the liquidation of human beings—whether in genocide or in euthanasia—often practiced by those who act in the name of their own sense of superior worth.

But even granting the soundness of the purpose—which I embrace wholeheartedly and without reservation—*asserting* that we all

---

* See, for example, the essay by Gilbert Meilaender in this volume.

have "equal dignity" does not, by itself, make it so. Mere assertion will not convince the skeptic nor refute the deniers of human dignity. We need to examine the grounds for thinking that all human beings—dignified or not in their conduct—actually have, or should be treated *as if they had*, full and equal human dignity.

The first—and perhaps best—ground remains practical and political, not theoretical and ontological. If you or your government (or my doctor or health maintenance organization) wants to claim that I am, for reasons of race or ethnicity or disability or dementia, subhuman, or at least not your equal in humanity, and, further, if you mean to justify harming or neglecting me on the basis of that claim, the assertion of universal human dignity exists to get in your way. The burden of proof shifts to you, to show why I am not humanly speaking your equal: *you* must prove why you are entitled to put a saddle and bridle on me and ride me like a horse, or to deny me the bread that I have earned with the sweat of my brow, or to dispatch me from this world because I lead a subhuman existence. You will, in fact, face an impossible task: you will be unable to prove that you possess God-like knowledge of the worth of individual souls or carry the proper scale of human worth for finding me insufficiently "weighty" to deserve to continue to breathe the air. In this approach to grounding basic human dignity, I offer not a metaphysically based proof but a rhetorically effective demonstration—shown precisely by my *asserting* my equal dignity—that I, like you, am a somebody, like you born of woman and destined to die, like you a member of the human species each of whose members knows from the inside the goodness of his own life and liberty.

Mention of life and liberty reminds us that, for Americans *as* Americans, the doctrine of human equality and equal humanity has its most famous and noblest expression in the Declaration of Independence. It is, in fact, to the principles of the Declaration that some people repair in seeking to ground the dignity of human being, and it makes some sense to try to do so. We Americans, in declaring ourselves a separate people, began by asserting our belief in the self-evident truth, "That all men are created equal." However human beings may differ in talent, accomplishment, social station, race, or religion, they are, according to the Declaration, self-evidently equal, at least in this: "That they are endowed by their Creator with certain unalienable rights, that among these are Life, Liberty, and the Pursuit of Happiness."

I yield to no one in my admiration of these passages, and they have always seemed to me to be, exactly as claimed, self-evidently true—neither requiring proof nor admitting of proof, yet evident on their face. But they do not go far enough in providing a ground for the *equal dignity* of human being as such. True, some interpreters of these passages, placing great weight on the words *"created"* equal and *"by their Creator,"* suggest that human beings have dignity because God, in creating humankind, *gave* it to them. But the Declaration does not say that the Creator gave all men dignity; indeed, it does not speak of equal dignity but of equal *rights*. The thrust of the assertion of human equality atop the list of self-evident truths (whose enumeration is ultimately intended to reach and establish a right of revolution against governments that fail to safeguard rights) falls forward onto the claim of equality of unalienable rights: all human beings *qua human* possess so-called natural rights—rights not dependent on positive law or human agreement— the rights to life, to liberty, and to pursue (that is, "practice") happiness as each person sees fit.

The relation between possessing rights and possessing human dignity is, however, still unclear. If one traces the pedigree of the idea of natural rights back to their sources in Hobbes and Locke, one discovers that these rights rest not on anything humanly lofty (such as dignity) but instead on something humanly low (namely, self-love). The natural "right to life" in its 18th-century meaning is not a right *to be* or *to stay alive* or even a right *not to be killed or harmed*. It is rather a right to practice active self-preservation, the right to defend, protect, and preserve your life not only against those who threaten your life but also in the face of those who would deny the rightfulness of your liberty to do so (for example, by insisting that you must "turn the other cheek"). The right to life is a (negative) right against interference with acts of self-preservation; and it rests, in short, on the precariousness of human life, the equal "kill-ability" of every human being, and especially on the self-conscious passion that each of us legitimately has for our own continued existence.

It follows that human dignity is *not* the foundation of these inalienable rights, nor is dignity ours by virtue of the mere fact that we possess them. Human dignity is to be found, rather, in *asserting* your rights, and, even more, in *standing up* for them, in defending your rights and the rights of fellow human beings against those who threaten or deny them or who interfere with their exercise. The true manifestation of dignity in the American Founding is found at the end of this revolutionary declaration, as the signers declare, "And for the support of this Declaration, with a firm reliance on the protection of Divine Providence, *we mutually pledge to each other our lives, our fortunes, and our sacred honor*" (emphasis added). *Having* equal natural rights is neutral (or less) with respect to dignity; *exercising* them in the face of their denial carries the dignity of self-assertion; *defending* with one's life and honor the rights of a whole people is high dignity indeed.

Some people suggest that our equal dignity resides not in our rights but in that more fundamental truth that makes rights necessary: our common mortal fate and our consciousness of this fact.\* But as was true with rights, so with vulnerability: our equal human dignity cannot reside in our equal mortality or our equal capacity to suffer. There is, truth to tell, *nothing* dignified in vulnerability as such or in the fact of suffering per se; a sufferer *as sufferer* merely undergoes, merely receives—as passive patient—what is inflicted by the active "agent," natural, human, or divine. To be sure, for Christians, Christ on the Cross may be regarded as the supreme exemplar of human dignity, notwithstanding the fact that the image of the crucified man-God is, deliberately, a complete inversion of what would ordinarily and everywhere be regarded as "dignified" or "elevated." But even here, it is not suffering *as such* but suffering understood and accepted as *sacrificial* and as *redemptive* that alone makes the crucified Jesus the epitome of dignity. Self-inflicted suffering or self-mutilation for no higher purpose is utterly undignified, and there is no dignity in being merely an object to which something happens, no dignity in being "a patient" in the sense of being passive. If there is dignity to be

---

\* Consider, for example, Pascal: "Man is but a reed, the most feeble thing in nature; but he is a thinking reed. The entire universe need not arm itself to crush him. A vapor, a drop of water suffices to kill him. But, if the universe were to crush him, man would still be more noble than that which killed him, because *he knows that he dies*, and the advantage which the universe has over him; the universe knows nothing of this. All our dignity consists, then, in thought." (Blaise Pascal, *Pensées*, William F. Trotter [New York: Dutton, 1958(1670)], pensée no. 347, p. 97; added.)

found in the vicinity of suffering, it consists either in the purpose for which suffering is borne or in the manner in which it is endured. The virtue of "patience" in the presence of suffering is itself anything but passive. Dignity with respect to suffering, like dignity with respect to rights, is a matter of virtue or strength of soul. Not everyone has it, and it therefore cannot be the basis of the equal dignity of human being.

A deeper ground for our equal human dignity—natural and ontological, not merely political—may perhaps be found in our equal membership in the human species.* All members of the class *Homo sapiens* are equally members of that class, and share thereby in whatever standing and dignity adheres to the class as a whole, especially, for example, in contrast with the dignity of other animals. There is surely something to this suggestion. Even when we condemn or show contempt for another person—and even when such condemnation and contempt are richly deserved, as, for example, for a Stalin or a Hitler—we cannot help but notice that he is, alas, "one of us." Indeed, the condemnation comes precisely from the great gap between his despicable deeds and what we have good reason to expect from another member of our species; we do not find fault with lions and tigers for *their* predatory and lethal conduct.

As it happens, the recognition of the human "species-form" or *gestalt*—upright posture, eyes to the horizon, hands fit for grasping, fingers for pointing, arms for embracing or cradling, and mouths fit for speaking and kissing no less than for eating—functions silently yet surely to elicit a primordial recognition from our fellow species members. Such mutual identification is the basis of hospitality to strangers, acts of good Samaritans, or even just a nod of recognized human kinship when we pass one another on the street. The salutary reminder of common humanity, even in the face of severe deformity or degradation, puts a limit on possible tendencies to banish another human being, in thought or in deed, from the realm of human concern and connectedness or even from the world of the living. Our almost untutored ability to recognize the *humanum* in the other prevents many an outrage and many a violation, and it encourages many a sympathetic word and many a charitable deed.

---

* For elaborations of this view, see the essays by Daniel P. Sulmasy and by Patrick Lee and Robert P. George in this volume.

So far so good. Yet once again, trouble comes if we are compelled to answer just what it is about membership in *Homo sapiens* that justifies allowing our "species pride" or sense of special worthiness to serve as guarantor of the inviolability of our life and being. The (higher) animals too are not without their special dignity and special standing.* Thus, the dignity that attaches to us as human beings cannot be grounded simply in our being alive or in being members of a closed interbreeding population; the same properties, to repeat, belong also to chimpanzees and cheetahs and kangaroos. Once again, the elevated moral status of the human species must turn on the special capacities and powers that are ours and ours alone among the creatures.

Thus, to speak of dignity as predicable of all human beings, say in contrast to animals, is to tie dignity to those distinctively human features of human animals, such as the capacities for thought, image-making, freedom and moral choice, a sense of beauty, love and friendship, song and dance, family and civic life, the moral life, and the impulse to worship. Yet once we introduce these material properties, we will be hard pressed not to assess the dignity of particular human beings in terms of the degree to which they *actually manifest* these attributes and activities of life. For the universal attribution of dignity to human beings on the basis of the specific attributes of our humanity pays tribute only to human *potentiality*, to the *possibilities* for human excellence. Because, as the scholastics rightly taught, "actuality" is prior—both in speech *and* in being—to "potentiality," *full* dignity, or dignity properly so-called, will depend on the *realization* of these possibilities.

For partisans of the "equal dignity of human being," the search for its content has reached a troubling point: the ground of our dignity lies in the humanly specific potentialities of the human species, but this basic dignity is not *dignity in full*, is not the *realized* dignity of fine human *activity*. Questions again arise regarding the dignity of those members of our species who have lost or who have never attained these capacities, as well as those who use them badly or wickedly. The horizontal ground of the egalitarian dignity of human

---

* For beautiful presentations of this point, see Adolf Portmann, *Animal Forms and Patterns* (London: Faber and Faber, 1964; paperback, New York: Schocken Books, 1967) and *Animals as Social Beings* (New York: Viking Press, 1961).

being appears to be shifting in the direction of the vertical scale of being (more and less) actually and actively human.

Having now come at human dignity from two directions—beginning the first time from the dignity of flourishing humanity at its heroic peak, and beginning the second time from the dignity of human life at its primordial level of mere existence—we note a curious coincidence: the more "aristocratic" account could not help but be universalized and democratized, once we learned how to find virtue and read worthiness in the doings of everyday life; and the more "egalitarian" account could not help but introduce standards of particular excellences, once we were forced to specify what *it is* about human beings that gives them special dignity. This convergence of the two accounts invites the suggestion that the two aspects of dignity actually have something to do with one another, indeed, that they may be mutually implicated and interdependent. The final section of this paper briefly offers several suggestions as to how and why this might be true.

## The Dignity of Being "In-Between": Human Aspiration, Transcendent Possibilities

Let me suggest three aspects of the relationship between the dignity of human being and the dignity of being human: mutual dependence; the ground of human aspiration; and intimations of transcendence.

First, the (lower) dignity of human being and the (higher) dignity of being human are mutually interdependent, but in different ways. The flourishing of human possibility—in each of its many admirable forms—depends absolutely on active human vitality, that is, on the goodness and worth of *life as such*. The humanly high depends *for its very existence* on the humanly low, on the mere existence and well-working of the enlivened human body. One image for this relation of dependence is that between ceiling and floor: no floor, no ceiling.*
But the architectural comparison is misleading, for it suggests independent and separate "structures" piled one atop the other. Instead,

---

\* I have myself used half of such an image, in speaking about "basic" dignity, the dignity of the base or foundation, though the counter-pole I have employed, "full dignity," is not architectural.

the living relation between the high and the low is—no surprise—*organic* and *integral*: the human being, in every stage of life and degree of health, is a psychophysical unity, with all its powers and all aspects of its activity grown-together and interconnected.

As a consequence, just as the higher human powers and activities depend upon the lower for their existence, so the lower depend on the higher for their standing; they gain their worth or dignity mainly by virtue of being integrated with the higher—because the *nature* of the being is *human*. What I have been calling the *basic* dignity of human *being*—sometimes expressed as the "sanctity of human life," or the "respect owed to human life" as such—in fact depends on the *higher* dignity of being *human*.

This mutual dependence of the two aspects of human dignity can be clearly illuminated if we ask why murder is wrong, why we (and all civilized people) hold innocent life to be inviolable—a subject I have explored elsewhere.[6] Particularly helpful is a philosophical examination of the biblical story of the Noahide law and covenant (*Genesis* 9), where a paradigmatic law against murder is explicitly promulgated for all humankind united, well before there are Jews or Christians or Muslims. Unlike the more famous enunciation of a similar prohibition in the Ten Commandments ("Thou shalt not murder"; *Exodus* 20), the earlier formulation offers a specific reason why murder is wrong.\*

The prohibition of murder—or, to be more precise, the institution of retribution for shedding human blood—is part of the new order following the Flood. Before the Flood, human beings lived in the absence of law or civil society. The result appears to be something like what Hobbes called the state of nature, characterized as a condition of war of each against all. Might alone makes right, and no one is safe; in consequence the world descends into chaos. The Flood washes out human life in its *natural* (that is, uncivilized) state, the remedy for which not nature but only reason and law can provide.

---

\* Non-religious readers may rightly express suspicion at my appeal to a biblical text for what I will claim is a universal or philosophical explanation of the taboo against murder. This suspicion will be further increased by the content of the text cited. Nevertheless, properly interpreted, I believe the teaching of the passage stands free of its especially biblical roots and offers a profound insight into the ground of our respect for human life.

Immediately after the Flood, primordial law and justice are instituted, and nascent civil society is founded.

At the forefront of the new order is a newly articulated respect for human life,* expressed in the announcement of the punishment for homicide:

> Whoever sheddeth man's blood, by man shall his blood be shed; for in the image of God was man made (9:6).

In this cardinal law, combining speech and force, the threat of capital punishment stands as a deterrent to murder and provides a motive for obedience. But the measure of the punishment is instructive. By equating a life for a life—no *more* than a life for a life, and the life only of the murderer, not also, for example, of his wife and children—the threatened punishment implicitly teaches the *equal* worth of each human life. Such equality can be grounded only in the equal *humanity* of each human being. Against our own native self-preference, and against our tendency to overvalue what is our own, blood-for-blood conveys the message of universality and equality.

But murder is to be avoided not only to avoid the punishment. That may be a motive, which speaks to our fears; but there is also a reason, which speaks to our minds and our loftier sentiments. The deep reason that makes murder wrong—and that even justifies punishing it homicidally!—is man's divine-like status.† Any man's *very being* requires that we respect his life. Human life is to be respected more than animal life—Why?—because man is more than an animal;

---

* This respect for human life, and the self-conscious establishment of society on this premise, separates human beings from the rest of the animals. This separation is made emphatic by the institution of meat-eating (9:1-4), permitted to men here for the first time. (One can, I believe, show that the permission to eat meat is a concession to human blood lust and voracity, not something cheerfully and happily endorsed.) Yet, curiously, even animal life must be treated with respect: the blood, which is identified as the life, cannot be eaten. Human life, as we shall see more clearly, is thus both continuous and discontinuous with animal life.

† The second part of verse 9:6 seems to make two points: man is in the image of God (that is, man is god-like), and man was made thus by God. The decisive point is the first. Man's creatureliness cannot be the reason for avoiding bloodshed; the animals too were made by God, yet permission to kill them for food has just been given. The full weight rests on man's *being* "in the image of God," on man's god-like-ness.

man is said to be god-like. Please note that the *truth* of the Bible's assertion does *not* rest on biblical authority: man's more-than-animal status is in fact performatively proved whenever human beings quit the state of nature and set up life under such a law—as only the god-like animal can do. The law that establishes that men are to be law-abiding both insists on, and thereby demonstrates the truth of, the superiority of man.

How is man god-like? *Genesis 1*—where it is first said that man is created in God's image—introduces us to the divine *activities* and *powers*: (1) God speaks, commands, names, and blesses; (2) God makes and makes freely; (3) God looks at and beholds the world; (4) God is concerned with the goodness or perfection of things; (5) God addresses solicitously other living creatures. In short: God exercises speech and reason, freedom in doing and making, and the powers of contemplation, judgment, and care.

Doubters may wonder whether this is truly the case about God—after all, it is only on biblical authority that we regard God as possessing these powers and activities. But even atheists recognize that we human beings have them, and that they lift us above the plane of a merely animal existence. Human beings, alone among the earthly creatures, speak, plan, create, contemplate, and judge. Human beings, alone among the creatures, can articulate a future goal and bring it into being by their own purposive conduct. Human beings, alone among the creatures, can think about the whole, marvel at its many-splendored form and articulated order, wonder about its beginning, and feel awe in beholding its grandeur and in pondering the mystery of its source.

A complementary, preeminently moral, gloss on the "image of God" is provided—quite explicitly—in *Genesis 3*, at the end of the so-called second creation story. Commenting on the significance of man's (disobedient) eating from the tree of the knowledge of good and bad, the Lord God comments:

> Now the man is become *like one of us* knowing good and bad....(3:22; emphasis added)*

---

* In the first creation-story, *Genesis* 1-2:3, man is created straightaway in God's likeness; in this second account, man is, to begin with, made of dust, and he *acquires* god-like qualities only at the end, and then only in transgressing.

Human beings, unlike the other animals, distinguish good and bad, have opinions and care about their difference, and constitute their whole life in the light of this distinction. Animals may suffer good and bad, but they have no notion of either. Indeed, the very pronouncement, "Murder is bad"—and the willingness to punish it—constitute proof of *this* god-like quality of human beings.

In sum, the human being has special dignity because he shares in the godlike powers of reason, freedom, judgment, and moral concern, and, as a result, lives a life freighted with moral self-consciousness—a life above and beyond what other animals are capable of. Speech and freedom are used, among other things, to promulgate moral rules and to pass moral judgments, first among which is that homicide is to be punished in kind because it violates the dignity of such a moral being. We reach a crucial conclusion: the *inviolability* of human life rests absolutely on the higher *dignity*—the god-like-ness—of human beings.

Yet man is, at most, only god*ly*; he is not God or a god. To be an image is also to be *different* from that of which one is an image. Man is, at most, a *mere* likeness of God. With us, the seemingly godly powers and concerns just described occur conjoined with our animality. God's image is tied to blood, which is the life.

The point is crucial, and (like the previous insight about man's superior dignity) stands apart from the text that teaches it: everything high about human life—thinking, judging, loving, willing, acting—depends absolutely on everything low—metabolism, digestion, respiration, circulation, excretion. In the case of human beings, "divinity" needs blood—or "mere" life—to sustain itself. And because of what it holds up, human blood—that is, human life—deserves special respect, beyond what is owed to life as such: the low ceases to be the low. (Modern physiological evidence could be adduced in support of this thesis: in human beings, posture, gestalt, respiration, sexuality, and fetal and infant development, among other things, all show the marks of the co-presence of rationality.) The biblical text elegantly mirrors this truth about its subject, subtly merging both high and low: though the *reason* given for punishing murder concerns man's *godliness*, the *injunction* itself concerns man's *blood*. Respect the god-like; don't shed its blood! Respect for anything *human* requires respecting *everything* human, requires respecting human *being* as such.

In a word, the wanton spilling of human blood is a violation and a desecration, not only of our laws and wills but of being itself. There is, finally, no opposition between the dignity of human *being* (or "the sanctity of life") and the dignity of being *human*. Each rests on the other. Or, rather, they are mutually implicated, as inseparable as the concave and the convex. Those who seek to pull them apart are, I submit, also engaged in wanton, albeit intellectual, violence.*

The dignity of being human depends not only for its *existence* on the presence and worth of human vitality; our dignity's full realization in admirable human activity depends for its *active pursuit* and *attainment*—the second aspect of their relationship—on human *aspiration*, which, although directed toward the high, is driven by sources in animate vitality itself. Everything humanly high gets its energizing aspiration from what is humanly low. Necessity is not only the mother of invention; it is also the mother of excellence, love, and the ties that bind and enrich human life. Human life is lived always with and against necessity, struggling to meet and elevate it, not to eliminate it. Like the downward pull of gravity without which the dancer cannot dance, the downward pull of bodily necessity and fate makes possible the dignified journey of a truly human life. It is a life that will use our awareness of need, limitation, and mortality to craft a way of being that has engagement, depth, beauty, virtue, and meaning—not despite our embodiment but *because* of it.† Human aspiration depends absolutely on our being creatures of need and finitude, and hence of longings and attachments. Pure reason and pure mind have no aspiration; the rational animal aspires in large part because he is an animal.

This discovery gives rise to what might seem to be a paradox: human dignity is ours in part because of our "animality," because we are not incorporeal minds, angels, or gods. Indeed, once again it is our in-between status—at once god-like *and* animal—that is the deep

---

* The rest of the essay, "Death with Dignity and the Sanctity of Life," goes on to explore the implications of this insight for specific ethical questions regarding end-of-life care and end-of-life decision-making. Arguments are made as to why euthanasia and assisted-suicide cannot be defended by appeals to human dignity.
† For an elaboration of these "blessings of mortality," see my "*L'Chaim* and Its Limits: Why Not Immortality?" in *Life, Liberty and the Defense of Dignity: The Challenge for Bioethics*.

truth about our nature, the ground of our special standing, and the wherewithal of our flourishing. Yet, at the same time, human dignity is not on all fours with the dignity of the other animals, even if it is linked to theirs and belongs to us only because we, like they, are embodied creatures.

Perhaps the most profound account of human aspiration is contained in Socrates' speech about *eros* in Plato's *Symposium*. *Eros*, according to Socrates' account, is the heart of the human soul, an animating power born of lack but pointed upward. *Eros* emerges as both self-seeking and overflowingly generative: it is said to be the longing "for the good to be one's own always," as well as "of giving birth and immortality." At bottom, *eros* is the fruit of the peculiar conjunction of and competition between two conflicting aspirations conjoined in a single living body, both tied to our finitude: the impulse to self-preservation and the urge to reproduce. The first is a self-regarding concern for our own personal permanence and satisfaction; the second is a self-forgetting—and, finally, self-denying—aspiration for something that transcends our own finite existence, and for the sake of which we spend and even give our lives.

Other animals, of course, live with these twin and opposing drives. And, as Socrates suggests, *eros* is a ruling power also in the lives of other animals. But *eros* in the other animals, who are *unaware* of the tension between these twin and opposing drives, manifests itself exclusively in the activity of procreation and the care of their offspring—an essential aspect of the dignity of all animal life. Socrates speaks of the noble self-sacrifice often displayed by animals on behalf of their young. And I would add that all animal life, by one path or another, imitates the "noble" model of the salmon, swimming upstream to spawn and die.

But *eros* comes fully into its own as the arrow pointing upward only in the human animal, who is conscious of the doubleness in his soul and who is driven to devise a life based in part on the tension between the opposing forces. Human *eros*, born of this self-awareness, manifests itself in explicit and conscious longings for something higher, something whole, something eternal—longings that are ours precisely because we are able to elevate the aspiration born of our bodily doubleness and to direct it upwards toward the good, the true, and the beautiful. In the human case, the fruits of "erotic giving-birth" are not only human children, but also the arts and crafts, song and story, noble deeds and customs, fine character, the search for wisdom, and a reaching for the eternal and divine—all conceived by resourcefulness to overcome experienced lack and limitation, and all guided by a divination of that which would be wholly good and lacking in nothing.

Aspiration, I am suggesting, is the mother of all aspects of the dignity of being human. Though born of our frailty and bodily neediness, it is sired also by a divine spark to which—miraculously—Being has prepared the human animal to recognize and pursue. This transcendent possibility is the third aspect of the relationship between what is humanly low and what is humanly high; indeed, it is a possibility that points us to what is high, indeed highest, simply.

Once again, an ancient story shows us the point. In the Garden of Eden, the serpent tempts the woman into disobedience, by promising her that if she eats from the forbidden tree of the knowledge of good and bad her eyes will be open and she "will be as gods, knowing good and bad" (*Genesis* 3:5). But, as the text comments with irony, when the human pair disobeyed "their eyes were opened and they saw that they were naked" (3:7). Far from being as gods, they discovered their own sexuality, with its shameful implications: their incompleteness, their abject neediness of one another, their subjection to a power within them that moves them toward a goal they do not understand, and the *un*godly bodily ways in which this power insists on being satisfied—not standing upright contemplating heaven but lying down embracing necessity.

As in Socrates' account, the discovery of human lowliness is the spur to rise, but here it comes in two stages, one purely human, the other something more. First, the human beings, refusing to take their shame lying down, take matters into their own hands: "and they sewed fig leaves and made themselves girdles" (3:7). Covering their nakedness, out of a concern for approbation one from the other, human lust is turned into *eros*, into a longing for something more than sexual satisfaction. Shame and love are born twins, delivered with the help of the arts of modesty and beautification.

But there is more. Immediately after covering their nakedness, reports the text, "they heard the voice of the Lord God walking in the Garden" (3:8), the first reported instance of human recognition of and attention to the divine. For it is only in recognizing our lowliness that we human beings can also discover what is truly high. The turn toward the divine is founded on our discovery of our own lack of divinity, indeed, of our own insufficiency.

It is a delicate moment: having followed eyes to alluring temptations, promising wisdom, human beings come to see, again through their eyes, their own insufficiency. Still trusting appearances but seeking next to beautify them, they set about adorning themselves, in order to find favor in the sight of the beloved. Lustful eyes gave way, speechlessly, to admiring ones, by means of intervening modesty and art. Yet sight and love do not alone fully disclose the truth of our human situation. Human beings must open their ears as well as their eyes, they must hearken to a calling, for which sight and the beautiful beloved do not sufficiently prepare them. The prototypical human pair, opened by shamefaced love, is in fact able to hear the transcendent voice.

Thus, *awe* is also born twin to shame, and it is soon elaborated into a desire to close with and to have a relationship with the divine. The dignity of being human, rooted in the dignity of life itself and flourishing in a manner seemingly issuing only in human pride, completes itself and stands tallest when we bow our heads and lift our hearts in recognition of powers greater than our own. The fullest dignity of the god-like animal is realized in its acknowledgement and celebration of the divine.

# Notes

[1] Leszek Kolakowski, "What Is Left of Socialism," *First Things* 126 (October 2002): 42-46.

[2] See, among other places, *Human Cloning and Human Dignity: An Ethical Inquiry* (2002), especially chapter 5, "The Ethics of Cloning-to-Produce-Children," and chapter 6, "The Ethics of Cloning-for-Biomedical-Research"; *Monitoring Stem Cell Research* (2004), especially chapter 3, "Recent Developments in the Ethical and Policy Debates"; *Beyond Therapy: Biotechnology and the Pursuit of Happiness* (2004), all chapters, and especially the discussion of "The Dignity of Human Activity" in chapter 3, "Superior Performance"; *Reproduction and Responsibility: The Regulation of New Biotechnologies* (2005), especially the section on "The Character and Significance of Human Procreation" in (the introductory) chapter 1, chapter 6 on "Commerce," and the section on "Targeted Legislative Measures" in chapter 10, "Recommendations"; *Being Human: Readings from the President's Council on Bioethics* (2004), especially chapter 10, "Human Dignity"; and *Taking Care: Ethical Caregiving in Our Aging Society* (2005), especially chapters 3 and 4, "The Ethics of Caregiving: General Principles," and "The Ethics of Caregiving: Principle and Prudence in Hard Cases." All of these books except for *Being Human* are available online at www.bioethics.gov.

[3] The readings in *Being Human* were collected and offered to provide the humanistic wherewithal for thinking about and responding to these and other inadequate views of our humanity. See especially the chapters on "The Pursuit of Perfection," "Are We Our Bodies," "Among the Generations," "Why Not Immortality," "The Meaning of Suffering," "Living Immediately," and, of course, "Human Dignity." This anthology has been republished by W. W. Norton, under the title *Being Human: Core Readings in the Humanities* (2004).

[4] See, among other places, *Life, Liberty and the Defense of Dignity: The Challenge for Bioethics* (San Francisco, California: Encounter Books, 2002), especially the Introduction, the discussion of the "Profundity of Sex" in chapter 5, "Cloning and the Post Human Future," chapter 6, "Organs for Sale: Propriety, Property, and the Price of Progress," chapter 8, "Death with Dignity and the Sanctity of Life," and chapter 9, "*L'Chaim* and Its Limits: Why Not Immortality"; *Toward a More Natural Science: Biology and Human Affairs* (New York: The Free Press, 1984), especially chapters 2, 3, and 4 on reproductive technologies and genetic screening, chapter 10, "Thinking About the Body," and most especially chapter 13, "Looking Good: Nature and Nobility"; an essay on "The Right to Life and Human Dignity," in *The New Atlantis* 16 (Spring 2007), pp. 23-40; *The Hungry Soul: Eating and the Perfecting of Our Nature* (New York: The Free Press, 1994; Chicago: University of Chicago Press, 1998), especially chapter 2, "The Human Form: Omnivorosus Erectus"; and *The Beginning of Wisdom: Reading Genesis* (New York: The Free Press, 2003; Chicago: University of Chicago Press, 2006), especially chapters 2 and 3 on the anthropology of the Garden of Eden story and chapter 6 on the Noahide Law and its foundations.

[5] *Der Blaue Engel* (*The Blue Angel*), directed by Josef von Sternberg, Universum Film and Paramount Pictures, 1930.

[6] "Death with Dignity and the Sanctity of Life," in *Life, Liberty and The Defense of Dignity*, and "Elementary Justice: Man, Animals and the Coming of Law and Covenant," in *The Beginning of Wisdom: Reading Genesis*, both cited above.

# 13

# Kant's Concept of Human Dignity as a Resource for Bioethics

Susan M. Shell

Is "human dignity" a vacuous concept—a mere placeholder for varying ethical commitments and biases—or has it a useful role to play in bioethics? The former impression is seemingly confirmed by the disparate uses to which "human dignity" is put by opposing sides in contemporary bioethical debates. For the liberal and secular left, it is generally associated with personal "autonomy" and expanded individual choice.* For the conservative and religious right, it is generally associated with the sanctity of "life" and related limits on such choice. Does the term "human dignity" merely encourage each side to talk past the other, or can it supply fruitful common ground?

The purpose of this paper is to explore Kant's concept of human dignity as a potential resource for contemporary bioethical debates. The name of Kant is frequently invoked in such discussions, but generally only in passing. On the one hand, Immanuel Kant is surely the philosopher who put the concept of human dignity on the map of

---

* Thus Ruth Macklin has urged that the concept be abandoned as "useless" on the grounds that it adds nothing to that of "autonomy," which itself suffices. See Macklin, "Dignity is a Useless Concept," *BMJ* 327 (2003): 1419-1420.

modern moral discourse. Few thinkers on either the right or left, and whether religious or secular, fail to pay him homage. Prevailing contemporary views concerning patient "autonomy" and informed consent surely reflect a clear Kantian provenance.[1] On the other hand, his thought can appear too rigidly dualistic to offer much practical guidance on more difficult and contentious issues, such as stem cell research and other matters that touch upon the limits of what is and isn't "human." My guiding hypothesis is that a more complete and fully rounded view of Kant's thought can indeed shed useful, non-question-begging light on such liminal questions. Despite his reputation as a rigid dualist, Kant's thought has much to offer bioethical debate in a liberal democratic context. As I hope to show, one need not be a strict Kantian to find many of his arguments helpful in supplying common ground to citizens of otherwise diverse moral and religious views. The key to such a retrieval lies in giving Kant's notion of "humanity" as *embodied* rationality the attention it deserves.

## Dignity and Embodied Rationality

Kant's concept of human dignity has two components: humanity and dignity. "Dignity" (*Würde*) designates a value that has no equivalent—i.e., that which is "beyond price." As he puts it in a famous passage of the *Groundwork of the Metaphysics of Morals*:

> What is related to general human inclinations and needs has a *market price*; that which, even without presupposing such a need, conforms with a certain taste...has a *fancy price*; but that which constitutes the condition under which alone something can be an end in itself has not merely a relative value, that is, a price, but an inner value, that is, *dignity*.... Morality, and humanity insofar as it is capable of morality, is that which alone has dignity.[2]

This manner of speaking has particular resonance in a commercial society like ours, in which almost all goods are commodified or seem capable of becoming so. The concept of "dignity" gains much of its moral force from its insistence upon an absolute limit to the fungibility of human goods. If something has intrinsic worth, or dignity, then not all values are homogenous. Hobbes had infamously insisted that "a man's worth" is the same as his "price," or the "amount that would be paid for the use of his power."[3] Kant's concept of human dignity is a direct rejoinder to that claim.

The ultimate basis of that rejoinder is what Kant calls the categorical imperative—the implicit moral command to which the voice of conscience, in his view, testifies. According to the first and most basic version of that imperative, one should act "only according to those maxims [or rules of action] that one could at the same time will to be a universal law." This version of the imperative is often criticized—first and most famously by Hegel—for its empty formalism, and I will not pause here to consider it. Instead, it will be more fruitful to move to a second version, which commands: *So act that you use humanity, whether in your own person or in the person of any other, always at the same time as an end, never merely as a means.*[4] Kant derives this second version from the fact that willing requires an end, and in the case of moral willing, an absolute end, or end in itself. Unlike ends that are "to be acquired by our action," and are thus "conditional" in value—either on our desires or on the contingencies of nature—an end in itself has objective value, or "dignity." Kant had earlier claimed that the only thing "good without limitation" that is possible to think is a good will. But a good will must have some objective end if it is not to be utterly empty. If morality is to be possible at all—if a "good will" is to have an objective end—then good will itself, or the rationality that makes it possible, is the only candidate that can fill the bill.

Such are the considerations behind the following exclamation on Kant's part:

> Now I say that the human being and in general every rational being *exists* not merely as a means to be used by this or that will at its discretion; instead he must in all his actions… always be regarded *at the same time as an end*.[5]

The idea of humanity as an "objective end" refers not to a goal to be achieved by our action (as in the usual meaning of an "end") but to an absolute limit that restricts our other ends and maxims, and the activities they prompt. An "end in itself" is not "an object that we of ourselves actually make our end"; it is, rather, in Kant's words, the "objective" end that serves as a "supreme [limiting] condition" upon whatever ends we have.[6]

The most clear-cut cases of Kantian "respect" for humanity involve not using others in ways whose ends they cannot formally share—i.e., by not acting on them without their own consent. The moral impermissibility of false promising (along with "assaults on the freedom and property of others") follows directly and unproblematically, in Kant's view, from this formula.[7] It is easy to see the attractiveness of Kant, from a liberal political perspective, given the congruence between his moral thought and traditional liberal insistence on the right to life, liberty, and the pursuit of property and/or happiness. The peculiar force and influence of Kantian principles in contemporary arguments for patient choice and informed consent is especially apparent.[8]

If matters rested here, it would be easy to conclude, with Macklin, that appeals to "human dignity" as such could be abandoned without much loss. Autonomy, in the sense of choice, and the deference that in her view it commands, would indeed suffice. Whatever adults consent to (with a somewhat hazier provision for children and other "dependents") would set the bioethical standard.

But Kant indeed has more to say. Duties toward oneself (and toward others in matters where consent is impossible or otherwise has no immediate bearing) are more complicated but no less essential to a full understanding of what the claims of "human dignity," in his view, require of us. One is obliged on Kant's account to treat humanity in oneself, no less than in others, as an "end in itself."[9] But to fully appreciate this point, one must turn from the second term in "human dignity" back to the first.

What, then, does Kant mean by "humanity"? Scholars, it must be said, differ on this point. For Christine Korsgaard, it is the sheer capacity to set ends;[10] for Allen Wood, it is that capacity joined with an ability to think systematically.[11] Kant himself seems to speak of it in two ways. On the one hand, humanity is the "subjective" side of rational nature—the way in which rational nature in us immediately and unmistakably impinges on our consciousness. Every human being "necessarily represents his own existence" as an end that needs no further justification. Every human being, in other words, naturally regards himself as his own center of reference, in terms of which all other goods express their value. Humanity, one might say (echoing Nietzsche) is the natural capacity of a being to think in terms of value—a capacity, so far as we know, that belongs to man alone of all earthly creatures. But humanity, as the "subjective" side of "rational nature," also points beyond itself. Man can regard his own existence as something that has *objective* value only through recognition of a law that applies equally to others.[12] Only to the extent that he gives full weight to that law (by "respecting humanity") can he rationally regard his own existence as worthy of "esteem." Humanity is thus the capacity that both enables us to think in terms of value at all and orients us toward (without physically necessitating) full-fledged moral autonomy—and its realm of objective worth or dignity.* Respect and esteem are at once distinct and intrinsically related to one another.

This consideration helps explain Kant's otherwise puzzling separation, in *Religion within the Boundaries of Bare Reason*, of "reason" from moral personality proper. Kant there asks us to imagine our human "endowments" as three-fold: physical, "human" (or "rational" in a strictly instrumental sense) and moral. A rational animal without a conscience—without an awareness, however primitive, of the moral law—is a thinkable possibility; but it is not *us*. Even human infants, in their crying—counterpurposive, Kant thinks, if one regards the end of humanity to be mere physical survival—"immediately announce" their "claim to freedom (an idea possessed by no other animal)." Although absent in the newborn, that idea is already present in some way by the time infants are capable of "crying":

> The newborn child certainly cannot have this outlook. But the tears that accompany his screaming a few months after birth reveal that his feeling of uneasiness comes, not from physical pain, but from an obscure idea (or a representation analogous to it) of freedom and its hindrance, injustice; they express a kind of exasperation when he tries to approach certain objects or merely to change his general position, and

---

\* In the *Metaphysics of Morals* Kant defines humanity as "the capacity to set oneself an end—any end whatever," a capacity unique to rational beings. See *Metaphysics of Morals* 6: 392; translation in Kant, *Practical Philosophy*, trans. Gregor, pp. 522-23.

feels himself hindered in it.—This impulse [*Trieb*] to have his own way [*seinen Willen zu haben*] and to take any obstacle as an affront is marked, especially by his tone, and manifests ill nature that the mother sees herself required to punish; but he retaliates by screaming even louder. The same thing happens when he falls, through his own fault. While the young of other animals play, children begin early to quarrel with one another; and it is as if a certain concept of justice (which is based on outer freedom) develops along with their animal nature, without having to be learned gradually.[13]

I linger over the passage because it touches with unusual directness on the relation between nature and freedom in man, and hence on the "dualism" with which Kant is so often taxed. Unlike Lucretius, who interprets such crying as apprehension on the young infant's part of the "dolefulness" of the life in store for him, Kant sees in it the (possible) irruption into nature of the "idea of freedom" as a genuinely moral cause. To be sure, the immediate consequences are *morally* doleful: the malevolent wish, expressed even by the young infant, to have one's way without granting similar sway to others. Still, as in Kant's other historical and religious writings, this fall into evil is the path human beings almost inevitably take in their progress toward earthly realization of the moral idea.

The point for our purposes is this: not the specifics of Kant's moral anthropology, but the larger claim about our need to make sense of our existence as embodied rational beings who are in nature but not fully of it. We are driven by our end-setting nature to make sense of the world both in relation to ourselves and as a whole. (Kant sometimes calls this our capacity for *a priori* principles of judgment.) But all the stories that we tell are riven by (partial) failure, beginning with the infant who angrily discovers that his claim to freedom is not externally supported. Our very efforts to make sense of the (natural) world, in their (initial) failure, orient us toward the demands of moral transcendence.

Whatever "embodied rationality" might mean for other beings elsewhere in the universe (and Kant kept up a lively openness to the possibility of life on other planets), it is inscribed, for us, within an experiential framework that is dialectical in character. The freedom that enables us to reason leads us to make demands upon the world that ultimately devolve upon ourselves if "only we are rationally consistent." Our "dignity" ultimately derives from our capacity to act upon the dictates of our own reason—i.e., from our autonomy as moral agents. The objective value that we claim is one that we ourselves cannot take to be rational, and hence cannot take seriously, unless we grant it to others who are similarly organized.

As this brief and inadequate sketch suggests, Kant's moral anthropology, broadly construed, is well positioned to support a regime of individual rights, or of "equal recognition," as Hegel will later call it. And this, indeed, is the use to which Kant is most often put, as we have seen, in today's bioethical debates. But "humanity," I am claiming, means more for Kant than the reciprocal freedom of consenting adults (or those who might become or might once have been so); it also imposes limits on the uses to which one may put one's own capacities. What, then, are those limits?

Here the story grows more complicated, as Kant himself admits. Still, certain fundamental principles are clear enough. In regarding ourselves as practical worldly agents—in "looking out" upon the world from a pragmatic standpoint—we cannot help thinking teleologically about our own capacities. Contrary to some contemporary accounts of liberal "self-ownership," our bodies are not things we own, items that are indistinguishable, in principle, from other sorts of alienable property. As the site of our own worldly agency, our bodies are at once more emphatically and irreducibly our own than any merely worldly "thing" and less available to manipulation by our arbitrary will. Certain organic necessities cannot be overcome, nor could we wish to do so without seeking to undermine basic feelings (like the difference between left and right, or between pain and pleasure) by which we orient ourselves. Such indispensable feelings, one could say, are the necessary polestars of living beings like ourselves who are (also) self-aware. The pleasant will always affect us differently than the painful, our left foot cannot become our right one. Of course, one can strive to render oneself relatively indifferent to both pain and pleasure; or to compensate, by strengthening one foot, for weakness in the other. But such orienting feelings remain, at least so long as we are in that rough state of organic functionality and wellness that we associate with human sanity.

Attention to our necessary ways of orienting ourselves in the world can help us to avoid certain absurdities to which certain "liberal" models of the self are otherwise all too prone. The sharp distinction between "persons" and "things" that liberalism encourages can, if wrongly applied, lead either to treatment of one's own body and its parts as if they were as "alienable" as, say, a suit of clothes (as in *Nip/Tuck*, a popular satire on the plastic surgery industry) or, alternatively, to confusion of the body's surface boundaries with those of self-hood proper (as in Andrea Dworkin's portrayal of the female body as a fortress that is, or ought to be, literally impregnable).

In the first case, one may be driven to regard such arrangements as the sale of body parts or maternal surrogacy as no more problematic than any other exchange of goods or services. But even the fiercest champions of untrammeled market freedom in such areas are sometimes brought up short by due recognition of the human consequences—consequences that would ultimately make markets as such impossible.[14] A recent example: our unease with the idea of transplanting faces, even to restore healthy function rather than for the sake of aesthetic "enhancement." As the very term "person" (derived from *persona*, the Latin word for "mask") suggests, the relation between individual identity and bodily appearance—especially the appearance of one's face—is neither accidental, on the one hand, nor perfectly straightforward on the other. Eighteenth-century physiognomists may have exaggerated the extent to which our inner character can be read in our faces; but that there is some reciprocal relation and effect seems undeniable. The face is a mask that both reveals us and permits us to hide, just as actors' masks allow them to assume, in highly stylized ways, identities other than their own. Still, a world in which faces, and the peculiar expressions that accompany them, were as exchangeable as hats does not seem to be one in which human life as we know it could easily exist.

In the second, admittedly rarer case, the body and the self become confused in such a way as equally to challenge the possibility of human life. In Dworkin's words:

> There is a never real privacy of the body that can co-exist with intercourse: with being entered.... The thrusting is persistent invasion. She is opened up, split down the center. She is

occupied—physically, internally, in her privacy.[15]

For Dworkin, for whom all intercourse is rape, the skin, as Jean Grimshaw notes, "is the boundary of the self." If one identifies the body and the self in Dworkin's way, "such that *any* 'invasion' of the boundaries of the body [voluntary or not] is invasive of the self," it is "difficult to see what space is left for giving an account of sexuality at all."[16] To this one could add that not only is sexuality (and human generation generally) written out of the equation; even basic acts like eating become morally repellent. The body, so construed, is a pure idea, without engagement with the world—life, as it were, without metabolism.

Whatever personal pathology Dworkin's argument may or may not reflect, its conceptual coherence remains, given the impoverished set of categories with which Dworkin, like many of her libertarian counterparts, sets out. Thus there is a singular advantage, if we are to arrive at a satisfactory and comprehensive liberal understanding of the world, in starting (like Kant), not with the abstract distinction between things and persons—a distinction in which human bodies as such disappear—but from our experience as embodied rational beings who make claims on one another and hence also on ourselves. It is that "pragmatic" starting point (as in the infant's own tearful cry—its initial act of worldly self-assertion) that in Kant's view gives rise, when we try to think it through consistently, to the conceptual distinction between things, persons, and a certain thing-like use of persons that falls somehow in between.*

Kant's pragmatic starting point, which begins with man and his deeds, bears the following fruit. Human consciousness is punctuated

---

* This category particularly pertains to marriage law, where bodies are in some sense reciprocally "owned" (see *Metaphysics of Morals* 6: 276-284; 357-362). However disagreeable Kant's infamous legal description of marriage as a mutual possession of sexual faculties, there is surely something to his insistence that sexual uses of the body have, at least potentially, a personal and moral significance different in kind from other uses. On the meaning of "pragmatic," see *Anthropology from a Pragmatic Point of View* 7: 119-122: "Physiological knowledge of man investigates what *nature* makes of him: pragmatic knowledge investigates what *man* as a free agent makes, or can and should make, of himself." For Kant, our practical knowledge of the world has a formally teleological character that ultimately points us toward moral purposes.

from the start by freedom and a related sense of justice and injustice, right and wrong. Our valuations are not only homogeneous but also hierarchical. Pleasure and esteem are related (e.g., in our judgment that those we esteem as just deserve also to be happy) and yet incommensurable. That observation permits us to make a three-fold distinction among human aptitudes: animal, rational (in an instrumental or calculative sense) and moral.* The original disposition (*Anlage*) to the good according to Kant, is threefold, consisting in:

1) the *Anlage* to animality (insofar as we are living beings);

2) the *Anlage* to humanity (insofar as we are living and also rational beings); and

3) the *Anlage* to personality (insofar as we are rational and also responsible beings).[17]

The usefulness for present purposes of this rank-ordering lies in its relative formality. On the basis of rather minimal assumptions about the character of human life—assumptions roughly congruent with the premises of liberalism itself—one can draw, as I will argue, some significant bioethical conclusions. That one can do so without appealing to the dogmatic claims of a specific religious tradition—claims that cannot fail to be politically problematic in a liberal society like ours—makes Kant's framework all the more promising.

His explicitly "pragmatic" starting point draws on our ordinary notions about health and sickness that are inseparably bound up with our most basic dealings in the world. That such notions have proved relatively immune to the ideological onslaughts of "value relativism" is not accidental. We may be willing to sacrifice our health for what we regard as a greater good; but we cannot regard it with indifference or as wholly arbitrary in its meaning. Kant analogically extends the

---

* To be sure, Kant's formalism here is not theoretically innocuous. In stressing, as he does, the conditions of experience rather than its particular content, Kant evades the immediate, concrete claims that may correspond to a specific way of life. His formalism here thus reflects a more fundamental difference between his own approach to moral matters and that shared by both classical philosophy and the Bible.

sort of reasoning we do with regard to health and sickness upward. Pleasure and pain serve as rough yet indispensable guides to health and illness. Pain and pleasure regulate the lives of animals instinctively. Human beings, in our capacity as calculative reasoners, can override the immediate demands of pain and pleasure with a view to maximizing our physical well-being deliberatively. By analogy, human beings can and should orient themselves with a view to moral health, or the subordination of physical well-being to a higher rational purpose.[18] Such an ideal of "moral" or "spiritual" life—an ideal that implies the complete organization of our physical, rationally calculative and moral being—is, admittedly, a construction on our part, that may or may not correspond to anything that we can (fully) realize. But it is not an *arbitrary* ideal nor one, in Kant's view, toward which we can remain indifferent. And it is an ideal whose formality can encompass, though not from their own point of view replace, moral and religious aspirations of a more traditional sort.

## Kant and Bioethics

How might such pragmatically informed reflections bear on contemporary questions of bioethics? Without entering fully into the many complexities involved, a few guiding principles can be educed. First, there is a certain teleological structure to human life that is anchored, at the lower end, by our primary experience of ourselves as worldly agents. By virtue of that experience, we are directed, first, toward physical well-being and, second, by demands upon others and ourselves that can be regulatively understood as the appearance in the world of a higher principle of life. Duties toward oneself seek a combination of physical and moral self-preservation that permits this higher principle to "take root."

Second, organized beings, though susceptible to scientific study, cannot in principle be fully comprehended. No Newton, as Kant famously put it, will ever arise who can explain a blade of grass.[19] By this Kant does not mean that biological inquiry cannot progress indefinitely, but rather that we are compelled to understand ourselves and, by analogy, all other living organisms in ways that ultimately transcend efficient causation. A physician or researcher informed by

Kantian principles will thus retain a sense of the ultimate mysteriousness of life—not on dogmatically religious grounds but as an extension of the speculative modesty that flows from a critical awareness of the necessary structure and limits of human cognition. We cannot help but understand our own organs and aptitudes as naturally purposive in a way we are not free to disregard. To be sure, such understanding does not meet the demands of objective scientific knowledge. That the eye is "for seeing" cannot be established on the basis of a mechanical science (or its contemporary equivalent). And yet this assumption is, in Kant's view, the indispensable subjective foundation of any objective scientific inquiry into the processes of vision.[20]

Man is not a brain in a vat; but he is also not a disembodied spirit free to use the matter in which it happens to be housed any way it chooses. Kant interprets this to mean that one must respect oneself "as an animal being," e.g., by not killing oneself or defiling oneself by lust. It also means that one ought not employ one's body in ways that strike us as counter-purposive: e.g., committing suicide for the sake of pleasure. Some of Kant's arguments in this regard are no doubt idiosyncratic, especially where sexual matters are concerned. Still, the general point seems both valid and of potential bioethical significance. Recognition of the impossibility, in principle, of reducing life to a mere mechanism argues for humility when confronted with new opportunities for genetic or other radical "enhancements" of the human organism. Wherever we strive to exceed the standard set by normal life functions (a standard roughly equivalent to "health"), we risk grave harms that we cannot in principle foresee. *Ethical compunction here conspires with ordinary prudence to urge the greatest caution in engaging in experiments that exceed what natural functions by themselves support.

A pragmatic orientation in Kant's sense no doubt suggests other ethical limits on uses of one's body—proscribing, for example, sale of organs or of services that drastically impinge on basic bodily processes.[21] Here fine distinctions may have to be drawn: selling one's hair or small quantities of blood differs from selling a kidney or contracting to become a maternal surrogate. Still the implicit ethical

---

* One example: according to one very recent study, disabling the cell's "aging" gene—a procedure undertaken in the hopes of extending its life expectancy—proves instead vastly to increase its susceptibility to cancer.

injunction—do not damage the functioning of the whole for the sake of a lesser and/or only partial good—remains.

There is a further way in which Kant's framework can be brought to bear on bioethical issues. From a strictly Kantian perspective, only duties of right are legally enforceable. Breaches of right (as distinguished from ethics) either violate the rights of other human beings or violate positive laws that are duly enacted to protect them. The state may certainly *discourage* unethical activities—e.g., by not granting licenses to doctors who fail to meet certain ethical standards—but it cannot punish them, unless they involve breaches to right (e.g., practicing medicine without a legal license to do so).

Current federal policy of withholding funding for certain medical procedures and kinds of scientific research that are nonetheless legal calls to mind this Kantian distinction between law and ethics. Present federal policy is designed to discourage an activity that many regard as ethically wrong but that the state cannot lawfully prevent, at least given the current political consensus. According to the weight of that consensus, destruction of an embryo for the sake of *in vitro* fertilization, or to conduct scientific inquiry into medical potential of stem cells, is not murder, nor should it otherwise constitute a legal crime. Still, in the view of many it is at least morally problematic and in the view of some ought in fact to be illegal.

In the remainder of this paper I should like briefly to consider how Kant's concept of human dignity might shed light on embryonic stem cell research and the political and moral controversy surrounding it. Here two issues come immediately to the fore: the ethical permissibility of allowing one's genetic material to be so used; and the legal *or* ethical permissibility of damaging or destroying the embryo for purposes of biological (medical) research.

On the first point (and without considering the moral status of the embryo as such): use of one's faculties should not flagrantly contradict its natural organic function, except in cases where a higher purpose (such as a desire to help others) is involved. This supports our ordinary moral intuition that donation of an organ may be permissible where its sale is not. To be sure, faculties related to generation have a peculiar ethical complexity, given the special moral and legal relations to which they may, and normally do, give rise. Extraction of genetic material—for purposes of enhancing one's own fertility or of advancing medical research—would seem to pass Kantian muster. Sale (rather than donation) of one's eggs appears more doubtful.

On the second and potentially more difficult question of the moral standing of the embryo: Kant's pragmatically informed moral teleology suggests a punctuated account of human development that avoids the extremes of granting the embryo full human status on the one hand, and no moral status whatsoever on the other. To be sure, the reflections that follow are highly speculative. Kant never commented directly on the moral status of the fetus or unborn child, though some of his remarks suggest that even newborns in his view may have lacked full moral standing.[22]

The traditional "natural law" position afforded complete human status to the fetus only with "quickening," taken for a sign of self-motion and hence "ensoulment." Modern embryology, it is sometimes claimed, shows that development is, in fact, continuous. Hence, the fetus must have either full human status from the moment of conception or none at all. But modern science also shows that the embryo in its earliest stages retains a certain plasticity of form. For the first ten days or so after conception the blastocyst may divide, becoming twins. Such a process is unusual but not abnormal in the sense of indicating the presence of some pathological factor or other defect. The embryo, at this early stage, is not yet a fully individuated human being. It does not yet have a unifying principle of development, a distinct soul (to speak in traditional terms) that is wholly its own. Pragmatically speaking, the moment at which such division is no longer possible thus represents the beginning of a new and qualitatively different stage in human development.

The punctuated character of early fetal development opens a window for potential uses of the fetus that might be juridically or ethically precluded at later stages. Embryonic stem cell research would seem to be one obvious candidate. One might still, for religious reasons, regard the blastocyst as fully human. But it becomes harder to make the case either on strictly philosophic grounds or on grounds of ordinary common sense.

What, then, of the limits that might apply to such uses? The blastocyst is (or must be viewed by us as) purposively directed toward fuller human development. It is not a mere "collection of cells" that we can injure or dispose of trivially.* Use of such embryonic cells for medical research—i.e., to enhance human health—may be permitted where other uses (e.g., for purely cosmetic purposes) are not. A new cure for cancer is one thing; an enhanced shade of lipstick is another. One can respect the human potential of the blastocyst in certain determinate ways, in other words, without granting it the status of a moral person.

None of this speaks directly to the contentious question of abortion and the moral status of the fetus more generally. But it does permit a helpful "bracketing" of the issue of embryonic stem cell research as such. Such considerations also suggest the wisdom of revisiting current federal policy. According to the most recent scientific findings, embryonic stem cells appear to have unique properties (e.g., with respect to longevity) that adult stem cells cannot duplicate. The federal government could support embryonic stem cell research more fully while preserving a sense of its ethical complexity and without begging the question of later-term abortion. Such a stance would not satisfy those for whom destruction of an embryo is murder. But current federal policy (and, indeed, most of our ordinary cultural and legal practices) does not so treat it.

In sum: human beings have dignity, for Kant, because they are capable of acting morally. But this capacity is only realized dialectically, through our pragmatic dealings with the world. A richer understanding of "humanity," informed by Kant's moral and pragmatic reflections, might offer fuller and politically more useful guidance to contemporary bioethical debates than that provided by the usual image of Kant as a rigid dualist. Kant's conception of human dignity draws primarily not on metaphysical abstractions but on the necessities that inform our everyday efforts to lead an effectual and morally decent life. As such it offers potential common ground in a field of contest where it is often all too rare.

---

* This claim does not depend on an argument that is sometimes made: namely, that nonhuman things (such as giant sequoia trees) may nonetheless have intrinsic value. Kant's argument preserves our sense that the special moral status of the embryo lies in its emerging "humanity."

# Notes

[1] For a thoughtful articulation of this point of view, see Onora O'Neill, *Autonomy and Trust in Bioethics* (Cambridge: Cambridge University Press, 2002); an alternative, non-Kantian argument for "informed consent" and related contemporary practices might be drawn from Plato's *Laws* 720a-e.

[2] Kant, *Groundwork of the Metaphysics of Morals* 4: 434-435; translation, slightly emended, in Kant, *Practical Philosophy*, ed. and trans. Mary J. Gregor (Cambridge, Cambridge University Press, 1996), pp. 84-85. Note: I cite Kant's works by volume and page number of the standard German edition, *Kants Gesammelte Schriften*, edited by the Royal Prussian (later German) Academy of Sciences (Berlin: George Reimer, later Walter de Gruyter & Co., 1900—); these numbers are found in the margins of most translations.

[3] Thomas Hobbes, *Leviathan*, chapter 10.

[4] *Groundwork* 4: 429; *Practical Philosophy*, p. 80.

[5] *Groundwork* 4: 428; *Practical Philosophy*, p. 79.

[6] *Groundwork* 4: 431; *Practical Philosophy*, p. 81.

[7] *Groundwork* 4: 430; *Practical Philosophy*, p. 80.

[8] For a thoughtful exploration of this topic, see Onora O'Neill, op. cit.

[9] *Groundwork* 4: 428; *Practical Philosophy*, p. 79.

[10] Christine Korsgaard, *Creating the Kingdom of Ends* (Cambridge: Cambridge University Press, 1996), pp. 17, 110; cited in Richard Dean, *The Value of Humanity in Kant's Moral Theory* (Oxford: Clarendon Press, 2006), p. 6.

[11] Allen W. Wood, *Kant's Ethical Thought* (Cambridge: Cambridge University Press, 1999), p. 119.

[12] *Groundwork* 4: 429.

[13] *Anthropology from a Pragmatic Point of View* 7: 268-269n.; translation in Kant, *Anthropology from a Pragmatic Point of View*, trans. Mary J. Gregor (The Hague: Nijhoff, 1974), pp. 136-137n.

[14] See, for example, Jennifer Roback Morse, *Love and Economics: Why the Laissez-Faire Family Doesn't Work* (Portland, Oregon: Spencer, 2001).

[15] Andrea Dworkin, *Intercourse* (London: Martin Secker & Warburg, 1987), p. 122; cited in Jean Grimshaw, "The Bodily Self: Privacy, Autonomy and Identity," in *Liberalism, Citizenship and Autonomy*, ed. David Milligan and William Watts Miller (Aldershot, England: Avebury, 1992), p. 194.

[16] Grimshaw, op. cit., p. 196.

[17] See Kant, *Religion within the Boundaries of Bare Reason* 6: 26; translation in Kant, *Religion and Rational Theology*, ed. and trans. Allen W. Wood and George di Giovanni (Cambridge: Cambridge University Press, 1996), p. 74.

[18] For an elaboration of this analogy, see Kant's "What it is to Orient Oneself in Thinking" and "On the Use of Teleological Principles in Philosophy."

[19] See Immanuel Kant, *Critique of Judgment*, trans. Werner Pluhar (Indianapolis, Indiana: Hackett, 1987[1790]), §75, pp. 282-283.

[20] Kant's argument is most fully worked out in Part Two of the *Critique of*

*Judgment.*
[21] For an alternative approach, based on highly modified Kantian arguments, to the question of body ownership see Deryck Beyleveld and Roger Brownsword, *Human Dignity in Bioethics and Biolaw* (Oxford: Oxford University Press, 2001), pp. 173-194.
[22] See *Metaphysics of Morals* 6: 327, 336.

# 14

# Human Dignity and Political Entitlements

## Martha Nussbaum

Human dignity is an idea of central importance today. It plays a key role in the international human rights movement, and it figures prominently in many documents that ground political principles for individual nations. It also plays a role in abstract theories of justice and human entitlement. I myself have given the idea a key role in my own political conception of justice, holding that a hallmark of minimum social justice is the availability, to all citizens, of ten core "capabilities," or opportunities to function. All citizens are entitled to a threshold level of these ten capabilities because, I argue, all ten are necessary conditions of a life worthy of human dignity.[1]

The idea of dignity, however, is not fully clear, and there are quite a few different conceptions of it, which can make its use to ground a political conception slippery. For this reason, John Rawls concluded that, all by itself, it could not play a grounding role: the idea only acquired determinate content through specific political principles.[2] I believe that Rawls was somewhat too pessimistic, and I also believe that he himself used the idea in at least some crucial parts of his argument, insisting that "Each person possesses an inviolability founded on justice that even the welfare of society as a whole cannot override."[3] We should agree with Rawls, however, in judging that the bare idea, without further philosophical clarification, does not do enough work to ground political principles. Some interpretations of the idea, indeed, might lead political thought seriously astray.

I propose, here, to articulate further the conception of human dignity that I have used in my account of social and global justice, and to show why it is preferable to some other conceptions of that idea. I shall begin historically, looking at the influential Stoic account of human dignity and at some of the problems inherent in it. These problems, I argue, should lead us to prefer an Aristotelian/Marxian account of dignity, which sees the dignity of the human being as squarely a part of the world of nature and does not posit a sharp split between rationality and other human capacities. I shall show how such an account might ground basic political entitlements (in a non-metaphysical way suited to a pluralistic society). Then I shall look at two challenges such an account has to face: the challenge of equal respect/inclusiveness, and the challenge of doing justice to the claims of other animals and the types of dignity that their lives exhibit. I conclude with some preliminary reflections on what a capabilities-based approach implies about some important questions of bioethics.

## The Stoic Account[4]

According to the Greek and Roman Stoics, the basis for human community is the worth of reason in each and every human being.[5] Reason (meaning practical reason, the capacity for moral choice), is, in the Stoic view, a portion of the divine in each of us. And each and every human being, just in virtue of having rational capacities, has boundless worth. Male or female, slave or free, king or peasant, all are alike of boundless moral value, and the dignity of reason is worthy of respect wherever it is found. Moreover, even if human beings vary in their moral attainments, moral/rational capacity is fundamentally equal, and a source of our equal worth across all that divides us.

Moral capacity is wonderful and worthy, so it ought to be respected. People usually give reverence and awe to the outward trappings of wealth and power. Instead, the Stoics argue, we should respect what is really worthy in us. Seneca is especially eloquent in his description of the beauty of the moral substance of humanity in each person and the attitude of quasi-religious awe with which he is inspired by his contemplation of a human being's rational and moral purpose. In a passage that seems to have profoundly influenced Kant, he writes:

> God is near you, is with you, is inside you.... If you have ever come on a dense wood of ancient trees that have risen to an exceptional height, shutting out all sight of the sky with one thick screen of branches upon another, the loftiness of the forest, the seclusion of the spot, your sense of wonder at finding so deep and unbroken a gloom out of doors, will persuade you of the presence of a deity.... And if you come across a man who is not alarmed by dangers, not touched by passionate longing, happy in adversity, calm in the midst of storm,...is it not likely that a feeling of awe for him will find its way into your heart?... Praise in him what can neither be given nor snatched away, what is peculiarly human. You ask what that is? It is his soul, and reason perfected in the soul. For the human being is a rational animal.[6]

Seneca speaks here of developed moral capacities, but his view is that those capacities all by themselves are proper objects of respect.

The Stoic view includes (and is perhaps the source of) the Kantian thought that we must test our principles to see whether they could be a universal law of nature, because that will show whether we have really given all human beings equal respect and concern, or whether we have unfairly favored our own case. It also includes, and is closely linked to, the Kantian thought that what respect for human dignity requires is to treat the human being as an end, rather than merely as a means to one's own purposes.[7] If one properly appreciates the worth of human moral and rational capacities, one will see that they must always be treated as ends, rather than merely as means; and one will also see that they require equal respect, rather than the exploitative attitude that is willing to make an exception to favor one's own case.

Indeed, one good general way of thinking about the intuitive idea of dignity is that it is the idea of being an end rather than merely a means. If something has dignity, as Kant put it well, it does not merely have a price: it is not merely something to be used for the ends of others, or traded on the market. This idea is closely linked to the idea of *respect* as the proper attitude toward dignity; indeed, rather than thinking of the two concepts as totally independent, so that we would first offer an independent account of dignity and then argue that dignity deserves respect (as independently defined), I believe that we should think of the two notions as closely related, forming a concept-family to be jointly elucidated. Central to both concepts is the idea of being an end and not merely a means.

## Problems in the Stoic Account

The Stoic account was of enormous importance in cultures accustomed to ranking and dividing people in accordance with outward markers of status. It had enormous influence on the history of philosophy, particularly the part of it dealing with international and cosmopolitan obligation, shaping the thought of Grotius, Kant, and many others. It is an attractive starting point in many ways, urging us to ignore the attributes that come to people through heredity and luck and to base our dealings with them on something more fundamental, something that is the inalienable property of every human being.

Nonetheless, the Stoic account contains several large problems that make it a bad basis for contemporary thought about political obligation. First is what I shall call the *animals problem*. The Stoics commend the worth of rational and moral capacities by arguing that they are what raise us above "the beasts." Their descriptions of human worth typically involve a pejorative comparison with nonhuman animals—which, it is implied, would be fine to use merely as means. Indeed, the Stoics did think that animals were brutish and unintelligent and that, in consequence, it was fine to use them merely as means. Their hostility to the ethical claims of animals was unusual in their cultures, and, sadly, this hostility had long and deep influence.[8] Stoics not only split humans off from other animals more sharply than the evidence supports, refusing to grant animals any share in intelligence, they also denied without argument that there is any dignity or end-like worth inherent in those human capacities in which animals also partake, such as sentience, everyday (non-moral) practical reasoning, emotion, and the capacity for love and care. Thus, the split not only slights the other animals, it also slights elements in human life that would appear to have worth, urging us to respect only a small sliver of ourselves.

Another grave difficulty concerns the Stoic doctrine of the worthlessness of "external goods." Money, honor, status—but also health, friendship, the lives of one's children and spouse—all these things, according to the Stoics, have no true worth, nor should they ever be the objects of eager attachment. One should recognize that only virtue and moral capacity deserve our reverence. Such externals may sensibly be pursued if nothing impedes us. Should they fail us, however, we are not to be upset. Paradigmatic is the Stoic father described by Cicero, who, being told of the death of his child, replied, calmly, "I was already aware that I had begotten a mortal."[9]

This doctrine does not look like a good basis for an energetic political stance that aims at securing to people important goods such as food, health, and education. Respect human dignity, the Stoics say. But it turns out that dignity, radically secure within, invulnerable to the world's accidents, doesn't really need anything that politics can give. So the appeal to dignity grounds a practical attitude that is either inconsistent or quietistic. The Stoics are quietistic when they make no objection to the institution of slavery, on the grounds that the soul is always free within.[10] They are inconsistent, I believe, when they argue, in the same breath, that respect for human dignity requires the master to refrain from beating slaves or using them as sexual tools:[11] for what is the harm of these things, if they do not affect what is most precious, and merely touch the body's morally irrelevant surface? Being raped is something to which one should be utterly indifferent, since it does not remove or damage the moral capacities; so what can be so bad about inflicting on someone something that is not real damage?

Why should the Stoics have taken such an extreme line? They believed, clearly, that in order to give human dignity its due reverence they had to show it to be radically independent of the accidents of fortune. If moral capacities are of equal and infinite worth, then they can't be the sort of thing that is tarnished or eclipsed by fortune: for otherwise the degree of people's human worth will be dependent on fortune, and the well-born and healthy will be worth more than the ill-born and hungry.

Suppose for a moment that we accept this move (though in fact we should not accept it without some further distinctions, as I shall later argue). So we grant that human dignity is inalienable, not damaged in itself by bad fortune. Why, still, we might ask, could the Stoics not have taken Aristotle's line (and, later, Kant's), drawing a distinction between virtue and happiness? Why should we not say that human dignity is necessary, but not sufficient, for the fullness of human flourishing, or *eudaimonia*? Here again, it appears that the Stoics are inspired by a kind of radical egalitarianism about human worth. Think of the person who suffers poverty or hardship. Now either this person has something that is beyond price, by comparison to which all the money and health care and shelter in the world is as nothing—or she does not have something that is beyond price, but virtue is just one piece of her happiness, a piece that can be victimized and held hostage to fortune, in such a way that she is needy and miserable, even though she has human dignity. That would mean that virtue is to be put in the balance with other things and is not the thing of infinite worth that we took it to be.

Let's put it this way. A virtuous person is hit by the blows of fortune. Now either she is lofty and beautiful, and at no time more beautiful than when she suffers the greatest loss[12]—or she is a pathetic victim, moaning and groaning, asking fate and her fellow men for help, childishly dependent. Plausibly, the Stoics don't want to depict virtue as flattering power. So they say: the virtuous person is complete, even though she lacks the whole world.

Before we reject this move utterly, we should think about people who are victims in our own society: let's say, victims of inequality based on race or sex or disability. There is a quite understandable tendency for such people to demand things from the powerful, saying, we need these things in order to live. But there is an equally understandable tendency for some members of that group to say, "We have our pride and strength. We are complete in ourselves. No whining and complaining for us. We are more beautiful, ultimately, than those who oppress us." Think of recent attacks on "victim feminism" in the name of "agency feminism." Naomi Wolf, for example, decries a "victim feminism" that "urges women to identify with powerlessness."[13] Similarly, the disability-rights movement strongly resists the notion that a disability is a deprivation. I think we see here the basic intuition behind the negative side of Stoicism: to conceive of people as helpless is to denigrate them, to fail to respect their dignity as agents. Nobody is ever a victim, because human dignity is always enough.

The Stoics have gotten one big thing right. We do want to recognize that there is a type of worth in the human being that is truly inalienable, that exists and remains even when the world has done its worst. Nonetheless, it does appear that human capacities require support from the world (love, care, education, nutrition) if they are to develop internally, and yet other forms of support from the world if the person is to have opportunities to exercise them (a suitable material and political environment). So we need a picture of human dignity that makes room for different levels of capability and functioning and that also makes room for unfolding and development. For this, we now turn to the Aristotelian tradition, with some help from the young Karl Marx.

## The Aristotelian/Marxian Alternative[14]

The basic idea in my own version of this tradition is that human beings have a worth that is indeed inalienable, because of their capacities for various forms of activity and striving. These capacities are, however, dependent on the world for their full development and for their conversion into actual functioning. I use the term *basic capabilities* for the untrained capacities, the term *internal capabilities* for the trained capacities, and the term *combined capabilities* for the combination of trained capacities with suitable circumstances for their exercise. (Thus, someone might have fully developed internal capabilities without having the associated combined capabilities, if, for example, she is an educated person capable of free speech and association but is living in a repressive regime that denies those freedoms.) Capacities have to be evaluated. Not all capacities that inhere in nature are the source of moral/political claims. The capacity for cruelty, for example, exerts no claim on others that it be developed because, when we consider that capacity, we do not conclude that it is necessary for living a life that is worthy of the dignity that human beings possess. This evaluative task is slippery and delicate, because we are moving back and forth between thinking of capacities and thinking of a flourishing life, and there is need both for sensitive imagination and for lots of cross-checking in the theory, as when we arrive at some political principles based upon our intuitive idea and then see how they look. (Following Rawls here, I urge a holistic account of justification, in which intuitions and political principles, and alternative accounts of both, are held up and scrutinized against our considered judgments until we reach, if we ever do, a reflective equilibrium.)

How exactly does my view address the Stoic contention that (untrained) capacities are all one needs to be complete? The Aristotelian view sees capacities as worthy of respect, but as yet unfulfilled, incomplete. They are dynamic, not static: they tend toward development and toward exercise, or at least the opportunity for exercise. They are preparations for something further, they demand space within which to unfold themselves. Human beings (like other sentient beings) are endowed with capacities for various forms of activity and striving, but the world can interfere with their progress toward development and functioning.

To see why these impediments are harms, despite the worth and dignity of the capacities, let us think of two images: imprisonment and rape. (These images were powerfully deployed by American philosopher Roger Williams in his 17th-century defense of liberty of conscience.[15]) Why is unjust imprisonment bad for a good person, given that it does not diminish the person's worth or dignity? Even though imprisonment does not diminish the worth of a good person, it is still a serious harm for a person to be unfairly imprisoned, because it deprives the person of the opportunity to exercise his or her good capacities. These capacities are preparations for activity, and it is necessary for a flourishing human life, a life worthy of those capacities, that there be opportunities to use them in activity.

Once again, why is rape bad? Why do we consider it a violation of human dignity, or even a "crime against humanity"?[16] We have long rejected the old bad view that rape really sullies a woman's worth. And yet we still believe that rape is a violation of a woman's dignity. Why? Rape violates the bodily, mental, and emotional life of a woman, affecting all her opportunities for development and functioning. Rape, we might say, does not remove or even damage dignity, but it violates it, being a type of treatment that inhibits the characteristic functioning of the dignified human being. It is inappropriate to use a human being as a mere tool in that way, because a human being should not be used as a mere tool: respect for human dignity prevents that. It would be a bit peculiar to force one's penis into a hole in a tree, but nobody would call this a violation of the dignity of the tree (I think). A woman, by contrast, has sentience, imagination, emotions, and the capacity for reasoning and choice: to force sexual intercourse on her is inappropriate, lacking in respect for the dignity that those capacities possess.

Roger Williams used the images of imprisonment and of "soul rape" to show what is wrong with the denial of religious liberty. For Williams, the conscience, that is, each person's capacity to search for the meaning of life, is a precious "jewel," whose worth is truly inalienable and grounds political claims. Nonetheless, this jewel-like entity can both be imprisoned (denied free religious activity) and also raped (denied free speech, subjected to forced conversion, etc.).[17] This is the sort of claim that my neo-Aristotelian view makes about all the major human capacities.

What do I mean, then, by saying that a life that does not contain opportunities for the development and exercise of the major human capacities is not a life worthy of human dignity? I mean that it is like imprisoning or raping a free thing whose flourishing (based on these capacities) consists in forms of intentional activity and choice. Such a life is a violation in much the way that rape and unjust imprisonment are violations: they give a thing conditions that make it impossible for it to unfold itself in a way suited to the dignity of those capacities. So the Stoics are wrong if they think that respect requires only a reverential attitude. It requires more: it requires creating the conditions in which capacities can develop and unfold themselves. (Similarly, we would say that a young child is a precious thing and that this preciousness is not itself an artifact of political arrangements while also thinking that it entails some very specific political obligations of respect and support.) Respect for human dignity is not just lip service, it means creating conditions favorable for development and choice.

Whose task is it to create the conditions? We now need an account of the purposes of political arrangement. On one very plausible account, it is the task of the "basic structure" of society to put in place the necessary conditions for a minimally decent human life, a life at least minimally worthy of human dignity, expressive of at least minimal respect. If we accept such an account (which I do accept but won't defend here), this yields the conclusion that government (meaning the basic structure of society) should support the central human capabilities.

## The Aristotelian Alternative and Political Liberalism

One can use the appeal to human dignity in a variety of different contexts, and it is extremely important to distinguish these. First of all, one may make a notion of human dignity central to a comprehensive ethical or religious doctrine. Many religions and many secular ethical conceptions (e.g., Kant's) have done so. But in modern pluralistic democracies it is inappropriate to base political principles on any particular comprehensive doctrine not shared by reasonable citizens, because that would itself be a failure of respect and a type of soul rape. If all consciences require space to search for meaning in their own way, then a state that builds its principle on a single religious (or secular) doctrine fails to accord conscience the right sort of space. Or rather, worse, it accords space to some, those who accept the preferred creed, and not to others. This insight was already well understood in colonial America, and is the underpinning for much in our constitutional tradition.[18]

Political principles have a moral content, and of course principles that make use of the idea of human dignity have an especially marked moral content. This content, however, can be affirmed from the point of view of many different comprehensive doctrines. The framers of the UN's *Universal Declaration of Human Rights* were conscious of their profound religious and philosophical differences. As Jacques Maritain writes, however, they could agree on the idea that the human being is an end and not merely a means, and their account of human rights embodied a practical political agreement deriving from this shared intuitive idea, which different religions would then interpret further in different ways (some in terms of the idea of the soul, and others eschewing that concept, for example).[19] Like Maritain, and following John Rawls's related notion of the "overlapping consensus,"[20] I think we ought to seek political principles that have a moral content but that avoid contentious metaphysical notions (for example, the notion of the soul) that would make them incompatible with some of the many reasonable comprehensive doctrines that citizens hold.

To make a dignity-based approach appropriate to the basis for political principles in a pluralistic democratic society, then, we must first work to develop it in a non-metaphysical way, articulating the relevant idea of dignity in a way that shows the ethical core of that idea but that does not insist on linking it to involved metaphysical or psychological doctrines concerning which the major religions and secular conceptions differ.

We must also, second, make adjustments in the way in which we talk about human capacities and their realization that move the conception away from Aristotle's comprehensive doctrine of human flourishing toward a political doctrine that can be accepted by many different religions and secular conceptions. I believe we can do this, but we have to be careful. To begin with, we should focus on (fullfledged, developed and institutionally prepared) capability rather than actual functioning as the political goal, leaving it to citizens to determine whether they wish to avail themselves of opportunities for functioning that politics gives them. A member of the Old Order Amish will not vote or participate in politics, but he or she can accept the *right* to vote as a fundamental entitlement of all citizens. An atheist would object to any required religious functioning, but he or she can happily accept religious liberty as a central political good. Another thing we must do, in order to show respect for the plurality of comprehensive doctrines, is to keep our list of fundamental entitlements relatively short and circumscribed, not a full account of a flourishing life but only some very central prerequisites of a life worthy of human dignity. In this way we leave lots of space for different religions to add different further specifications to which their adherents will attend. All of this is thoroughly un-Aristotelian, since Aristotle thought it was just fine to base political arrangements on a single comprehensive conception of the flourishing life. So it is important to understand that my dignity-based approach not only draws from Kant as well as Aristotle in its articulation of the idea of dignity, it also puts that idea to work in ways of which Aristotle would not have approved. I believe that we have learned a lot since Aristotle (or, rather, that the West has learned, since India had these ideas of inter-religious respect since the time of Ashoka, only a little later than Aristotle), and that we now understand that it is itself violative of human dignity to base political arrangements on a single comprehensive doctrine.

## Dignity and Its Basis

Let us now return to the Stoic approach and its excessive rationalism, and let us try to define the proper role for a notion of "basic capabilities" in the articulation of a dignity-based capability approach. This is a question on which my views have evolved over time, and I welcome this opportunity to discuss the shift. In early formulations of the idea, I said that the ground of political entitlements lay in a set of "basic capabilities," undeveloped powers of the person that were the basic conditions for living a life worthy of human dignity. I acknowledged that the potential for abuse in assessing which children of human parents have the basic capabilities was very high, and that many groups (women, members of minority races, people with a variety of disabilities) had been prematurely and wrongly said not to have some major basic capabilities (rationality, the capacity for choice, and so forth). So in practical terms I took the line that it was always best to proceed as if everyone was capable of all the major internal capabilities, and to make tireless efforts to bring each one up above the threshold. I still believe that this practical approach is essentially correct. I do think, however, that it is quite crucial not to base the ascription of human dignity on any single "basic capability" (rationality, for example), since this excludes from human dignity many human beings with severe mental disabilities. Even if we should shift to some different capacity, such as the capacity for social interaction or care, many human beings would still be excluded.

On the one hand, then, we want an account of the basis of human dignity that is respectful of the many different varieties of humanity and that doesn't rank and order human beings. On the other hand, however, the intuition I have tried to articulate, concerning the dynamic nature of human capacities and the harm done by penning them up or failing to develop them, seems to me quite central and part of what we must retain, if we want to have an account of why we have political obligations to human beings and not to rocks. I believe that the best way to solve this complex problem is to say that full and equal human dignity is possessed by any child of human parents who has any of an open-ended disjunction of basic capabilities for major human life-activities. At one end, we would not accord equal human dignity to a person in a persistent vegetative state, or an anencephalic child, since it would appear that there is no striving there, no reaching out for functioning. On the other end, we would include a wide range of children and adults with severe mental disabilities, some of whom are capable of love and care but not of reading and writing, some of whom are capable of reading and writing but severely challenged in the area of social interaction. So the notion of "basic capabilities" still does some work in saying why it is so important to give capacities development and expression, but it is refashioned to be flexible and pluralistic, respectful of human diversity.

In general, when we select a political conception of the person we ought to choose one that does not exalt rationality as *the* single good thing and that does not denigrate forms of need and striving that are parts of our animality. Indeed, it is crucial to situate rationality squarely within animality, and to insist that it is one capacity of a type of animal who is also characterized by growth, maturity, and decline, and by a wide range of disabilities, some more common and some less common. There is dignity not only in rationality but in human need itself and in the varied forms of striving that emerge from human need.

On the other hand, I would continue to insist that the political entitlements of all citizens are equal and the same, and that they include all the (developed) major capabilities on the list. I believe that if we say anything else, we fail to respect people with disabilities as fully equal citizens. To say that this person will have property rights and that one will not, that this one will be able to vote and that one will not, seems an intolerable violation of *equal* respect for human dignity. Moreover, if we start fashioning different levels of political entitlement we lose a strong incentive that my single conception gives us for making every effort we can to develop the capacities of people with disabilities to the point at which they are able to exercise these entitlements on their own.

The list of entitlements in that way tracks the idea of the human species. This is reasonable, because the human community is the community within which all citizens, with and without various unusual physical and mental disabilities, live their lives. Sometimes philosophers make comparisons between human children with mental retardation and chimpanzees. This comparison is profoundly misleading for political purposes. A human child with profound mental retardation has no option of going off to live happily with the chimps in the forest. Her life will be lived with human beings. Human beings are her parents, her caregivers. If she ever has a sexual life, it will be with human beings. If she has children, they will be human children. Relationships with other species may be very important in her life (as they are on my capabilities list), but they do not constitute the overall environment for her life. So, she should have the entitlements of an equal human being, and that means, I think, all the same ones that every other human being has.

So, on the "basic capabilities" my approach is flexible and pluralistic, but on the political goal it is single and demanding. What, then, becomes of individuals who, after our best efforts, cannot attain the capabilities on the list because of a disability? Here I insist that they still have these capabilities, for example the right to vote and the right to own property, but that these capabilities in some cases will have to be exercised in a relationship with a guardian. It is always preferable to use guardians in as few areas of life as possible: thus I defend a flexible multi-layered approach to legal guardianship. Moreover, even with guardianship it is always better if the guardian can act as a facilitator rather than a substitute. Thus, a young woman with profound mental retardation has a guardian in matters of voting. If at all possible, the guardian will consult her and try as best she can to make the choice that coheres with what she knows of the young woman's preferences. Where that is simply not knowable, however, the young woman still gets a vote and the guardian will vote for her as best she can.

I should add that the species norm also tells us that certain abilities are not equally valuable in all species. Thus language is an extremely valuable capacity for life in the human community, and we should make maximal efforts to teach language to all human children.

Many chimps are capable of learning language, but, by contrast, in the chimp community it is a frill rather than something central to their life, so we would not think of ourselves as required to spend money to teach all chimps language, even if we accept the idea that we have obligations to develop and promote the capabilities of non-human animals.

## Extending the Notion of Dignity: Animal Entitlements

If we take the line that I have recommended, refusing to ground dignity in rationality alone, and insisting on grounding it in a varied set of capacities that are all elements in the life of a type of animal being, we can easily move onward to recognize that the world contains many distinct varieties of dignity, some human and some belonging to other species. What I have said about dignity in humans goes as well for most animals (at least all those who move from place to place and have complex forms of sentience—I am not going to comment here on sponges and other related "stationary animals"). Namely, animals have capacities that are dynamic and not static, that seek expression in a characteristic form of life. They reach out, as it were, for those types of functioning and are frustrated and made vain if the animal is not permitted to develop them further internally and/or is denied suitable external conditions for their expression. It would seem that these capacities too inspire awe and should be objects of respect. Respecting animal capacities would seem to require, at the very least, undertaking not to impede animals' chances to grow up and lead flourishing lives.

These are controversial issues, and there is no space here to give them the argument they deserve. One-third of my book *Frontiers of Justice* is devoted to these questions, first arguing that our relationship to nonhuman animals raises issues of justice, and then trying to extend the capabilities approach to deal with these questions. Clearly, the Aristotelian-Marxian account is suited for such extension in a way that the Stoic rationalistic account of dignity is not. And I argue, too, that it does better than Utilitarianism, because it can recognize worth in a wide variety of distinct capacities for functioning, and is not single-mindedly focused on pain and pleasure, which are very important, but not the only issues. In the book I try to show how the approach will have to be modified to deal well with these cases, and I then ask what obligations this yields for human beings.

Advocates for human beings with disabilities are often edgy about the animal rights movement, or even hostile to it. It seems to me that it would be helpful if I can show how my approach may be able to defuse that sense of rivalry to at least some degree. One reason for edginess is that Utilitarians frequently make comparisons between human individuals with disabilities and animals with similar powers, suggesting that we have exactly the same ethical obligations to both. My approach comes to no such conclusion. I have argued that the comparison is thoroughly misleading, given that each creature lives, above all, in most of the central functionings of life, as a member of her own species community. I have also argued that, given the importance of *equal* respect and regard, a human being with major disabilities has all the same political entitlements as a so-called "normal" person. So, there need be no fear that my account will conclude that a human child with mental retardation doesn't have the right to an education, just because education would not be particularly important or useful for a chimpanzee. Nor need there be any worry that such a human will be denied property rights or voting rights, on the grounds that chimpanzees don't have them or need them. So that reason for edginess can relatively easily be dispelled by stating precisely what the role of the species norm is in my conception.

The other source of edginess is more practical. It is that, once we recognize a wide range of entitlements to animals, we will be dividing our resources in ways that will take them away from the protection and development of humans with disabilities. I believe that this worry, too, is basically ill-founded. To protect the capabilities of animals in the way that my conception requires, we will surely have to stop the factory farming industry and lots of other cruel abuses of animals. (I argue that one can reasonably be agnostic about the painless killing of some animals for food, after a decent life, on the grounds that most animals don't have the type of interests that are frustrated by death, an argument proposed by both Bentham and Peter Singer, though still controversial.) We have to stop hunting and fishing for sport, the desecration of the habitat of animals "in the wild," and lots of other practices in which our world currently engages. Some people will lose money if those practices are stopped, as the protection of endangered species already shows. But there is no reason to think that the protection of animal life is so prohibitively costly that it will take needed resources away from our children, especially those with disabilities.

Medical research is a more difficult matter, since research using animal subjects does have benefits for many humans (as well as many animals). For this reason, I do not recommend ending all such research immediately, but, instead, working as hard as we can to develop methods of research (e.g. computer simulation) that do not require animal subjects, while ending the unnecessarily cruel treatment of animals used in research.

Animals other than human beings possess dignity for the very same reason that human beings possess dignity: they are complex living and sentient beings endowed with capacities for activity and striving. It seems to me morally unacceptable to harp on the importance of human dignity while denying this dignity to other animals. We could rescue ourselves from inconsistency if we were to return to the Stoic account, arguing that dignity resides in rationality. I have argued, however, that such an account is unacceptable even if we focus only on the human community. If we do accept the Aristotelian account I recommend, it seems very difficult to draw a sharp line between our species and other species, and much more ethically responsible to reflect long and hard about the reasons we have to change our behavior to other species.

## Directions for Bioethics?

What lessons does the human-capability conception I have developed here offer to bioethics? I firmly believe that one should not simply apply philosophical principles to a case. Instead, my approach to philosophical justification suggests that we ought to make a long and close study of the new case, asking both how the principles developed so far would help us to approach it, and also whether the case itself poses any challenge to the practical principles so far articulated. Justification is in that way holistic, not top-down, or so I argue.[21] Then too, I have not devoted sustained study to any of the prominent dilemmas of bioethics, and do not know enough biology to read the literature on them with the sort of understanding that I hope I have achieved concerning the strivings of poor people in developing nations, concerning the demands of people with disabilities, and concerning the current bad treatment of animals. Given that there exists an international Human Development and Capability Association, many of whose members have expertise that I do not have, I think it reasonable to view this as a case of shared intellectual labor, where others with biological knowledge will work on those problems and see what guidance my principles offer, and whether that guidance seems helpful.

I can, however, make a few preliminary general observations concerning the directions in which my principles (should they be kept in their present form and not modified by confrontation with the new cases) would steer bioethics.

It is very important to notice that the view I defend makes capability, not actual functioning, the appropriate political goal. Thus, a just society offers people the opportunity to vote, but it does not require them to vote. (Voting is not acceptable to some religions, for example the Old Order Amish. We respect them by working for capability, not function.) A just society offers people freedom of religion, but it does not dragoon all citizens into mandatory religious functioning, which would be violative of the commitments of the atheist, the agnostic, or whoever does not share the sort of religion that the state has chosen. With children I make an exception, defending compulsory education on the grounds that it is necessary for the development of many adult capabilities.

This preference for capability as goal is supported by two closely related considerations. First, practical reason and choice are extremely important capabilities on the list, and I have argued that (along with sociability) they have an architectonic function, pervading and organizing all of the others. That is to say, if one has adequate nutrition, but without the opportunity to exercise practical reason and choice in the use of nutrients, one has not been shown respect for one's dignity. (Note that it is the *opportunity* for practical reason and choice, not its actual exercise, that is valued here: politics does not denigrate people who prefer to live in an authoritarian religious community, or in the military.) So also with health more generally: to be in a healthy condition, without having any opportunity to exercise practical reason and choice with regard to one's health, is to have an incompletely human healthy condition, one that is not worthy of one's human dignity.

The second reason why capability, not functioning, is the appropriate political goal is that the conception is defended as a form of political liberalism in Rawls's sense: that is, it ought to be, or to become, the object of an overlapping consensus among people who hold different comprehensive views of the good human life. If we required all the types of functioning that the list suggests, we would clearly show deficient respect for people whose comprehensive doctrine does not endorse one of them. Many people can sign on to a set of goals understood as capabilities, even when they don't think it right to use one or more of them, without feeling violated. Things would be different if the political conception announced that its functions were essential to a life with human dignity: the Amish citizen, the citizen who belongs to an authoritarian religion, and many more would then feel violated.

Sometimes it is very difficult to know when the absence of a given functioning signals the absence of a capability. If certain groups and people don't vote, is this a sign that they lack political capability, or is it just a sign that they don't care to vote? We should feel nervous if the failure to vote correlates with class, or gender, or race, or any other marker of subordinate status: we should then consider whether there may not be subtle obstacles to choosing that function. If women work the famous "double day," working a full-time job and then doing all or most of the housework and child care, is this because they choose not to have play and recreation, or is it because they are being pushed into leaving that out of their lives? Again, we should be skeptical here, seeing that the failure to play, in many if not most of the world's countries, is strongly correlated with traditional subordination.

It is important to notice that one could have a capability-based political conception without accepting, or without accepting across the board, my contention that capability, not functioning, is the appropriate political goal. For example, Richard Arneson argues that I ought to make an exception for health, and say that there the appropriate goal is healthy functioning, so that it is legitimate for government to push citizens into healthy lifestyles. I take issue with him for the reasons given, reasons deriving from the equal respect we owe to people's choices of a comprehensive doctrine.[22]

Although I reject Arneson's argument, I myself make a significant exception in the area of public humiliation. Here I observe that the government could say to citizens, "If you pay ten cents, we'll treat you with respect. We'll even give you the dime ourselves. But it's your choice. If you choose to use the dime for something else, we will publicly humiliate you." I say that offering choice in this area goes counter to the entire purpose of the conception, for the whole idea is that government should be showing equal respect to all citizens and should offer humiliating treatment to nobody. Private humiliation is a different matter, and I see no reason why government should step in to prevent people from choosing a humiliating friendship, or even marriage, short of recognized criminal violations. (Of course to refuse to offer divorce on grounds of psychological humiliation would make government an accomplice to the private humiliation and would not be acceptable to me.)

All right, so what does this mean about health? It means that the respectful government promotes health capabilities, not healthy functioning. That is, it should make sure that all citizens have adequate health insurance and access to good medical facilities. It should also make sure that all citizens have access to healthy nutritional and lifestyle choices, for example by focusing on building more parks and recreational facilities in urban areas. It should also make sure that all citizens have access to accurate health information. But it should not penalize citizens if they prefer to live unhealthy lives. Policies that would be supported by my program include bans on smoking in public places, but only because of secondary smoke. They include the extensive program of bicycle paths, underpasses, and sheds that Chicago's Mayor Daley has recently been constructing, many of them in poorer neighborhoods, so that poor people can have what the rich typically have already, access to the recreational facilities of the lakeshore, and the ability to go to work on a bike. They include, further, Mayor Daley's deliberate construction of public parks that are interesting and fun, so that people will actually want to go there and walk around in them, rather than seeing them as boring displays of opulence. And of course they include Chicago's recent improvements to public transportation, so that people will be able to commute to work on buses and trains, thus walking more than they would had they taken their cars (a move that obviously has big environmental payoffs as well).

In short, the approach should focus on disseminating information and promoting genuine choice, not on penalizing people who make choices doctors and politicians don't like.

I also believe that my approach entails the decriminalization of recreational, as well as therapeutic, drug use. Children certainly should be taught the dangers of drugs, and it is entirely legitimate to make drugs, like cigarettes, off-limits to children. It is also legitimate to inform adults aggressively of the dangers of recreational drugs, as is done with cigarettes. But I see no reason why Americans should remain so phobic and dictatorial about drugs. Our current policy is not only blatantly inconsistent in itself (permitting alcohol, one of the most damaging and dangerous drugs, to remain legal), it is also inconsistent when we think of the issue of personal risk more generally. Americans have many hobbies that involve health risks, including mountain climbing, sailing, and playing basketball. There are some sports that are clearly far more risky than is marijuana use—boxing, for example, which remains legal. So it is a mystery (philosophically, for historically it is probably easy enough to understand) why Americans are so phobic about drugs. I myself happen to be personally very phobic about drugs, and I am probably one of the very few baby boomers who never tried marijuana even once. Yet I would think it most disrespectful to inflict those preferences on other people, and I do not understand why our government has so strenuously insisted on doing so.

Favoring the decriminalization of recreational drugs does not entail opposing the regulation of drugs in sports, where the issue is one of fair competition. Anyone who stages a competition is entitled to set rules for fair participation. The important thing is that these rules should apply equally and fairly to all. Some forms of drugging (such as blood doping) are not per se dangerous; they are bad simply because they are unfair, when some get away with them and others don't. (And of course the rules here are quite arbitrary, since sleeping in an oxygen-deprivation tent is permitted, whereas injecting red blood cells is not.)

Fairness, however, is not the only issue to consider. If a given drug (e.g., anabolic steroids) has a bad effect on health and its use appears to be a necessary condition of successful competition when lots of people are using it, then such a regime probably puts undue pressure on participants to make an unhealthy choice, effectively removing their choice-capability. I think banning steroids is rather like requiring boxing gloves and other protective gear: it sets up some reasonable health-parameters for the sport so that its participants are not forced to make unhealthy choices that they don't want to make. Once that protective standard is in place, fairness kicks in, since allowing the one who really, really wants to use steroids to do so would give that person an unfair advantage.

In all such debates, the rhetoric of "nature" is singularly unhelpful. There is nothing wrong with the use of "unnatural" enhancements in sports. Indeed sports depend thoroughly on the non-natural: on tennis rackets, poles for vaulting, skis for skiing, hi-tech running gear, fancy wet suits, and, in addition, on protective gear of many kinds. Both steroids and boxing gloves are unnatural. The latter are good and should be, as they are, required; the former are dangerous, and should be banned for the reasons I have given.

In *Sex and Social Justice*[23] I defended a similar position concerning sex work: that it ought to be decriminalized, and that the focus of government should be on making sure that poor women have education and a range of employment options, and that all workers, including sex workers, have access to adequate health care and to protection from violence. Putting that employment choice utterly off limits is not only inconsistent (since we permit types of factory work that are at least as risky in health terms, and we permit boxing, which is more risky), but also not adequately respectful of the choice-capabilities of working women.

In short, respecting human dignity requires informing people about their choices, restricting dangerous choices for children, but permitting adults to make a full range of choices, including unhealthy ones—with the proviso that competitive sports need to set reasonably safety conditions so that unwilling participants are not dragooned into taking a health risk that they don't want to take.

For similar reasons related to the importance of practical reason and choice, and the importance of respect for comprehensive conceptions of the good, I would tentatively favor a limited right of access to physician-assisted suicide, as a way of showing respect for people whose overall view of life may strongly favor suicide in the case of a terminal illness. This looks like an easy case for the person who focuses on respect for choice, and suicide all by itself is, for me, an easy case: each person should have that choice, free from penalty to the estate or to insurance benefits for survivors, and then each will make it in accordance with his or her religious or secular comprehensive doctrine. To impose the comprehensive doctrine of a particular variety of Christianity on all citizens is to violate their dignity. Suicide hot lines and counseling to deter people from suicide are extremely important, because many suicidal people are temporarily depressed and have not deliberated fully; they recover and are happy that their lives were saved. At the end of life especially, however, the choice to end life, by a mentally fit person, should be respected. Assisted suicide is more difficult than this, however, because it usually involves a doctor, whose commitment to the patient's life is in *prima facie* tension with the act of suicide. And yet, I would favor such a right, *if* it is hedged round with sufficient safeguards to prevent manipulation and pressure. That seems to me the really difficult issue here, because we know that our society undervalues aging people and that relatives are therefore not to be trusted to have respect for the aging person's life. When we add that relatives often cannot afford the cost of care, we have a situation where abuse can easily occur. The danger of abuse is the only good reason I can think of to refuse to make assisted suicide illegal.

As for when human dignity begins to assert its ethical claims, I have so far argued that sentience is a necessary condition of moral considerability. Thus, I have argued that animals who do not appear to have the capacity to feel pleasure and pain (some insects and shellfish, for example) are not moral subjects in the way that most animals are. Nor are plants moral subjects, despite their possession of life. I have no very solid argument for this position, and I have for some years urged the young members of the Human Development and Capability Association to work out alternative positions on the question, "Whose capabilities count?"

I shall not apply this criterion to the question of abortion, because I myself do not know enough about when the capacity to feel pain begins, but I suspect that very late-term abortions would be rendered problematic under this principle. That does not mean, however, that they would be forbidden, since I do not categorically forbid all killings of animals. Instead, like Jeremy Bentham and Peter Singer, I say that the nature of a creature's plans, emotions, and desires affects what can be a harm for it, and that some painless killings of animals who do not have future-directed plans are permissible. This may or may not be a correct position: I am quite torn about it.

If I give up, as I might, the position that some killings of sentient animals are permissible, I would still not be required to apply this conclusion directly to the case of the fetus, since I would need to consider, first, the equality arguments that legal theorists have put forward, when they argue that the denial of an abortion right requires an already subordinated group, namely women, to bear a burden of life support that males are not required to bear. They compare this case to a hypothetical society in which all and only African Americans were required to donate their kidneys for the support of people who need kidneys, and they point out that such a law would be plainly unconstitutional, inflicting a burden of life support unequally on a disadvantaged class. I am inclined to think that these equality arguments are the strongest arguments we have in favor of an abortion right, and they do not support a limitless right to abortion—for example, were women ever fully equal in a society, they would not defend an abortion right for that society. But this is one of those areas in which a great deal more thought is required before I can arrive at a conclusion.

As for stem cell research, my position on sentience as a necessary condition of moral considerability entails that it is not morally problematic. Indeed, I find it rather extraordinary that people are up in arms about the putative dignity of a non-sentient clump of cells, while the same people are happy to eat for dinner meat raised in the foulest and most degrading, as well as painful, conditions. I do not believe that such a sharp separation between the human and the non-human case can be defended in a pluralistic society. Only a religious or metaphysical comprehensive doctrine about the specialness of the human would lead one to make such a sharp split. If we go by what science tells us and what our daily experience tells us, trying not to bring our religious comprehensive doctrines into the picture, we will be bound to concede that many animals share many features with human beings, and that those features include sentience, emotional capacities, perceptual and motor capacities, a wide range of types of thinking, and, in the case of chimpanzees, dolphins, and elephants, a conception of the self. So I would like to hear the factory farming industry discussed by Congress at the same time as the comparable question of stem cell research. To countenance today's horrendous abuses of complexly sentient animals while waxing metaphysical over a clump of cells seems to me very odd.

As for human cloning, I cannot understand why it is thought to violate human dignity. Identical twins are not lacking in human dignity, and I am not sure why a clone, whose life will be much more different from its clonee's life than one twin's from another (because of generational differences) should be thought to be lacking in human dignity. There are many potential abuses in this area, and we will need to be vigilant. We might bring into the world humans who would not be able to live full lives, because the science of cloning is immature. We might also begin to create clones as an underclass to provide organs for the privileged elites, as Kazuo Ishiguro imagined in his wonderful novel *Never Let Me Go*. Both of these would be horrible, and so we should be reluctant to go forward until we have reason for confidence that these problems will not arise. (Thus my position is similar to my position on assisted suicide.) But the sheer fact of cloning does not seem to pose any threat to human dignity as I conceive it, since the basis of dignity is the person's strivings, or basic capabilities, and clones have these as much as the clonees.

My contribution to the edited collection on human cloning put together by me and Cass Sunstein was a short story whose point was to show that the big dangers of cloning are the same dangers we face now when we have biological children, such as: the danger of using a child as a surrogate for a loved one who has died; the danger of loving not the child but an ideal image of the child; the danger of egoism and greed. But surely we do not remove these dangers from human life by restricting human cloning. They are endemic to most nuclear families, in one or another form, since we are imperfect beings.[24]

And what about the question of death? Is it somehow contrary to human dignity to seek to prolong life? Once again, the use of the term "natural" seems to me to do great harm, as when people talk about extending life "beyond the natural lifespan," or, as I heard on NPR yesterday, "beyond our allotted threescore years and ten"—as if that figure were given by the stars or fate, rather than by conventional human experience.

People used to have a life expectancy at birth of around 35 years. (That seems to have been the situation in ancient Greece, where the effects of a healthy climate were greatly undercut by persistent warfare.) In the developing world today, average life expectancy at birth is still under 40 in many nations. Many people in those nations, especially those with no literacy, probably believe, then, that it is "natural" to die early, just as they may believe that it is "natural" that a majority of one's children will die before age five. We know, however, that the low life expectancy in many nations is an artifact of poverty and the unequal distribution of medical care and sanitation. On a recent visit to West Bengal, for example, I attended a workshop on the high rate of maternal mortality in one populous rural district. The primary causes of death mentioned were anemia, unsafe drinking water, and the sheer distance a woman would have to travel to find medical facilities. None of these is "natural" in the sense of "given, inevitable, unable to be changed."

We should say that what is wrong with this situation is not the fact that life expectancy in the richer nations is now around 80 years. What is wrong is the fact that food, medical care, and life-saving technologies are so unequally distributed around the globe. Seeking to prolong life for a privileged few while ignoring the low life-capabilities of the many is morally wrong, a violation of the dignity of those who are treated as if they were of unequal human dignity. That is why my capability approach urges ample redistribution from richer to poorer nations, as well as from rich to poor within each nation.[25] It is morally bad to focus on how one's own life can be extended while totally ignoring these global inequalities. (That doesn't mean waiting to do research about extending life until all global inequalities are corrected, since we learn a great deal from basic research, and it often has unexpected dividends in other areas.) The sheer fact of prolonging life is a very good thing, and should be encouraged, up to the point where life becomes nothing like a human life at all, such as when someone enters a persistent vegetative state—or, up until the point when the person, mentally fit and free from undue pressure, chooses not to live.

As I have said, each of these cases needs a deeper examination. Such scrutiny would not simply fit the principles more precisely to the cases. It would also ask whether there is something in the cases that ought to cause us to have doubt about the principles we have so far espoused. Perhaps, however, this sketch will offer a small glimpse of what a capability-based approach might offer for a future philosophical research program in bioethics.

## Appendix: The Central Human Capabilities

1. *Life.* Being able to live to the end of a human life of normal length; not dying prematurely, or before one's life is so reduced as to be not worth living.

2. *Bodily Health.* Being able to have good health, including reproductive health; to be adequately nourished; to have adequate shelter.

3. *Bodily Integrity.* Being able to move freely from place to place; to be secure against violent assault, including sexual assault and domestic violence; having opportunities for sexual satisfaction and for choice in matters of reproduction.

4. *Senses, Imagination, and Thought.* Being able to use the senses, to imagine, think, and reason—and to do these things in a "truly human" way, a way informed and cultivated by an adequate education, including, but by no means limited to, literacy and basic mathematical and scientific training. Being able to use imagination and thought in connection with experiencing and producing works and events of one's own choice, religious, literary, musical, and so forth. Being able to use one's mind in ways protected by guarantees of freedom of expression with respect to both political and artistic speech, and freedom of religious exercise. Being able to have pleasurable experiences and to avoid non-beneficial pain.

5. *Emotions.* Being able to have attachments to things and people outside ourselves; to love those who love and care for us, to grieve at their absence; in general, to love, to grieve, to experience longing, gratitude, and justified anger. Not having one's emotional development blighted by fear and anxiety. (Supporting this capability means supporting forms of human association that can be shown to

be crucial in their development.)

6. *Practical Reason.* Being able to form a conception of the good and to engage in critical reflection about the planning of one's life. (This entails protection for the liberty of conscience and religious observance.)

7. *Affiliation.*

A. Being able to live with and toward others, to recognize and show concern for other human beings, to engage in various forms of social interaction; to be able to imagine the situation of another. (Protecting this capability means protecting institutions that constitute and nourish such forms of affiliation, and also protecting the freedom of assembly and political speech.)

B. Having the social bases of self-respect and non-humiliation; being able to be treated as a dignified being whose worth is equal to that of others. This entails provisions of non-discrimination on the basis of race, sex, sexual orientation, ethnicity, caste, religion, national origin.

8. *Other Species.* Being able to live with concern for and in relation to animals, plants, and the world of nature.

9. *Play.* Being able to laugh, to play, to enjoy recreational activities.

10. *Control over one's Environment.*

A. Political. Being able to participate effectively in political choices that govern one's life; having the right of political participation, protections of free speech and association.

B. Material. Being able to hold property (both land and movable goods), and having property rights on an equal basis with others; having the right to seek employment on an equal basis with others; having the freedom from unwarranted search and seizure. In work, being able to work as a human being, exercising practical reason and entering into meaningful relationships of mutual recognition with other workers.

# Notes

[1] Nussbaum, *Women and Human Development: The Capabilities Approach* (Cambridge: Cambridge University Press, 2000), and Nussbaum, *Frontiers of Justice: Disability, Nationality, Species Membership* (Cambridge, Massachusetts: Harvard University Press, 2006). For my list of the Central Human Capabilities, see the Appendix at the end of my essay.

[2] John Rawls, *A Theory of Justice* (Cambridge, Massachusetts: Harvard University Press, 1971), p. 586.

[3] Ibid., p. 2.

[4] For a fuller historical discussion, see my "Kant and Stoic Cosmopolitanism," *Journal of Political Philosophy* 5 (1997): 1-25, also in *Perpetual Peace*, ed. Matthias Lutz-Bachmann and James Bohman (Cambridge, Massachusetts: MIT Press, 1997), pp. 25-58, and "The Worth of Human Dignity: Two Tensions in Stoic Cosmopolitanism," in *Philosophy and Power in the Graeco-Roman World: Essays in Honour of Miriam Griffin*, ed. Gillian Clark and Tessa Rajak (Oxford: Clarendon Press, 2002), pp. 31-49.

[5] I discuss these matters at greater length in Nussbaum, *The Therapy of Desire: Theory and Practice in Hellenistic Ethics* (Princeton, New Jersey: Princeton University Press, 1994), chapter 9, with references to many texts.

[6] Lucius Annaeus Seneca, *Epistulae morales ad Lucilium* 41, in *Letters From a Stoic*, trans. Robin Campbell (London and New York: Penguin Classics, 1969), hereafter cited as Seneca, *Epistulae morales*.

[7] These thoughts are most fully brought out in Cicero's *De Officiis*; see my "Duties of Justice, Duties of Material Aid: Cicero's Problematic Legacy," *Journal of Political Philosophy* 8 (2000): 176-206.

[8] Richard Sorabji, *Animal Minds and Human Morals: The Origins of the Western Debate* (Ithaca, New York: Cornell University Press, 1995).

[9] Cicero, *Tusculan Disputations* 3.30.

[10] Seneca, *Epistulae morales* 47.

[11] Ibid.

[12] Seneca, *Epistulae morales* 41.

[13] Naomi Wolf, *Fire With Fire: The New Female Power and How to Use It* (New York: Fawcett, 1993), p. 136.

[14] For a fuller description of the Aristotelian and Marxian themes in my writings, see my "Nature, Function, and Capability: Aristotle on Political Distribution," in *Oxford Studies in Ancient Philosophy*, Supplementary Volume (1988): 145-184, reprinted in *Marx and Aristotle*, ed. George E. McCarthy (Lanham, Maryland: Rowman and Littlefield, 1992), pp. 175-212; "Aristotle on Human Nature and the Foundations of Ethics," in *World, Mind, and Ethics: Essays on the Philosophy of Bernard Williams*, ed. James E. J. Altham and Ross Harrison (Cambridge: Cambridge University Press, 1995), pp. 86-131; "Aristotelian Social Democracy," in *Liberalism and the Good*, ed. R. Bruce Douglass, Gerald M. Mara, and Henry S. Richardson (New York and London: Routledge, 1990), pp. 203-252, reprinted in *Aristotle and*

*Modern Politics*, ed. Aristide Tessitore (Notre Dame, Indiana: University of Notre Dame Press, 2002), pp. 47-104; and *Women and Human Development: The Capabilities Approach* (New York: Cambridge University Press, 2000).

[15] Roger Williams, *The Bloudy Tenent of Persecution, for the Cause of Conscience* (London, 1644).

[16] This was held by the Indian Supreme Court in a case of gang-rape.

[17] Roger Williams, op. cit.

[18] See my *Liberty of Conscience: In Defense of Religious Equality* (New York: Basic Books, forthcoming).

[19] Jacques Maritain, *Man and the State* (Washington, D. C.: Catholic University of America Press, 1951).

[20] John Rawls, *Political Liberalism* (New York: Columbia University Press, expanded paperback edition 1996).

[21] See my *Women and Human Development*, chapter 2, and *Frontiers of Justice*, preface.

[22] See my "Aristotle, Politics, and Human Capabilities: A Response to Antony, Arneson, Charlesworth, and Mulgan," *Ethics* 111 (2000); 102-140.

[23] New York: Oxford University Press, 1998.

[24] "Little C: A Fantasy," in *Clones and Clones: Facts and Fantasies About Human Cloning*, ed. Martha C. Nussbaum and Cass R. Sunstein (New York: Norton, 1998).

[25] *Frontiers of Justice*, chapters 4 and 5.

# Commentary on Nussbaum, Shell, and Kass

## Diana Schaub

The repellent results of a focus on developed quality-of-life capabilities without an acknowledgment of either the equality of human rights or the unique dignity of the human being are on display in Martha Nussbaum's essay. She characterizes her approach as "Aristotelian/Marxian" (with a soupçon of Kant)—a philosophic mutation that the thinkers themselves (as she freely admits) would not have recognized or thought viable.

On the assumption that the proof is in the pudding, let me cut straight to the policy outcomes she envisions. Nussbaum tells us that it is impermissible for government to strive to rid communities of the scourges of drugs and prostitution that destroy the lives of individuals and families; however, the heroin-addled "sex workers" do have a political entitlement to bicycle paths to promote their "health capabilities." It's unclear whether helmets will be required, but should you wind up in a bad state (brain-injured, or persistently vegetative from all those legal drugs, or just terminally old and unhappy), the health workers will be there to ease you off. As Nietzsche said of Zarathustra's last man: "A little poison now and then: that makes for agreeable dreams. And much poison in the end, for an agreeable death." As Nussbaum sketches the future, there will be a choice of

381

ways to kill yourself, and even quite a few ways to kill your fellows, so long as they are the sort who don't have any "future-directed plans." Although factory farming of sentient nonhuman animals won't be allowed, factory farming of human embryos for tissues and organs would be unproblematic.

I don't want to leave the impression that I'm opposed to bicycle paths or in favor of the mistreatment of farm stock. In fact, I am very sympathetic to the call to reconsider our obligations to the natural world; both animal husbandry and environmental stewardship should be part of our bioethical inquiries. Nonetheless, it seems to me perverse to create entitlements to niceties for those beings, whether human or nonhuman, who are in their prime with certain functional capabilities, while refusing to protect the inalienable right to life of each and every human being. But bicycle paths and public parks (including, I assume, dog parks for our highly sensitive and complexly communicative canine companions) are "interesting and fun," whereas protecting human life is burdensome.

Protecting human life is especially burdensome for women. Accordingly, Nussbaum is receptive to the argument (while cagily withholding a final endorsement) that women should not be made to "bear a burden of life support that males are not required to bear." Since pregnancy and motherhood are not fairly distributed among males and females—and, thus, certainly couldn't pass constitutional muster—mothers must have the option to abort their children. That is the legal remedy for nature's (or God's) injustice to women. Should a woman come to regret the choice she has made, the drugs, recreational and/or lethal, will be there for her. According to Nussbaum, she could even clone herself and start afresh.

Unlike Nussbaum who treats the works of the philosophers as brightly colored scraps to be stitched together in a policy quilt of her own liking, Susan Shell conscientiously uncovers the thought of a particular philosopher. In most serious discussions of bioethics, reference is bound to be made to Immanuel Kant. Shell seeks to go beyond this obligatory acknowledgment of Kant's influence on our doctrines of personal autonomy and informed consent. She argues that a fuller understanding of Kant—including elements of what might be called a non-Kantian Kant—could continue to deepen and guide our bioethical reasoning, even correcting (by limiting) the doctrine of autonomy.

In his essay, Leon Kass delivers a powerful critique of Kant's approach to dignity which he regards as too abstract and disembodied:

> Precisely because it dualistically sets up the concept of "personhood" in opposition to nature and the body, it fails to do justice to the concrete reality of our embodied lives, lives of begetting and belonging no less than of willing and thinking. Precisely because it is universalistically rational, it denies the importance of life's concrete particularity, lived always locally, corporeally, and in a unique trajectory from zygote in the womb to body in the coffin.[1]

Shell seeks to counter this impression of Kant as a "rigid dualist" by explicating "Kant's notion of 'humanity' as embodied rationality."

Interestingly, all three of these authors (Nussbaum, Kass, and Shell), in their quest for the sources of human dignity, insist on the meaning to be found in our embodiment. For Nussbaum this leads to a reconsideration of the worth of "those human capacities in which animals also partake, such as sentience, everyday (non-moral) practical reasoning, emotion, and the capacity for love and care"—a reconsideration that ends by extending entitlements to other animals (most of them at least, although Nussbaum isn't so sure about nondynamic "sponges"). Kass, although an admiring analyst of animal beauty and nobility, does not turn to the body in order to invert hierarchies or contest man's place. Rather, he argues that only by understanding human life as "a grown-togetherness of body and soul" can we achieve and maintain our special dignity: "The defense of what is humanly high requires an equal defense of what is seemingly 'low.'" For Kass, natural desires are only "seemingly" low since they are, in effect, transmuted and elevated by being pursued in certain (humanly dignified) ways. Feeding can become dining and procreation can become family life. Shell's presentation of Kant similarly aims for a more full-blooded and integrated view of human life—although I doubt that it will be enough for Nussbaum and Kass to retract the reservations they both express against Kant.

Nonetheless, by drawing attention to Kant's notion of embodiment, Shell is able to show that Kant does not grant an unrestricted license to "the reciprocal freedom of consenting adults." She sketches the limits upon autonomy that follow from the requirement "that one must respect oneself 'as an animal being.'" Whereas Nussbaum's view seems to be that only government can debase human beings (by failing to provide the necessary entitlements for developing one's capabilities), Shell highlights the possibility of self-degradation and the Kantian obligation "to treat humanity in oneself, no less than in others, as an 'end in itself.'" There would doubtless be prostitutes in Kant's world, since human beings fail in their obligations to self and others, but there could not be the government-enabled sex workers that Nussbaum approves.

The Kantian bioethics that Shell articulates emphasizes caution, restraint, and due humility in our treatment of our bodies. But, according to Shell, these limits may not apply universally. Near the end of her essay, she suggests that Kant offers a "punctuated account of human development," which means that moral standing is not inherent to all human beings at all stages of life, but rather is an accrued quality linked to the acquisition of specific faculties—in the case of Kant, the faculty of moral reasoning. In applying this notion of accrued moral status to bioethics, Shell indicates that Kant himself might have regarded even newborns as lacking full moral standing. While Shell is not prepared to join Kant (and Peter Singer) in this opinion, she does wonder whether this notion of accrued moral status might not make embryo-destructive stem cell research permissible. She herself draws the line of personhood very early at the developmental moment that the twinning of the embryo is no longer possible. She argues that the possibility of identical twins from what was initially one embryo shows that a fully individuated being was not yet present.

Since neither of us is expert in embryology, let me offer a counterinterpretation from someone who is. According to Stanford biologist and Council member William Hurlbut, monozygotic twinning results from a disruption of normal development that provokes a restoration of integrity within two distinct trajectories. Hurlbut states that "twinning is not evidence of the absence of an individual, but of an extraordinary power of compensatory repair that reflects more fully the potency of the individual drive to fullness of form."[2] Twinning is a profound testament to the presence and the resilience of the organizing principle of life. The human being can double only because a human being was present from the beginning.

Whereas Nussbaum sarcastically dismisses "the putative dignity of a non-sentient clump of cells," Shell is clear that the early embryo "is not a mere 'collection of cells' that we can injure or dispose of trivially." Nonetheless, she wants to find some narrow window ("the first ten days or so after conception") during which these entities "purposively directed toward fuller human development" might be put to good use, might be treated as a means rather than an end, might be, so to speak, non-trivially disposed of. In a way, I find Shell's position harder to comprehend than Nussbaum's. What does it mean "to respect the human potential of the blastocyst…without granting it the status of a moral person"? For Shell, it seems to mean using early human embryos only for noble purposes like curing cancer.

Despite marked differences, both Nussbaum and Shell in the end agree that humanity is an acquired not an inherited quality—a matter of becoming not being. Those who haven't become enough may be judged unworthy of continued existence. In fairness to Shell, it should be noted that Nussbaum, despite her evident concern for the severely disabled, puts many more folks in this category than does Shell. While Nussbaum wants legal guardians to cast votes on behalf of the profoundly retarded (it's not hard to predict that they will vote for the party of entitlements), she declares that "we would not accord equal human dignity to a person in a persistent vegetative state, or an anencephalic child, since it would appear that there is no striving there, no reaching out for functioning."

While I understand the impulse to define humanity in exclusionary terms, it also seems to me that the case for the embryo—the case for the embryo's human standing—has never been easier to make, and that it is science itself, the science of embryology, that best makes the case. Both Nussbaum and Shell suggest that it could only be religion that would lead one to regard the early human embryo as human in the respect-worthy sense. And yet, it is undeniable that each and every post-natal human being has passed through the identical stages of embryonic and fetal development. We were all blastocysts once. That clump of cells is us at that stage of our life. The embryo is not just potentially a member of the human kind. It is human. From conception (or to use more technical language, from the moment of syngamy), the human zygote has 46 chromosomes and can be distinguished from embryos of other species. It is recognizably one of us—recognizable not to the naked eye, but to the scientifically trained eye. Moreover, the embryo is not like other cells or tissues. In the words again of Stanford biologist William Hurlbut, "it possesses an inherent organismal unity and potency that such other cells lack."[3] Because of this "unified organismal principle of growth," nothing external is added to its biological essence over time. Our unique being unfolds continuously from within. Along the way we develop and manifest various capacities, sensory and cognitive, but there isn't one of those capacities whose acquisition suddenly makes us human. There are many phases and stages of a human life, but the being—the unique human being—is there from beginning to end, from conception to death. Of course, certain externals need to be present for this human life-in-process to continue its self-directed growth, but that is true of every phase of human life. We are self-directed, but not self-sufficient. Knowledge of our earliest beginnings, and of the dynamic developmental process of the human organism as it matures, can awaken a sense of awe and respect. Knowledge of our origins does not destroy wonder; it deepens it.

In a letter written by Thomas Jefferson just 10 days before his death, he expressed the conviction that it is "the unbounded exercise of reason" and "the general spread of the light of science" that will open men's eyes to the truth that all men are created equal and endowed with inalienable rights. I hope he is right. I hope that the knowledge supplied by the science of embryology will lead us to question the moral legitimacy of embryo-destroying research. Perhaps we will realize that we are not at liberty to divest our posterity of their right to life, liberty, and the pursuit of happiness.

## Notes

[1] Leon R. Kass, "Defending Human Dignity," p. 313 above.
[2] The President's Council on Bioethics, *Human Cloning and Human Dignity: An Ethical Inquiry* (Washington, D.C.: Government Printing Office, 2002), p. 313.
[3] Ibid., p. 310.

# 15

# The Irreducibly Religious Character of Human Dignity

## David Gelernter

Human dignity has often been mentioned in recent controversies over bioethics. Some find the concept indispensable—most notably the President's Council itself. Others, such as Ruth Macklin, argue that it is either useless, because it simply means "autonomy," or dangerous, because it introduces religious ideas by stealth into the deliberations of a liberal democratic society, where (allegedly) they don't belong. Most defenders of the Council have responded that dignity is neither reducible to autonomy nor a Trojan horse for religion.

I'll argue that "human dignity" doesn't matter much in itself—but the hunt for its definition surely does, a great deal. It's a strange sort of hunt. We know how the term is used by thinkers on both sides of a large range of bioethical questions; they might disagree violently over conclusions, yet they often seem to agree (at least in general terms) on the meaning of "human dignity." Nonetheless, definitions are scarce. We need to guess what the implied meaning really is. The answer will be revealing. Modern academics seem to rely on a definition that, at its core, is irreducibly religious. But they don't like speaking about religion. The resulting discussion has the bizarre tone of a conversation where the adults don't want the children to catch on to the real topic. (But the kids usually do anyway.) I'll argue here that Macklin is right to see the religious underpinnings of "dignity," but that she (and the Council's defenders who want to keep dignity and religion separate) are wrong to think that religious ideas are bad for a liberal democracy. Modern scholarship suggests that *without* religious ideas, there would be no such thing as liberal democracy.[1] But leaving history aside, it seems to me that we can't even protect autonomy, much less avoid such horrors as human cloning, without the support of religion.

A pattern in modern thought: thinkers repeatedly find themselves wanting the effects of religion without the cause. In former generations, philosophy tried and repeatedly failed to achieve "religion within the limits of reason." It has long since quit that game and gone home. To most modern thinkers (me included), the game seems unwinnable and pointless. Yet modern philosophers still find themselves wanting what they can't have: religious effects without religious causes. Unfortunately, there's no free lunch, and it's no good trying to conjure one up by deep thinking.

One way to approach bioethical problems is to think of a foreground and a background, and "human dignity" as the bridge leading from one to the other. The foreground is the problem itself: designer babies, human cloning, the death of Terry Schiavo. (Obviously the foreground can vary greatly in specificity.) The background is your ethical system. Most bioethical discussion takes for granted that you approach such questions like a typical academic philosopher, armed with a strictly secular "ethics of human rights." The "ethics of human duty" is an alternative that is usually (though not always) associated with Judeo-Christian religion—and unthinkingly dismissed. In fact the "ethics of human duty" is rarely considered, rarely discussed, rarely even present in our bioethical debates.

In this informal essay I'll approach "human dignity" by way of the background problems of secular versus religious morality, and of a "morality of rights" versus a "morality of duties," and I'll discuss a few foreground cases. Of course there is no "religious morality" in the abstract, so I'll discuss parts of traditional Jewish morality—and try to explain what makes it, in certain cases, more humane and kindlier than the modern secular variety.

Finally I'll argue that erecting the vast intellectual structure of the modern age on the ethics of human rights—"they are endowed by their Creator with certain unalienable rights," not "unalienable duties"—was a tragic mistake. Obviously the mistake can't be undone; in itself there's no point discussing it. But bioethicists can choose any assumptions they like. They can choose an ethics of human duty for their own use; and if they do, they will be choosing wisely. (Unconventionally, but wisely.)

## Secular vs. Religious Morality

First, what right do I have introducing religion—quotations from the Talmud no less—into the clean, rational, sterile domain of western philosophy?

Let's start by considering what *secular* ethics has to say nowadays. Obviously there is no single answer. But here is one example, for concreteness. Modern ethics points us towards "an increased sensitivity" to various things—"to the environment, to sexual difference, to gender, to people different from ourselves in a whole variety of ways...." Modern ethics suggests that we must be "careful, and mature, and imaginative, and fair, and nice, and lucky."[2]

I am quoting from the last page of the last chapter of a respected recent introduction to ethics by Simon Blackburn, whose suggestions sound like a parody of left-wing thinking. They ask for nothing noble, uplifting or even difficult. They do *not* call on us to be generous or just, decent, good, honest, kind, gracious, merciful or loving. One thinks of a famous proclamation by the prophet Micah: "Man, it has been told you what is good, and what the Lord requires of you: only to do justice, love mercy and walk humbly with your God" (*Micah* 6:8). Justice, mercy, humility—tall orders, yet man *is* capable of filling them. We all know men and women (at least a few) who have done it. These are no pie-in-the-sky demands.

Modern ethics falls short of human capacities. It asks too little. It's too small for the human soul. We ought to send it back and demand something roomier. (Speaking of roomy, what does the medieval Christian art of the Gothic cathedral tell us about man's capacities? "Be great! Be worthy of the sublime grandeur and beauty of this place that man and God built together. Be humble: there are regions of this building beyond your grasp, and—all the more so—regions of this cosmos." The architecture is more articulate than modern ethics without speaking one word.)

I will show you, as an alternative, a few fragments of a religious viewpoint. Of course a philosopher might say, "*I* am using my brain; you're merely consulting some arbitrary authority." But philosophers and their reasoning power are (for me) an arbitrary authority. Few modern philosophers still believe that reason alone can reveal universal moral truth. They merely try their best, knowing that some will disagree and that, in the foreseeable future, virtually everyone might. Suppose one person relies on a consensus of academic philosophers and another on the ethical traditions of his religious or national community, based ultimately on the communal scriptures. Both are appealing to external authority. Both are relying on a consensus of learned and intelligent people—a consensus that is bound to change. (Christian and Jewish theologians, for example, do not see the world or interpret Scripture today as they did a century or ten centuries ago.)

Arguably the person who follows *his own* reasoning is making the best methodological choice. My reasoning tells me that anyone who believes in absolute, compulsory standards of behavior for the whole world believes, *ipso facto,* in God. And it seems to me that nearly everyone *does* believe in such absolute, compulsory standards. If you were to see someone who is about to commit murder, you would *compel* him (if you could) to submit to your view of murder even if he had an elaborately-reasoned defense of the contrary position. (He might be a Nazi, a euthanasia enthusiast, or the like. And he might, for that matter, be better at arguing than you.)

By compelling a person to submit to your standards whether he agrees or not—by proclaiming (in other words) the existence of absolute moral standards that are compulsory for everyone—you proclaim, implicitly, your belief in God. And not just any God; you have proclaimed your belief in the God of *your* standards. For most western peoples, that means the God of Judaism and Christianity.

This seems like a simple, obvious argument and is, but we don't hear it often because—after all—it is not an argument that God exists; it's merely an argument that you think He does. It's an argument, in other words, that all believers in absolute moral standards believe in God too, *ipso facto.*

As Abraham Lincoln said of the Bible: "But for it we could not know right from wrong."[3]

I've asserted that anyone who believes in absolute, compulsory standards of behavior for all the world must believe in God. Again, I'm not proposing a proof that God exists, which seems to me impossible given the nature of the proposition. I'm only asserting that most people in modern society *believe* that He does—probably a large majority, including many who call themselves agnostics or atheists.

Here's my argument. Let's suppose you are a "reasonable person"; being reasonable, you have "inner promptings" that provide you with moral guidance. They tell you, for example, not to commit murder. Accordingly you don't. Even if you somehow found yourself in a position where you could murder in cold blood a person you had every right to hate, in such a way that no one would ever find out—you still wouldn't do it.

So far there's no need to mention God. There might be all sorts of purely rational or psychological grounds for this inner prompting.

But now suppose you come upon *someone else* who is about to commit murder. (For concreteness, suppose the potential murderer has pinned the intended victim underfoot and is about to smash in his head with a sledgehammer.) Presumably you would see it as your duty to compel the would-be murderer to desist. Whether you actually do anything would probably depend on the presence or absence of onlookers, the tools at hand, and your own bravery. But you'd *want* to stop the murder, whether or not you are able to put this desire into effect.

Now, what gives you the right to compel another person to obey *your own personal* inner promptings?

You might answer that "my inner promptings tell me not only that *I personally* must not murder but that I must compel *all other* potential murderers to desist." But remember: you're a reasonable person. As such, you can't deny that the potential murderer has his own inner promptings, which might tell *him* that murder (or at least this particular murder) is good or even mandatory. If you insist that *your own* behavior must be governed by *your own* inner promptings, why shouldn't *this other person's* behavior be governed by *his own* inner promptings?

Since you are a reasonable person, your only rational conclusion is that each person has a right to obey his own inner promptings—insofar as they don't collide with anyone else's. But when they do collide with someone else's, you have no basis for asserting that *your* inner promptings are right and the other person's are wrong (leaving the law aside, which is irrelevant for our purposes). In other words: when a collision exists, you no longer have any rational basis for obeying your own inner promptings. It's reasonable for you to refrain personally from committing murder. It is unreasonable for you to compel others to do the same.

But let's leave reason aside and return to reality. In fact you *would* compel that would-be murderer to stop, if you could. (And you'd do so even if you found yourself in a lawless totalitarian state where there was—in effect—no law against murder.) But *what gives you the right* to compel that would-be murderer to stop? To compel another person to obey *your* inner promptings instead of his own? What gives you the authority to carry out this act of compulsion? Not reason. The answer must lie elsewhere, in some authority beyond reason.

We know two things about this authority. First, it must hold sway over (or set bounds to the behavior of) every human being on earth—because your wish to halt that murder had nothing to do with the murderer's identity. Second, the authority must outlaw murder and any other crimes or sins concerning which you believe yourself empowered to act.

In short: unless you are proclaiming yourself supreme ruler of mankind, you must believe in God. And not just any God. Most modern, ethically-minded people will find their "inner promptings" more or less in agreement with the Ten Commandments and the Holiness Code of *Leviticus* 19:

> Thou shalt leave [the gleanings of your fields] for the poor and the stranger....Ye shall not steal, neither shall ye deal falsely, nor lie to one another.... The wages of a hired servant shall not abide with thee all night until the morning. Thou shalt not curse the deaf, nor put a stumbling block before the blind.... In righteousness shalt thou judge thy neighbor. Thou shalt not go up and down as a talebearer among thy people; neither shalt thou stand idly by the blood of thy

neighbor.... Thou shalt not hate thy brother in thy heart.... Thou shalt not take vengeance.... But thou shalt love thy neighbor as thyself... (*Leviticus* 19:9-19).

In other words: your belief that you have the duty and authority to stop a murderer before he starts suggests that you believe, implicitly, in the God of Israel.

## Dignity and Humanity

So—what *does* bioethics mean by "human dignity"? We all know that dignity has two related meanings. It's a property we notice in some people more than in others, having to do with gravity, seriousness, unflappability, wisdom and (formerly) rank or position. It's also a property all human beings are said to possess, by virtue of which they are to be treated decently no matter what. The second property is the one we are discussing here.

Adam Schulman gives us a valuable starting point when he defines human dignity as "our essential and inviolable *humanity*."

Granted, "humanity" in the sense of humane-ness is easy to understand, and only humans have it. But the definition is problematic. (In discussing these problems, my goal is *not* to take pot-shots at Schulman's definition; it was intended as a starting point for discussion, and is serving exactly that purpose.)

If human dignity is the quality of humanity or humane-ness (as in the Yiddish "he's a *mensch*"—which means "man" in German too, but not in this sense), why should we preserve it if scientists can cook up something better? Why should the question of human dignity even arise when the topic is human cloning? Why should human dignity be "inalienable," given that "our essential humanity" is *not* inviolable—given that human beings sometimes act with inhuman cruelty?

Humanity or humane-ness is good—but many genetic engineers believe that they will be able to produce "better" humans eventually, better in all sorts of ways: smarter, stronger, tougher, better-looking, healthier. So isn't it possible that they will be able to cook up more humane humans too? Shouldn't we let them try?

Some bioethicists say, by all means. But others rely on "human dignity" to fend off the engineers who want to reshape human nature like children fooling with Play-Doh.

Not only might engineers be able to roll humans out of their labs who are more humane than we; they might be able to produce qualities that are more important—that trump our humane-ness. A genetically-engineered masterpiece with less humanity than I but twice the IQ might solve problems that I can merely commiserate over. (On similar lines, surgeons are renowned for their abrasiveness; but if you need an operation, you'll almost certainly choose a talented, obnoxious surgeon over a sweeter but less-talented specimen.)

Defining human dignity as "our essential humanity" has other problems too. Some bioethicists (perhaps most?) approve enthusiastically of human cloning. But some attack the idea and call it offensive to human dignity. Yet if human dignity means "our essential humanity," cloning a human being produces *more* of the stuff, more "essential humanity." At least so it would seem. No doubt a contrary argument is possible, but it's certainly not *obvious* why human cloning should raise the issue of human dignity at all.

And surely human dignity defined this way is not "inalienable." People can and do *lose* their "essential humanity." If Hitler had appeared at the Nuremberg trials, surely he'd have had no human dignity to stand on. He had ground out every trace of humanity he ever possessed as you grind out a cigarette underfoot. The same questions arose (on a vastly smaller scale) in the case of Saddam Hussein. Yet bioethicists like to treat "human dignity" as an attribute that all humans possess unless and until it's taken away by force.

## Dignity and Sanctity

Here is a different way to define human dignity. We begin by looking up the word "sacred" in (for example) the *Oxford English Dictionary*. The definitions rest on "set apart" in many forms—"set apart for or dedicated to some religious purpose"; "regarded with or entitled to respect or reverence"; "secured by religious sentiment, reverence, sense of justice, or the like, against violation, infringement, or encroachment."[4]

It seems to me that "human dignity" as bioethics understands it is actually a sanitized version of "human sanctity"—one that has been purified of all traces of religion. In bioethics, human dignity means (implicitly) that all human beings are "set apart or dedicated to some (higher) purpose," "regarded with or entitled to respect," "secured by sense of justice, or the like, against violation, infringement, or encroachment," to read the *OED*'s definitions with religion left out. Human dignity means that humans are *set apart*.

*Violation, infringement, or encroachment*—designer babies *infringe* or *encroach on* the human species even if they turn out to be more humane (or otherwise better) than we; human beings are and must remain *set apart* and are not to be tinkered with as we have always tinkered with other species. It's arguable that when a life is dominated by pain and suffering, the sick or hurt person's human dignity has been *violated, infringed,* or *encroached on*. (And when that happens, perhaps he is entitled to end his life.) And in many other cases, "set apart, not to be encroached on" seems like the essence of human dignity.

Yet we sacrifice something when we switch from "human sanctity" to "human dignity." *Deleting religion has a cost*—a truth the modern academic doesn't want to acknowledge. Human sanctity carries a built-in explanation of its existence. Humans are set apart because, no matter what they make of themselves, *God* made them in His own image. Human dignity implies no such explanation. (Unless, perhaps, you accept the Kantian idea that human beings are intrinsically set apart by their ability to conjure up the entire moral universe merely by reasoning. But nowadays almost nobody does.)

Saddam Hussein might have retained "human sanctity" because he was created in God's image. But why should he have retained "human dignity" when he has done his best to wipe out any and all differences between himself and the lower animals?

When we switch from sanctity to dignity, we switch from a world in which *the unique set-apartness of man* is grounded in our ideas (or perceptions) of God to a world in which *the unique set-apartness of man* isn't grounded in anything, is indeed merely *asserted*. And the fact that human dignity amounts to a mere bald assertion leaves some bioethicists so uncomfortable that they would rather not define the term at all. Furthermore, "man's unique set-apartness" sounds like a religious idea, even if God never comes up. In sum, many bioethicists would rather go on using the term while forgetting the definition—why rent a car when you can borrow one?—all the while assuring us that man is merely one species among many and hence entitled to nothing special.

I've claimed that human sanctity is grounded in the idea of God's having created man in His image, and I've referred to this as a "religious" argument. But I don't really mean it—don't mean religion in a general sense; I mean Biblical religion. (I include Islam insofar as it acknowledges the Bible's truth and has in principle many close connections to Judaism.) Indeed, man's being created in the image of God is the basic, defining characteristic of Biblical as opposed to other religions; everything else flows from this seminal assertion in *Genesis*. This becomes clear when we compare the revolutionary assertion in *Genesis* to the pagan view it replaced. Pagans believed that the gods were made in *man's* image. (Of course I don't want to call the great religions of the east "pagan"; but from certain angles they resemble pagan more than Biblical religion, and particularly in this respect.) What was the meaning and force of Judaism's startling assertion that *man* had been made in *God's* image instead of vice versa? If man is made in God's image, man's goal must be *not* to accept his animal nature but to transcend it; not to "blend into" nature or "become one with" nature or with the universe but to raise himself above nature; not to be himself but to be *better* than himself. Hence he must struggle toward goodness and sanctity. He can never reach that goal, not entirely, any more than he can become the deity he (in some sense) resembles, any more than Moses (in the most powerful metaphor in the Bible) was able to reach the Promised Land. But he must try.

This seems like a lot of religious doctrine to swallow. Surely such things could only be germane to devout Jews and Christians (and perhaps to Muslims). But when and if we accept (explicitly or otherwise) the Ten Commandments and the Holiness Code as the basis of our ethics, this is the God and the story we implicitly accept.

"Human sanctity" has other properties that make it useful in bioethics—at least to some bioethicists. The hardest bioethical problems often involve the creation of human life: for example, abortion, cloning, designer babies, and other related topics. Some thinkers are unwilling to cede control over the creation of human beings to science and technology. Can they convincingly explain *why not,* if "human dignity" is all they have to work with? Isn't it fundamentally a *religious* impulse (specifically a Judeo-Christian impulse) that drives many of them? Whatever good thing is at the root of "human dignity," scientists can make it better or provide more—at least they can try!—unless your vision of "human dignity" has no utilitarian handle to grab hold of at all. Unless you mean that the *essence of human-ness must not be tampered with,* no matter what. And isn't that a *Judeo-Christian* idea?

## Rights vs. Duties

But I've claimed that the "background" and "foreground" ultimately determine the role played by "human dignity." Let me explain.

"Background" means our basic approach to ethics; but here we find two competing alternatives: the antique religious "ethics of duty" versus the "ethics of rights" that has been assumed by most thinkers for centuries. Philosophers like to argue that these two worldviews are complementary. In fact they are contradictory. Each yields an all-inclusive blueprint for society, with no room for further contributions.

Granted, it's convenient to speak of one's "duty" to help the poor and one's "right" of self-defense. No contradiction there. But think it over and you will see that, by laying out everyone's duties explicitly, you lay out everyone's rights implicitly and vice versa. You have a right to self-defense—or, to put it differently, a duty to use no violence except (among other cases) in self-defense. Both formulas reach the same destination by different routes. By means of an "ethics of duty," you shape society as a sculptor carves stone; with an "ethics of rights," you shape it as a sculptor models clay. Two different, contradictory techniques.

The ethics of duty originated in Judeo-Christianity, the ethics of rights in Roman jurisprudence. The Hebrew tradition knows about rights—but only in the context of covenants, where two parties each acquire rights and responsibilities simultaneously.

A *right* ordinarily "confers an advantageous position," to put it formally; having a right means that your will is favored over someone else's. Rights-morality centers on what is coming to you. Duty-morality centers on what is *required* of you.

The Declaration of Independence says that "We hold these truths to be self-evident, that all men are created equal, that they are endowed by their Creator with certain unalienable Rights, that among these are Life, Liberty and the pursuit of Happiness. That to secure these rights, Governments are instituted among Men...."

It could also have said, "We hold these truths to be self-evident, that all men are created equal, that they are endowed by their Creator with certain unalienable Duties, that among these are safeguarding Life, Liberty and the pursuit of Happiness. That to make sure of these duties, Governments are instituted among Men...."

What's the difference? Jefferson's version is famous for eloquence, and only a lunatic would suggest that it ought to have been written differently. But this is a thought-experiment, not a proposed rewrite.

Jefferson's is easier to understand—though of course we are considerably more familiar with it.

But when we speak of rights, we tend to speak of *the individuals immediately concerned* on the one hand, and the *vast vague public* on the other. To achieve, on the other hand, the *effect* of granting a right by using the *mechanism* of duty, it's natural to impose specific duties on the whole public—you have a *right* to life and liberty versus a *duty to safeguard* life and liberty. In the first case, we award a right without saying how we will deliver it; "the government will take care of things" is a bad idea to propose to the citizenry, and over the generations (although mainly in the 20th century) we have seen the United States government grow bigger and more powerful, and its citizens more passive, while "rights" have proliferated. There are many causes. But the morality of rights must be one.

In the second version, we have imposed a specific duty on every citizen. (You have a duty to safeguard your fellow citizen's life, liberty, and pursuit of happiness.) Even the dutiful citizen will have a hard time carrying out these duties without the government's doing most of the work. But at least the government and the citizen pull in the same direction. Instead of one being the passive recipient and the other an all-powerful Fairy Godmother, the citizen and his government share the same duties. (Some have argued that police duties must be forbidden to the public—but that's a different question.)

Does the public actually *care* about any duties except mandatory legal ones? Surely it doesn't care about "philosophical duties"? But "Uncle Sam wants *you* for the United States Army" was a highly successful recruiting poster. When vague desiderata are translated into concrete duties—"only you can prevent forest fires"—the public takes note.

Of course we could say that "granting an individual some right *implies* imposing on the whole public or its representatives a corresponding duty." True. But the idea that the public will draw a conclusion just because the inference is logically possible is one of the great absurdities of academic philosophy. The public has other things to do than sift through known propositions looking for inferences to draw.

## The Foreground of Human Dignity

I've now discussed two of the "background" questions pertaining to human dignity—secular versus religious morality, and a "morality of rights" versus a "morality of duties"; on to a few cases.

First, some passages from the Bible and the Talmud that deal with treatment of the sick, the weak, the unprotected—the sort of problem bioethics frequently deals with. Then some modern problems suggested by bioethics directly.

In Judaism as in Christianity, the basis for all assertions regarding the proper treatment of our fellow men are the verses in which man is said to be created in the image of God. "And God said, Let us make man in our image, after our likeness" (*Genesis* 1:26, cf. 5:1-3 and 9:5-7). Judaism is a system of duties imposed on the Jewish people. Many deal with the treatment of fellow human beings. To give some idea of the character of these duties, I cite the Talmud and other classic rabbinic writings—which play roughly the same role in Judaism as the New Testament does in Christianity. (You can no more understand Judaism without the Talmud than you can Christianity without the New Testament. In fact the Talmud emerged from roughly the same community during roughly the same period as the New

Testament.) Practicing Jews don't consult the Talmud to learn their duties; they consult their rabbis or more recent legal writings that are ultimately based on the Talmud. But that is a detail. It's enough to say that observant Jews, although they are only a small minority of *all* Jews (who are a small enough minority themselves, God knows), are rigorous in keeping the commandments; and the Talmud provides a detailed guide to how these commandments are to be obeyed.

A Talmudic passage: "As to him who has nothing but refuses to take [charity], let him first be asked to give a pledge and let him *then* be asked to take, so that his mind will be cheered" (*Ketuvot* 67b).

At first, the passage seems strongly in keeping with "inalienable rights" and human dignity. Everyone has a right to sustenance, delivered in a way that doesn't compromise his self-respect. The rabbinic tradition is obsessed with giving charity *and* with giving it in the right way: "He who gives charity in secret [anonymously] is greater than Moses" (*Baba Basra* 9b). In a famous passage, Maimonides lists eight degrees of charity, where the greatest consists of giving someone a job, setting him up in business, or otherwise making him self-supporting.

But the charity-case in this passage has *refused* to take charity. He'd rather starve than be a public burden.

How could the Talmud's instructions be re-phrased in the language of rights? "The poor have a right to refuse charity, and then to be approached by someone who suggests that what is actually charity should be treated as a loan against collateral"? A strange-sounding right. We can fine-tune a *duty* more accurately and with greater subtlety than a *right*—because we are addressing those who will actively deliver, not those who will passively receive. (I can tell you how to throw a curve ball but *not* how to have one thrown at you.)

And notice that to approach a situation in terms of rights drains away all ethical content. "You have a right to be supported if you can't support yourself; you have a right to be supported in such-and-such a way." No good deeds or ethical achievements are contemplated.

(The Talmud's instructions are based—arguably—on something like "human dignity"—but is human dignity a strong enough idea to justify this sort of aggressive help? When you give charity tactfully, you show respect for human dignity. When you help a man who has refused charity, it's arguable that your motivation is human *sanctity*.)

Human beings rise (or sink) to the occasion.

Again: we can fine-tune a duty more accurately and with greater subtlety than a right, because we are addressing those who will actively deliver, not those who will passively receive. Another Talmudic passage: "Rav Yonah said: It is not written, Happy is he who gives to the poor, but Happy is he who *considers* the poor (*Psalms* 41:1)—that is, he who ponders how to fulfill the command to help the poor" (*Talmud Yerushalmi*).[5] This instruction tells would-be charity-givers to *think*. It says, in effect, "We can and will give you detailed instructions, but you must apply them thoughtfully, not by rote." In the language of rights we would have to say, "You are entitled to have someone think about how to help you"—another implausible-sounding right, impossible to enforce.

There are endless Talmudic instructions (based on Biblical verses) that enjoin care for and kindness to the sick, young, old, unprotected. But these are all subsumed in a general instruction that is even more important: one must perform "acts of loving-kindness." "Shim'on the Just used to say, The universe stands on three things: on Torah, on worship, and on acts of loving-kindness" (*Mishnah Avos*). "Rav Elazar said: Giving charity is greater than all sacrifice…. But acts of loving-kindness are greater than giving charity" (*Sukkah* 49b). Such duties cannot possibly be rephrased in rights-language. ("You are entitled to live in a world in which some people are duty-bound to perform acts of loving-kindness"?)

In all these cases, rights-based language is opaque and passive and sometimes impossible.

Let's consider some modern cases. Terry Schiavo's death was a tragic watershed that will be discussed for years. (Briefly, Mrs. Schiavo was either comatose or mostly but not entirely comatose, depending on whom you believe; she was unable to feed herself; although her parents pleaded for her life, legal authorities ordered that she be starved to death.) I will consider just one aspect of the case: certain elected officials tried to intervene on behalf of Mrs. Schiavo's parents. But polls suggested that the public regarded the case as none of its business and wanted politicians to butt out.

Ordinarily, refusing to feed someone who can't feed herself is murder. And virtually all ethical systems require us to help the weak and the sick, not starve them. There was plenty to argue about in this case; it's conceivable (at least remotely) that Mrs. Schiavo actually left instructions that her life should be ended if she were comatose, and it's certainly conceivable that she *was* comatose; and there are many other debatable points. One thing that is *not* debatable is that the public should have been part of the debate. When murder enters the picture, the public is automatically involved. Murder is a crime against the public. Why on earth would the public have regarded this case as none of its business?

Perhaps because of the warped viewpoint yielded by rights-language and rights-morality? If we speak only of *rights*, we have a case in which a woman's right to live is in question, along with her right to human dignity, and a husband's versus a parent's right to speak for someone who can't speak for herself. Where is the public in all this? The public's only role is the usual vague one of ensuring (in some unspecified way) that all rights be enforced. I am not speaking here of *laws* or *absolutes* that are hard-wired into the ethics of rights versus duties. I am discussing *tendencies*. When we speak of rights, we *tend* to speak of *the individuals immediately concerned* on the one hand and the *vast vague public* on the other.

But if we translate rights-language to duty-language, "you have a right to life" becomes "you have a duty to safeguard life." Instead of "you have the right as a husband to speak for your incapacitated wife," we get "you have a duty to listen to a husband if his wife is incapacitated."

How *should* the Terry Schiavo case have been decided? We notice first that "human dignity" doesn't help. But common sense might have. Suspected criminals must be guilty "beyond a reasonable doubt." Was Mrs. Schiavo wholly comatose and unresponsive, *beyond a reasonable doubt*? Was it more consistent with human dignity to kill her than to continue helping her to live, *beyond a reasonable doubt*? Was the public's duty to safeguard life overridden by other factors in this case, *beyond a reasonable doubt*? These are simple questions—but if anyone discussed them, I missed it.

There's a more specific issue too, suggested by duty-morality versus rights-morality. In the Judeo-Christian view, if you have a *right* to live, you also have a *duty* to live. Except in terribly abnormal circumstances (which are recognized in Jewish law), it is unlawful in Judaism to take your own life or to instruct anyone else to take it. But what good is it to stay alive if you are comatose, suffering; blind? Could Milton possibly have been *right* when he told us, in *On his blindness*, that "they also serve who only stand and wait?" Could Shakespeare have been right when, in one of the most extraordinary passages in *Lear*, Gloucester's loving son says to him (after Gloucester has been cruelly abused, tormented and blinded), "Thy life's a *miracle*!"?

To remain alive and serve God and man the best you can when you really want life to be over is profoundly inspiring—to man and (probably) to God. But what about a Terry Schiavo, evidently unable to do *anything*? She *was indeed* able to do something—maybe only one thing, but maybe the most important. She was able to inspire love. And when the topic is love, we need all the education we can get. "The Torah *for its own sake* is a law of love" (*Sukkah* 49b). (When the Talmud insists that one must grapple with Torah *for its own sake*, it foreshadows Kant's insistence that duty done *for its own sake* equals human freedom. In Judaism you achieve sanctity—in Kant freedom—by doing your duty simply *to do it*.)

Consider two of the horrors of human cloning and "designer babies." Any technology gets better; children of parents who order up the smartest possible babies in year *n* will easily be outclassed by younger children whose parents do the same ten years later (while probably paying a lot less for much spiffier models). Designer children will grow obsolete, just like PCs. (Bill McKibben discusses this possibility in *Enough*.[6])

Here's an even more horrifying possibility. I've heard and read several times (on cable TV and in ordinary newspapers) this justification for human cloning: consider parents whose child has contracted a fatal disease or been killed in an accident. Those parents could use tissue from the doomed or dead child to clone an exact duplicate—which would make the loss of the original less hard to bear.

But imagine the thoughts of the doomed original. "I'm sick and dying, but my parents have no need to grieve too much. Do they even need to grieve at all? Before long I'll be replaced by an exact duplicate, and life will carry on exactly as before, for everyone *except me*."

"Someone else will wear my clothes, sit at my place, speak my lines and impersonate me; he will make people believe I am still alive. Everyone will enjoy the performance—but I won't."

*Thanks to modern technology, my death won't matter.* And the thought that your own beloved child could die and you are then solaced by a genetic duplicate is deeply obscene. (Yet it's possible that some parents would buy it.)

These cases are (again) beyond the realm of rights. If we say "you have a right to a death that matters," doesn't this right apply to unloved children too?—maybe orphans, maybe children of parents who don't care? And what about unloved adults? Or the elderly who have no children or living spouse or relatives? The right in itself is good; who could disapprove? But it is also ridiculous, because even if we grant it there is no conceivable way to enforce it, to *deliver* on this promise.

Once again, duty-morality seems more appropriate than rights-morality. And even though we are attempting to prevent crimes against human dignity, it's more accurate to say that our goal is to prevent crimes against human *sanctity*. We are dealing with the creation of human life. We are ordering man not to take this business out of God's hands—or out of nature's, if you prefer. (But why *shouldn't* he take it out of "nature's" hands? The reason not to take it out of God's is that "human sanctity" means "created in God's image"—not in some image cooked up by human engineers.)

In short, secularized, sanitized ideas are too weak for the task at hand. "Human sanctity" is a stronger idea than "human dignity." An ethics based on universal, permanent rights is weaker, more opaque, and more passive than an ethics based on universal duties.

I myself believe that "dignity" in the end is a religious idea, and that we can't be rational *and* moral animals unless we acknowledge the God of Israel. But the ethics of duty is another matter. Although it barely exists on philosophy's agenda, there are reasons to believe that the ethics of duty is intrinsically superior to the ethics of rights—more precise and more expressive—regardless of your views on religion. (In fact, we might trace the actual decline of religion not to Darwin and modern science but to the rise of rights-talk versus the old duties-talk, which preceded Darwin by more than a century. Most people don't want duties but welcome rights. If duties are imposed on them, they demand to know—reasonably enough—on whose authority; and the only plausible answer comes down to "on God's authority." But if someone awards you a right, why ask questions?)

In any event, modern life is secularized, and that can't be undone. But Americans are *not* secularized. Many are Christian (some actively Christian); a few are actively Jewish.

Bioethics touches every life. This field can't possibly be allowed to develop in the secular ghetto where modern intellectuals lives. Bioethics *needs* Judeo-Christian ideas: *must understand* human sanctity and not just dignity, *must understand* the world of duties and not only of rights. Even atheists might gain from a broader, more tolerant, more *multi-cultural* approach to the hard questions of the human spirit.

## Notes

[1] See Michael Novak, *On Two Wings: Humble Faith and Common Sense at the American Founding* (San Francisco, California: Encounter, 2002); Jonathan Jacobs, "Return to the Sources: Political Hebraism and the Making of Modern Politics," *Hebraic Political Studies*, volume 1, number 3 (Spring 2006), pp. 328-342; Fania Oz-Salzberger, "The Political Thought of John Locke and the Significance of Political Hebraism," *Hebraic Political Studies*, volume 1, number 5 (Fall 2006), pp. 568-592.

[2] Simon Blackburn, *Being Good: A Short Introduction to Ethics* (New York: Oxford University Press, 2003).

[3] Abraham Lincoln, "Reply to Loyal Colored People of Baltimore upon Presentation of a Bible," September 7, 1864 in *Collected Works of Abraham Lincoln*, ed. Roy P. Basler (New Brunswick, New Jersey: Rutgers University Press, 1953), volume 7, p. 543.

[4] *Oxford English Dictionary*, 2nd ed. (Oxford: Oxford University Press, 1989).

[5] Cited in *A Rabbinic Anthology*, ed. Claude J. G. Montefiore and Herbert M. J. Loewe (Philadelphia: Jewish Publication Society, 1960).

[6] Bill McKibben, *Enough: Staying Human in an Engineered Age* (New York: Holt, 2003).

# Part V.
# Theories of Human Dignity

# 16

# The Nature and Basis of Human Dignity

## Patrick Lee and Robert P. George

Some people hold that all human beings have a special type of dignity that is the basis for (1) the obligation all of us have not to kill them, (2) the obligation to take their well-being into account when we act, and (3) even the obligation to treat them as we would have them treat us. Indeed, those who hold that all human beings possess a special type of dignity almost always also hold that human beings are equal in fundamental dignity. They maintain that there is no class of human beings to which other human beings should be subordinated when considering their interests or their well-being, and when devising laws and social policies.

Other thinkers deny that all human beings have a special type of dignity. They maintain that only some human beings, because of their possession of certain characteristics in addition to their humanity (for example, an immediately exercisable capacity for self-consciousness, or for rational deliberation), have full moral worth. In this paper we defend the first of these two positions. We argue that all human beings, regardless of age, size, stage of development, or immediately exercisable capacities, have equal fundamental dignity.

Let us begin by offering a few preliminary thoughts on the general concept of *dignity*. Dignity is not a distinct property or quality, like a body's color, or an organ's function. Although there are different types of dignity, in each case the word refers to a property or properties—different ones in different circumstances—that cause one to *excel*, and thus elicit or merit respect from others. Our focus will be on the dignity of a person or personal dignity. The dignity of a *person* is that whereby a person excels other beings, especially other animals, and merits respect or consideration from other persons. We will argue that what distinguishes human beings from other animals, what makes human beings *persons* rather than *things*, is their rational nature. Human beings are rational creatures by virtue of possessing natural capacities for conceptual thought, deliberation, and free choice, that is, the natural capacity to shape their own lives.

These basic, natural capacities to reason and make free choices are possessed by every human being, even those who cannot immediately exercise them. One's existence as a person thus derives from the kind of substantial entity one is, a human being—and this is the ground for dignity in the most important sense. Because personhood is based on the kind of being one is—a substantial entity whose nature is a *rational* nature—one cannot lose one's fundamental personal dignity as long as one exists as a human being.

There are other senses of the word "dignity." First, there is a type of dignity that varies in degree, which is the *manifestation* or *actualization* of those capacities that distinguish humans from other animals. Thus, slipping on a banana peel (being reduced for a moment to a passive object), or losing one's independence and privacy (especially as regards our basic bodily functions), detract from our dignity in this sense. However, while this dignity seems to be compromised in certain situations, it is never completely lost. Moreover, this dignity, which varies in degree, is distinct from the more basic dignity that derives from simply being a person.

Second, it is important also to distinguish one's *sense of* dignity. Something may harm one's *sense of* dignity without damaging or compromising one's real dignity. People who become dependent on others often *feel* a certain loss of dignity. Yet their personal dignity, and even their manifestation of that dignity, may not have been harmed at all. Often one's sense of dignity can be at variance with one's real dignity. Those who are sick, and who bear their suffering in a courageous or holy manner, often inspire others even though they themselves may *feel* a loss of dignity.

Third, a person may be treated in a way at odds with his or her personal dignity. Human beings may be enslaved, they may be killed unjustly, raped, scorned, coerced, or wrongly imprisoned. Such treatment is undignified, yet it too, like a person's low sense of dignity, does not diminish a victim's personal dignity; the slave or the murder victim are wronged precisely because they are treated in a way at odds with their genuine personal dignity.

In truth, all human beings have real dignity simply because they are persons—entities with a natural capacity for thought and free choice. *All* human beings have this capacity, so all human beings are persons. Each human being therefore deserves to be treated by all other human beings with respect and consideration. It is precisely this truth that is at stake in the debates about killing human embryos, fetuses, and severely retarded, demented, or debilitated human beings, and in many other debates in bioethics.

To explain the basis of human dignity, and how human beings inherently possess dignity, we will first explain more precisely the problem of the basis of human dignity; then we will examine proposals that deny that every human being has an intrinsic dignity that grounds full moral worth; then we will present and defend our position; finally, we will show how the feature (nature) that grounds full moral worth is possessed by human beings in all developmental stages, including the embryonic, fetal, and infant stages, and in all conditions, including severely cognitively impaired conditions (sometimes called "marginal cases").

## The Problem of Moral Status

The general problem regarding the ground of moral status can be expressed as follows. It seems that it is morally permissible to *use* some living things, to consume them, or to experiment on them for our own benefit (without their consent, or perhaps when they are unable to give or withhold consent), but that it is not morally permissible to treat other beings in this way. The question is: where do we draw the line between those two sorts of beings? By what criterion do we draw that line? Or perhaps there just is no such line, and we should always seek to preserve *all* beings, of whatever sort.

But we must eat, we must use some entities for food and shelter, and in doing so we inevitably destroy them. When we eat we convert entities of one nature into another and thus destroy them. Moreover, no one claims that we should not try to eradicate harmful bacteria (which are forms of life). That is, we should kill harmful bacteria in order to protect ourselves and our children. And it seems clear that we must harvest wheat and rice for food, and trees for shelter. So, plainly it is permissible to kill and use some living things. Given that it is not morally permissible to kill just any type of being, it follows that a line must be drawn, a line between those entities it is morally permissible to use, consume, and destroy, and those it is not permissible to use, consume, and destroy. How can the line be drawn in a non-arbitrary way?

Various criteria for where the line should be drawn have been proposed: sentience, consciousness, self-awareness, rationality, or being a moral agent (the last two come to the same thing). We will argue that the criterion is: having a rational nature, that is, having the natural capacity to reason and make free choices, a capacity it ordinarily takes months, or even years, to actualize, and which various impediments might prevent from being brought to full actualization, at least in this life. Thus, every human being has full moral worth or dignity, for every human being possesses such a rational nature.

While membership in the species *Homo sapiens* is sufficient for full moral worth, it is not in any direct sense the criterion for moral worth. If we discovered extra-terrestrial beings of a rational nature, or if we found that some other terrestrial species did have a rational nature, then we would owe such beings full moral respect. Still, all members of the human species do have full moral worth, because all of them do have a rational nature and are moral agents, though many of them are not able immediately to exercise those basic capacities. One could also say that the criterion for full moral worth is *being a person*, since a person is a rational and morally responsible subject.\*

---

\* Boethius's definition of *person*, especially as interpreted by St. Thomas Aquinas, is still valid: "An individual substance (that is, a unique substance) of a rational nature." So, neither a nature held in common by many, nor a part is a person. But every whole human being performing its own actions, including actions such as growth toward the mature stage of a human, *is* a person. See Boethius, *De Duobus*

The other suggestions listed above, we believe, are not tenable as criteria for full moral worth, and, worse yet, often have the practical effect of leading to the denial that human beings have full moral worth, rather than simply adding other beings to the set of beings deserving full moral respect.[1] Hence it is vital to explain how "being a person"—that is, being a distinct substance with the basic natural capacities for conceptual thought and free choice—is the ground for the possession of basic rights.

## The Capacity for Enjoyment or Suffering as a Criterion

Animal welfarists argue that the criterion for moral worth is simply the ability to experience enjoyment and suffering. Peter Singer, for example, quotes Jeremy Bentham: "The question is not, Can they *reason*? nor Can they *talk*? but, Can they *suffer*?"[2] Singer then presents the following argument for this position:

> The capacity for suffering and enjoyment is *a prerequisite for having interests at all*, a condition that must be satisfied before we can speak of interests in a meaningful way.... A stone does not have interests because it cannot suffer. Nothing that we can do to it could possibly make any difference to its welfare. The capacity for suffering and enjoyment is, however, not only necessary, but also sufficient for us to say that a being has interests—at an absolute minimum, an interest in not suffering.[3]

In short, Singer's argument is: All and only beings that have interests have moral status; but all and only beings that can (now) experience suffering or enjoyment have interests; therefore, all and only beings that can (now) experience suffering or enjoyment have moral status.

The major difficulties with Singer's position all follow from the fact that his proposed criterion for moral status involves the possession of an accidental attribute that varies in degree. Both the capacity for suffering and the possession of interests are properties that

---

*Naturis,* and St. Thomas Aquinas, *Summa Theologiae,* Pt. I, q. 29, a. 1.

different beings have in different degrees, and the interests themselves are possessed in varying degrees. As we shall show, this feature of Singer's theory leads to untenable conclusions.

Although Singer has made famous the slogan, "All animals are equal," this theory actually leads to *denying* that all animals, including all humans, have equal moral worth or basic rights. Singer means that "all animals are equal" in the sense that all animals are due "equal consideration." Where the interests of two animals *are* similar in quality and magnitude, then those interests should be counted as equal when deciding what to do, both as individuals and in social policies and actions. However, as Singer himself points out, on this view, some animals can perform actions that others cannot, and thus have interests that those others do not. So the moral status of all animals is not, in fact, equal. One would not be required to extend the right to vote—or to education in reading and arithmetic—to pigs, since they are unable to perform such actions. This point leads to several problems when we attempt to compare interests. According to this view, it is the *interests* that matter, not *the kind of being* that is affected by one's actions. So, on this view, it would logically follow that if a human child had a toothache and a juvenile rat had a slightly more severe toothache, then we would be morally required to devote our resources to alleviating the rat's toothache rather than the human's.

Moreover, a human newborn infant who will die shortly (and so does not appear to have long-term future interests) or a severely cognitively impaired human will be due *less* consideration than a more mature horse or pig, on the ground that the mature horse or pig will have richer and more developed interests. Since the horse and the pig have higher cognitive and emotional capacities (in the sense of immediately or nearly immediately exercisable capacities) than the newborn infant (that will die shortly) and the severely cognitively impaired human, and since it is the interests that directly count morally, not the beings that have those interests, the interests of the horse and the pig should (on this account) be preferred to the interests of the newborn or the severely cognitively impaired human.[4]

On the other hand, when we note the differences between types of interests, then Singer's position actually implies an indirect moral elitism. It is true that according to this position no individual animal is greater than another solely on the ground of its species (that is, according to its substantial nature). Still, one animal will be due more consideration—indirectly—if it has capacities for higher or more complex mental functions. As Singer puts it: "Within these limits we could still hold that, for instance, it is worse to kill a *normal* adult human, with a capacity for self-awareness, and the ability to plan for the future and have meaningful relations with others, than it is to kill a mouse, which presumably does not share all of these characteristics...."[5] But this difference between degrees of capacity for suffering and enjoyment will also apply to individuals within each species. And so, on this view, while a human will normally have a greater capacity for suffering and enjoyment than other animals, and so will have a higher moral status (indirectly), so too, more intelligent and sophisticated human individuals will have a greater capacity for suffering and enjoyment than less intelligent and less sophisticated human individuals, and so the former will have a higher moral status than the latter. As Richard Arneson expressed this point, "For after all it is just as true that a creative genius has richer and more complex interests than those of an ordinary average Joe as it is true that a human has richer and more complex interests than a baboon."[6]

These difficulties are all due to the selection of a criterion of moral worth that varies in degree. If the moral status-conferring attribute varies in degree—whether it be the capacity for enjoyment or suffering, or another attribute that comes in different degrees—it will follow that some humans will possess that attribute to a lesser extent than some nonhuman animals, and so inevitably some interests of some nonhuman animals will trump the interests of some humans. Also, it will follow that some humans will possess the attribute in question to a higher degree than other humans, with the result that not all humans will be equal in fundamental moral worth, i.e., *dignity*. True, some philosophers bite the bullet on these results. But in our judgment this is too high a price to pay. A sound view of worth and dignity will not entail such difficulties.

On such a view, the criterion for moral worth must be the possession of a property that does not itself vary in degree—it must, that is, be the possession of a *nature*. Being of moral worth must be grounded in an entity's existence as a substance of a certain sort (we discuss what sort in more detail below) rather than in the possession of a set of accidental or variable properties.

This view explains why our moral concern is for persons, rather than for their properties. After all, when dealing with other persons it is clear that the locus of value is the persons themselves. Persons are not mere vehicles for what is intrinsically valuable: one's child, one's neighbor, or even a stranger, are not valuable only because of the valuable attributes they possess. If persons were valuable as mere vehicles for something else—some other quality that is regarded as what is *really* of value—then it would follow that the basic moral rule would be simply to maximize those valuable attributes. It would not be morally wrong to kill a child, no matter what age, if doing so enabled one to have two children in the future, and thus to bring it about that there were two vehicles for intrinsic value rather than one.

On the contrary, we are aware that persons themselves—the substantial entities they are—are intrinsically valuable. But if that is so, then it would make sense that what distinguishes those entities that have full moral status (inherent dignity) from those that do not should be the type of substantial entity they are, rather than any accidental attributes they possess. True, it is not self-contradictory to hold that the person himself is valuable, but only in virtue of some accidental attributes he or she possesses. Still, it is more natural, and more theoretically economical, to suppose that *what* has full moral status, and *that in virtue of which* he or she has full moral status, are one and the same.

Moreover, this position more closely tracks the characteristics we find in genuine care or love. Our genuine love for a person remains, or should remain, for as long as that person continues to exist, and is not dependent on his or her possessing further attributes. That is, it seems to be the nature of care or love that it be unconditional, that we continue to desire the well-being or fulfillment of one we love for as long as he or she exists. Of course, this still leaves open the question whether continuing to live is always part of a person's well-being or fulfillment; we do maintain that a person's life always *is* in itself a good, but that is a distinct question from the one being considered just now.

We shall argue below that being a substance *with a rational nature* is the criterion for moral worth. But the point now is that, whatever the specific criterion is, it involves existing as a type of *substance*—being a certain type of thing—rather than possessing a set of accidental or variable properties. In consequence, every substance of that sort will have full moral worth, and any substance of that sort will have a higher and different type of moral worth than entities that are not of that type.[7]

Moreover, the argument for sentience, or the ability to experience suffering and enjoyment, as *the* basic criterion of moral status, supposes that only such beings have interests. However, although rocks do not seem to have interests, the same cannot be said about plants. It is not true that only beings with feelings or some level of consciousness can be reasonably considered to have interests. It is clear that living beings are fulfilled by certain conditions and damaged by others. As Paul Taylor, who defends a biocentrist view (according to which *all* living beings have moral worth), explains,

> We can think of the good of an individual nonhuman organism as consisting in the full development of its biological powers. Its good is realized to the extent that it is strong and healthy.[8]

One can then say that what promotes the organism's survival and flourishing is *in its interest* and what diminishes its chances of survival or flourishing is *against its interests*. Further, while it may be initially plausible to think that all animals have rights because they have interests, it is considerably less plausible to think that all living beings (which include wheat, corn, and rice, not to mention weeds and bacteria) have rights. But the interest argument would lead to that position.

Finally, the arguments advanced by Singer and Taylor do not actually attempt to establish that nonhuman animals and other living things have moral rights in the full sense of the term. We think it is true of *every* living being, in some way, that we should not *wantonly* destroy or damage it.* With sentient beings, whether their life goes

---

* Could this be true of every being, living or not? It is hard to see what the good or fulfillment of a non-living being is, since on that level it is hard to know just what are the basic, substantial entities as opposed to aggregates of entities. Thus, when we breathe we convert oxygen and carbon molecules into carbon dioxide molecules—have we destroyed the oxygen in that process or have we only rear-

well or badly for them will significantly include their pleasure, comfort, or lack of suffering. And so their flourishing includes pleasure and lack of pain (though it also includes other things such as their life and their activities). Yet it does not follow from these points that they have full basic and inherent dignity (moral worth) or rights.[9] There simply is no conceptual connection between pleasure and pain (enjoyment and suffering) on the one hand, and full moral worth (including genuine rights), on the other hand.[10]

However, almost no one actually argues that these beings have basic dignity or full moral rights. Rather, biocentrists argue that all living things merit *some* consideration, but also hold that human beings are due *more* consideration (though not, apparently, different in kind).[11] In effect, instead of actually holding that all living beings (in the case of biocentrists) or all animals (in the case of animal welfarists) have *rights*, they have simply denied the existence of rights in the full sense of the term.* Instead, they hold only that all living beings (or animals or higher mammals) deserve some varying degree of respect or consideration. We agree with this point, but we also maintain that every human being is a subject of rights, that is, every human being should be treated according to the golden rule, and it is absolutely wrong intentionally to kill any innocent human being or intentionally to deprive any innocent human being of any basic, intrinsic good.† In other words, we grant that we should take account of the flourishing of living beings, and the pleasures and pains of nonhuman animals. But we are not morally related to them in the same way that we are related to other beings who, like ourselves, have a rational nature—beings whom (out of fairness) we should treat as we would have them treat us.

But one might argue for animal rights starting from our natural empathy or affection for them (though most people's natural empathy or affection, notably, does *not* extend to all animals, for example, to spiders or snakes). If one identifies what is to be protected and pursued with what can be felt, that is, enjoyed or suffered in some way,

---

ranged the atoms in their constitution? It is hard to say.

* Peter Singer acknowledges that he is "not convinced that the notion of a moral right is a helpful or meaningful one, except when it is used as a shorthand way of referring to more fundamental considerations."

† We are simply abstracting from the issue of capital punishment in this essay.

then one might conclude that every entity that can have pleasure or pain deserves (equal?) consideration. If the only intrinsic good were what can be enjoyed, and the only intrinsic bad were suffering, then it would not be incoherent to hold that sentience is the criterion of moral standing, that is, that every entity with sentience has (some degree of) moral standing. In other words, it seems that one can present an *argument* for animal rights that begins from natural feelings of empathy only by way of a hedonistic theory of value. We can think of no other arguments that begin from that natural empathy with, or affection for, other animals.

But hedonism as a general theory of value is mistaken. The good is not exhausted by the experiential—the key tenet of hedonism. Real understanding of the way things are, for example, is pleasurable because it is fulfilling or perfective of us, not vice versa. The same is true of life, health, or skillful performance (one enjoys running a good race because it is a genuine accomplishment, a skillful performance, rather than vice versa). So, as Plato and Aristotle pointed out, hedonism places the cart before the horse.

Our desires are not purely arbitrary: we are capable of desiring certain things while other things leave us unmoved, uninterested. So, prior to being desired, the object desired must have something about it that makes it *fitting*, or *suitable*, to being desired. What makes it fitting to us is that it would *fulfill* or *perfect* us in some way or other. Thus, what makes a thing good cannot consist in its being enjoyed, or in its satisfying desires or preferences. Rather, desires and preferences are rational only if they are in line with what is genuinely good, that is, genuinely fulfilling.* So, hedonism is mistaken. It cannot

---

* Thus, the pleasures of the sadist or child molester are in themselves bad; it is false to say that such pleasures are bad only because of the harm or pain involved in their total contexts. It is false to say: "It was bad for him to cause so much pain, but at least he enjoyed it." Pleasure is secondary, an aspect of a larger situation or condition (such as health, physical, and emotional); what is central is what is really fulfilling. Pleasure is not a good like understanding or health, which are goods or perfections by themselves—that is, are good in themselves even if in a context that is overall bad or if accompanied by many bads. Rather, pleasure is good (desirable, worthwhile, perfective) if and only if attached to a fulfilling or perfective activity or condition. Pleasure is a good: a fulfilling activity or condition is better with it than without it. But pleasure is unlike full-fledged goods in that it is not a genuine good apart from some other, fulfilling activity or condition. It is a good if and only

then provide support for the view that sentience (or the capacity for suffering and enjoyment) is the criterion of full moral worth. While it is wrong to damage or kill a plant wantonly, still it can be morally right to do so for a good reason. Similarly, it is wrong wantonly to damage or kill a non-rational animal, but it can be morally right to do so for a good reason.*

## The Difference in Kind Between Human Beings and Other Animals

Human beings are fundamentally different in kind from other animals, not just genetically but in having a rational nature (that is, a nature characterized by basic natural capacities for conceptual thought, deliberation and free choice). Human beings perform *acts of understanding*, or conceptual thought, and such acts are fundamentally different kinds of acts than acts of sensing, perceiving, or imaging. An act of understanding is the grasping of, or awareness of, a nature shared in common by many things. In Aristotle's memorable phrase, to understand is not just to know water (by sensing or perceiving this water), but to know what it is to be water.[12] By our senses and perceptual abilities we know the individual qualities and quantities modifying our sense organs—this color or this shape, for example. But by understanding (conceptual thought) we apprehend a nature held in common by many entities—not this or that instance of water, but what it is to be water. By contrast, the object of the sensory powers, including imagination, is always an individual, a *this* at a particular place and a particular time, a characteristic, such as this red, this shape, this tone, an object that is thoroughly conditioned by space and time.

---

if attached to another condition or activity that is already good.

* It is worth noting that nonhuman animals themselves not only regularly engage in killing each other, but many of them (lions and tigers, for example) seem to depend for their whole mode of living (and so their flourishing), on hunting and killing other animals. If nonhuman animals really did have full moral rights, however, we would be morally required to stop them from killing each other. Indeed, we would be morally required to invest considerable resources—economic, military, even—in order to protect zebras and antelopes from lions, sheep and foxes from wolves, and so on.

The contrast is evident upon examination of language. Proper names refer to individuals or groups of individuals that can be designated in a determinate time and place. Thus "Winston Churchill" is a name that refers to a determinate individual, whereas the nouns "human," "horse," "atom," and "organism" are common names. Common names do not designate determinate individuals or determinate groups of individuals (such as "those five people in the corner"). Rather, they designate *classes*. Thus, if we say, "Organisms are composed of cells," the word "organisms" designates the whole class of organisms, a class that extends indefinitely into the past and indefinitely into the future. All syntactical languages distinguish between proper names and common names.

But a class is not an arbitrary collection of individuals. It is a collection of individuals that have something in common. There is always some feature (or set of features), some intelligible nature or accidental attribute, that is the criterion of membership for the class. Thus, the class of organisms includes all, and only those, beings that have the nature of *living bodily substance*. And so, to understand the class as such, and not just be able to pick out individuals belonging to that class, one must understand the nature held in common. And to understand the class as a class (as we clearly do in reasoning) one must mentally apprehend the nature or features (or set of features) held in common by the members of the class and compare this to those individual members. Thus, to understand a proposition such as, "All organisms require nutrition for survival," one must understand a nature or universal content designated by the term "organisms": the term designates the nature or feature that entities must have in them in order to belong to that class.

Human beings quite obviously are aware of classes as classes. That is, they do more than assign individuals to a class based on a perceived similarity; they are aware of pluralities as holding natures or properties in common.[13] For example, one can perceive, without a concept, the similarity between two square shapes or two triangular shapes, something that other animals do as well as human beings. But human beings also grasp the criterion, the universal property or nature, by which the similars are grouped together.[14]

There are several considerations tending to confirm this fact. First, many universal judgments require an understanding of the nature of the things belonging to a class. If I understand, for example, that every organism is mortal, because every composite living thing is mortal, this is possible only if I mentally compare the nature, *organism*, with the nature, *composite living thing*, and see that the former entails the latter. That is, my judgment that every composite living thing can be decomposed and thus die, is based on my insight into the nature of a composite living thing. I have understood that the one nature, *subject to death*, is entailed by the other nature, *composite living being*, and *from* that knowledge I then advert to the thought of the individuals that possess those natures. In other words, I judge that individual composite living beings must be included within the class of individuals that are subject to death, but I judge *that* only in virtue of my seeing that the nature, *being subject to death*, is necessitated by the nature, *composite living being*. This point is also evident from the fact that I judge that a composite living being is *necessarily* capable of dying.* By the senses, one can grasp only an individual datum. Only by a distinct capacity, an intellect, only by apprehending *the nature* of a thing, can one grasp that a thing is *necessarily* thus or so.†

---

* True, something extrinsic could preserve it from death, but it is the sort of thing that is, by its nature, subject to death. This is the basis for the major premise in the classic example of a syllogism: All men are mortal; Socrates is a man; therefore, Socrates is mortal.

† Another example will illustrate this point. When children arrive at the age at which they can study logic, they provide evidence of the ability to grasp a nature or property held in common by many. They obviously do something qualitatively distinct from perceiving a concrete similarity. For example, when studying elementary logic, the child (or young man or woman) grasps the common pattern found in the following arguments:

    A. If it rains then the grass is wet.
       The grass is not wet.
       Therefore, it is not raining.
    B. If I had known you were coming, I would have baked you a cake.
       But I did not bake you a cake.
       So, (you can see that) I did not know you were coming.

We understand the difference between this type of argument, a *modus tollens* argument, and one that is similar but invalid, namely, the fallacy of affirming the consequent (If A then B, B, therefore A). But, what is more, we understand *why* the fallacy of affirming the consequent is invalid—namely, some other cause (or antecedent) could be, or could have been, present to lead to that effect. A computer, a mechanical device, can be programmed *to operate according to* the *modus tollens* and to react differently to (give a different output for) words arranged in the

The capacity for conceptual thought in human beings radically distinguishes them from other animals known to us. This capacity is at the root of most of the other distinguishing features of human beings. Thus, syntactical language, art, architecture, variety in social groupings and in other customs,[15] burying the dead, making tools, religion, fear of death (and elaborate defense mechanisms to ease living with that fear), wearing clothes, true courting of the opposite sex,[16] free choice and morality—all of these, and more, stem from the ability to reason and understand. Conceptual thought makes all of these specific acts possible by enabling human beings to escape fundamental limitations of two sorts. First, because of the capacity for conceptual thought, human beings' actions and consciousness are not restricted to the spatio-temporal present. Their awareness and their concern go beyond what can be perceived or imagined as connected immediately with the present.[17] Second, because of the capacity for conceptual thought, human beings can reflect back upon themselves and their place in reality, that is, they can attain an objective view, and they can attempt to be objective in their assessments and choices. Other animals give no evidence at all of being able to do either of these things; on the contrary, they seem thoroughly tied to the here and now, and unable to take an objective view of things as they are in themselves, or to attempt to do so.[18]

The capacity for conceptual thought is a capacity that human beings have in virtue of the kind of entity they are. That is, from the time they come to be, they are developing themselves toward the mature stage at which they will (unless prevented from doing so by disability or circumstances) perform such acts. Moreover, they are structured—genetically, and in the non-material aspect of themselves—in such a way that they are oriented toward maturing to this stage.* So,

---

pattern of the fallacy of affirming the consequent. But *understanding* the arguments (which humans do) and merely *operating according to* them because programmed to do so (the actions of computers) are entirely different types of actions. The first does, while the second does not, require the understanding or apprehending of a form or nature as distinct from its instances. (This is not to say that the nature exists separately from the individuals instantiating it, or as a universal, outside the mind. We hold that the nature exists in the mind as a universal but in the real as individuated.)

* The genetic (and epigenetic) structure orients them toward developing a complex brain that is suitable to be the substrate for conceptual thought; that is, it is

every human being, including human infants and unborn human beings, has this basic natural capacity for conceptual thought.*

Human beings also have the basic natural capacity or potentiality to deliberate among options and make free choices, choices that are not determined by the events that preceded them, but are determined by the person making the choice in the very act of choosing. That is, for some choices, the antecedent events are not sufficient to bring it about that these choices be made in this way rather than another way. In such choices, a person could have chosen the other option, or not chosen at all, under the very same conditions. If a choice is free, then, given everything that happened to the person up to the point just prior to his choice—including everything in his environment, everything in his heredity, everything in his understanding and in his character—it was still possible for him to choose the other option, or not to choose at all. Expressed positively: he himself in the very act of choosing determines the content of his willing. Human beings are ultimate authors of their own acts of will and partial authors (together with nature and nurture) of their own character.[19]

How, then, does a person finally choose one course of action rather than another? The person by his own act of choosing directs his will toward this option rather than that one, and in such a way that he

---

capable of providing the kind of sense experience and organization of sense experience that is suitable for data for concepts. Since the object of conceptual thought is not restricted to a particular place and time, this is evidence that the power of conceptual thought is non-material. So, we hold that human beings have a non-material aspect, the powers of conceptual thought and free choice.

* It is not essential to the defense of human dignity to argue that *only* humans have this power of conceptual thought and (to be discussed in a moment) free choice. However, there is no evidence of such conceptual thought or free choice in other animals. It is sometimes argued that perhaps some nonhuman animals do have minds like humans do, only at a diminished level. Perhaps, it is speculated, it is only the complexity of the human brain, a difference only in degree, that distinguishes humans from other animals. Perhaps other primates are intelligent but they have lacked the opportunities to manifest their latent intelligence. But such speculation is misguided. While intelligence is not directly observable, it is unreasonable to think that an intelligence of the same type as human intelligence, no matter how diminished, would fail to manifest itself in at least some of its characteristic effects. If a group of beings possesses a power, and possesses that power over many years (even decades or centuries), it is implausible to think that such a power would not be actualized.

could, in those very same circumstances, have chosen otherwise.[20]

A good case can be made to support the position that human beings do make free choices.[21] First, objectively, when someone deliberates about which possible action to perform, each option (very often, in any case) has in it what it takes to be a possible object of choice. When persons deliberate, and find some distinctive good in different, incompatible, possible actions, they are free, for: (a) they have the capacity to understand the distinct types of good or fulfillment found (directly or indirectly) in the different possible courses of action, and (b) they are capable of willing whatever they understand to be good (fulfilling) in some way or other.[22] That is, each alternative offers a distinct type of good or benefit, and it is up to the person deliberating which type of good he will choose.

For example, suppose a student chooses to go to law school rather than to medical school. When he deliberates, both options have a distinctive sort of goodness or attractiveness. Each offers some benefit the other one does not offer. So, since each alternative has some intelligible value in it (some goodness that is understood), then each alternative *can* be willed. And, second, while each is good to a certain extent, neither alternative (at least in many situations) is good, or better, in *every respect*. Here the role of conceptual thought, or intellect, becomes clear. The person deliberating is able to see, that is, to *understand*, that each alternative is good, but that none is best absolutely speaking, that is, according to every consideration, or in every respect. And so, neither the content of the option nor the strength of one or another desire, determines the choice. Hence there are acts of will in which one directs one's will toward this or that option without one's choosing being determined by antecedent events or causes. Human persons, then, are fundamentally distinct from other animals in that they have a nature entailing the potentialities for conceptual thought and free choice.

## Having a Rational Nature, or Being a Person, Is the Criterion for Full Moral Worth

Neither sentience nor life itself entails that those who possess them must be respected as ends in themselves or as creatures having full moral worth. Rather, having a rational nature is the ground of full moral worth.

The basis of this point can be explained, at least in part, in the following way. When one chooses an action, one chooses it for a reason, that is, for the sake of some good one thinks this action will help to realize. That good may itself be a way of realizing some further good, and that good a means to another, and so on. But the chain of instrumental goods cannot be infinite. So, there must be some ultimate reasons for one's choices, some goods that one recognizes as reasons for choosing that need no further support, that are not mere means to some further good.

Such ultimate reasons for choice are not arbitrarily selected. Intrinsic goods—that is, human goods that as basic aspects of human well-being and fulfillment provide more-than-merely-instrumental reasons for choices and actions—are not just whatever we happen to desire, perhaps different objects for different people.* Rather, the intellectual apprehension that a condition or activity is *really fulfilling* or *perfective* (of me and/or of others like me) is at the same time the apprehension that this condition or activity is a fitting object of pursuit, that is, that it would be worth pursuing.† These fundamental

---

* The Humean notion of practical reason contends that practical reason begins with given ends that are not rationally motivated. However, this view cannot, in the end, make sense of the fact that we seem to make objective value judgments that are not contingent on, or merely relative to, what this or that group happens to desire—for example, the judgment that murder or torture is objectively morally wrong. Moreover, the Humean view fails to give an adequate account of how we come to desire certain objects for their own sake to begin with. A perfectionist account, on the contrary, one that identifies the intrinsic goods (the objects desired for their own sake) with objective perfections of the person, is able to give an account of these facts. For criticism of the Humean notion of practical reason, see: Joseph Boyle, "Reasons for Action: Evaluative Cognitions that Underlie Motivations," *American Journal of Jurisprudence* 46 (2001): 177-197; R. Jay Wallace, "How to Argue About Practical Reason," *Mind* 99 (1990): 355-387; Christine Korsgaard, "Skepticism about Practical Reason," in her *Creating the Kingdom of Ends* (Cambridge: Cambridge University Press, 1996); David Brink, "Moral Motivation," *Ethics* 107 (1997): 4-32; John Finnis, *Fundamentals of Ethics* (Washington, D.C.: Georgetown University Press, 1983), pp. 26-79; and Joseph Raz, *The Morality of Freedom* (New York: Oxford University Press, 1986), pp. 288-368.

† The idea is this: what is to be done is what is perfective. This seems trivial and perhaps is obvious, but it is the basis for objective, practical reasoning. The ques-

human goods are the actualizations of our basic potentialities, the conditions to which we are naturally oriented and which objectively fulfill us, the various aspects of our fulfillment as human persons.[23] They include such fulfillments as human life and health, speculative knowledge or understanding, aesthetic experience, friendship or personal community, and harmony among the different aspects of the self.*

The conditions or activities understood to be fulfilling and worth pursuing are not individual or particularized objects. I do not apprehend merely that *my* life or knowledge is intrinsically good and to be pursued. I apprehend that life and knowledge, whether instantiated in me or in others, is good and worth pursuing. For example, seeing an infant drowning in a shallow pool of water, I apprehend, without an inference, that a good worth preserving is in danger and so I reach out to save the child. The feature, *fulfilling for me or for someone like me,* is the feature in a condition or activity that makes it an ultimate reason for action. The question is: In what respect must someone be like me for his or her fulfillment to be correctly viewed as worth pursuing for its own sake in the same way that my good is worth pursuing?

The answer is not immediately obvious to spontaneous, or first-order, practical reasoning, or to first-order moral reasoning. That is, the question of the extension of the fundamental goods genuinely worthy of pursuit and respect needs moral reflection to be answered. By such reflection, we can see that the relevant likeness (to me) is that others too rationally shape their lives, or have the potentiality of doing so. Other likenesses—age, gender, race, appearance, place of origin, etc.—are not relevant to making an entity's fulfillment

---

tion, "What is to be done?", is equivalent to the question, "What is to be actualized?" But what is to be actualiz*ed* is what actualiz*es*, that is, what is objectively perfective. For human beings this is life, knowledge of truth, friendship, and so on.

* Once one apprehends such conditions or activities as really fulfilling and worthy of pursuit, the *moral* norm arises when one has a choice between one option the choice of which is fully compatible with these apprehensions (or judgments) and another option that is not fully compatible with those judgments. The former type of choice is fully reasonable, and respectful of the goods and persons involved, whereas the latter type of choice is not fully reasonable and negates, in one way or another, the intrinsic goodness of one or more instances of the basic goods one has already apprehended as, and recognized to be, intrinsically good.

fundamentally worth pursuing and respecting. But being a rational agent *is* relevant to this issue, for it is an object's being worthy of *rational* pursuit that I apprehend and that makes it an ultimate reason for action, and an intrinsic good.[24] So, I ought primarily to pursue and respect not just life in general, for example, but the life of rational agents—a rational agent being one who either immediately or potentially (with a *radical* potentiality, as part of his or her nature) shapes his or her own life.[25]

Moreover, I understand that the basic goods are not just good for me as an individual, but for me acting in communion—rational cooperation and real friendship—with others. Indeed, communion with others, which includes mutual understanding and self-giving, is itself an irreducible aspect of human well-being and fulfillment—a basic good. But I can act in communion—real communion—only with beings with a rational nature. So, the basic goods are not just goods for me, but goods for me and all those with whom it is possible (in principle, at least) rationally to cooperate. All of the basic goods should be pursued and respected, not just as they are instantiable in me, but as they are instantiable in any being with a rational nature.

In addition, by reflection we see that it would be inconsistent to respect my fulfillment, or my fulfillment plus that of others whom I just happen to like, and *not* respect the fulfillment of other, immediately or potentially, rational agents. For, entailed by rational pursuit of my good (and of the good of others I happen to like) is a demand on my part that others respect my good (and the good of those I like). That is, in pursuing my fulfillment I am led to appeal to the reason and freedom of others to respect that pursuit, and my real fulfillment. But in doing so, consistency, that is, reasonableness, demands that I also respect the rational pursuits and real fulfillment of other rational agents—that is, any entity that, immediately or potentially (that is, by self-directed development of innate or inherent natural capacities), rationally directs his or her own actions. In other words, the thought of the Golden Rule, basic fairness, occurs early on in moral reflection. One can *hope* that the weather, and other natural forces, including any non-rational agent, will not harm one. But one has a moral *claim* or *right* (one spontaneously makes a moral *demand*) that other mature rational agents respect one's reasonable pursuits and real fulfillment. Consistency, then, demands that one respect reasonable pursuits and real fulfillment of others as well. Thus, having a rational nature, or, being a person, as traditionally defined (a distinct subject or substance with a rational nature) is the criterion for full moral worth.

## Marginal Cases

On this position every human being, of whatever age, size, or degree of development, has inherent and equal fundamental dignity and basic rights. If one holds, on the contrary, that full moral worth or dignity is based on some accidental attribute, then, since the attributes that could be considered to ground basic moral worth (developed consciousness, etc.) vary in degree, one will be led to the conclusion that moral worth also varies in degrees.

It might be objected against this argument, that the basic natural capacity for rationality also comes in degrees, and so this position (that full moral worth is based on the possession of the basic natural capacity for rationality), if correct, would also lead to the denial of personal equality.[26] However, the criterion for full moral worth is having a nature that entails the capacity (whether existing in root form or developed to the point at which it is immediately exercisable) for conceptual thought and free choice—not *the development* of that natural basic capacity to some degree or other (and to what degree would necessarily be an arbitrary matter). The criterion for full moral worth and possession of basic rights is not *having* a capacity for conscious thought and choice, but *being* a certain kind of thing, that is, having a specific type of substantial nature. Thus, possession of full moral worth follows upon being a certain type of entity or substance, namely, a substance with a rational nature, despite the fact that some persons (substances with a rational nature) have a greater intelligence, or are morally superior (exercise their power for free choice in an ethically more excellent way) than others. Since basic rights are grounded in being a certain type of substance, it follows that having such a substantial nature qualifies one as having full moral worth, basic rights, and equal personal dignity.

An analogy may clarify our point. Certain properties follow upon being an animal, and so are possessed by every animal, even though in other respects not all animals are equal. For example, every animal has some parts that move other parts, and every animal is subject to death (mortal). Since various animals are equally animals—and since being an animal is a type of substance rather than an accidental attribute—then every animal will equally have *those* properties, even though (for example) not every animal equally possesses the property of being able to blend in well with the wooded background. Similarly, possession of full moral worth follows upon being a person (a distinct substance with a rational nature) even though persons are unequal in many respects (intellectually, morally, etc.).

These points have real and specific implications for the great controversial issues in contemporary ethics and politics. Since human beings are intrinsically valuable as subjects of rights at all times that they exist—that is, they do not come to be at one point, and acquire moral worth or value as a subject of rights only at some later time—it follows that human embryos and fetuses are subjects of rights, deserving full moral respect from individuals and from the political community. It also follows that a human being remains a person, and a being with intrinsic dignity and a subject of rights, for as long as he or she lives: there are no subpersonal human beings. Embryo-destructive research, abortion, and euthanasia involve killing innocent human beings in violation of their moral right to life and to the protection of the laws.

In sum, human beings constitute a special sort of animal. They differ in kind from other animals because they have a rational nature, a nature characterized by having the basic, natural capacities (possessed by each and every human being from the point at which he or she comes to be) for conceptual thought and deliberation and free choice. In virtue of having such a nature, all human beings are persons; and all persons possess the real dignity that is deserving of full moral respect. Thus, every human being deserves full moral respect.

## Notes

1 See Jenny Teichman, *Social Ethics: A Student's Guide* (Oxford: Blackwell, 1996).
2 Peter Singer, "All Animals are Equal," in *Morality in Practice*, 4th edition, ed. James P. Sterba (Belmont, California: Wadsworth, 1994), p. 478, quoting Jeremy Bentham's *Introduction to the Principles of Moral and Legislation* (1789), chapter 17.
3 Peter Singer, op. cit., p. 441.
4 Jeff McMahan, whose views are in other respects more complex than Singer's, still holds that only interests are of direct moral concern, and explicitly recognizes and accepts this logical consequence. See his *The Ethics of Killing: Problems at the Margin of Life* (New York: Oxford University Press, 2002), pp. 205-206.
5 Peter Singer, op. cit., p. 484, emphasis added.
6 Richard Arneson, "What, If Anything, Renders All Humans Morally Equal?" in *Singer and his Critics*, ed. Dale Jamieson (Malden, Massachusetts: Blackwell, 1999), pp. 103-127, at p. 105.
7 This is our solution to what Richard Arneson calls "the Singer problem." See Richard Arneson, loc. cit.
8 Paul Taylor, "The Ethics of Respect for Nature," in *Morality in Practice*, 4th edition, ed. James P. Sterba (Belmont, California: Wadsworth, 1994), p. 488.
9 Cf. Louis G. Lombardi, "Inherent Worth, Respect, and Rights," *Environmental Ethics* 5 (1983): 257-270.
10 David Oderberg, *Applied Ethics: A Non-Consequentialist Approach* (Oxford: Blackwell, 2000), p. 101.
11 For example, Taylor, op. cit.
12 Aristotle, *De Anima* III.4.
13 See Joel Wallman, *Aping Language* (Cambridge: Cambridge University Press, 1992), especially chapters 5 and 6.
14 Cf. Richard J. Connell, *Logical Analysis: An Introduction to Systematic Learning* (Edina, Minnesota: Bellwether Press, 1981), pp. 87-93; John Haldane, "The Source and Destination of Thought," in *Referring to God: Jewish and Christian Philosophical and Theological Perspectives*, ed. Paul Helm (New York: St. Martin's Press, 2000); Mortimer Adler, *Intellect: Mind Over Matter* (New York: Macmillan, 1990); Russell Pannier and Thomas D. Sullivan, "The Mind-Marker," in *Theos, Anthropos, Christos: A Compendium of Modern Philosophical Theology*, ed. Roy Abraham Varghese (New York: Peter Lang, 2000); James F. Ross, "Immaterial Aspects of Thought," *Journal of Philosophy* 89 (1992): 136-150.
15 Mortimer Adler noted that, upon extended observation of other animals and of human beings, what would first strike one is the immense uniformity in mode of living among other animals, in contrast with the immense variety in modes of living and customs among human beings. See Mortimer Adler, op. cit.
16 Cf. Roger Scruton, *Sexual Desire: A Moral Philosophy of the Erotic* (New York: The Free Press, 1986).
17 This point is developed in James B. Reichmann, *Evolution, 'Animal Rights,' and*

*the Environment* (Washington, D.C.: Catholic University of America Press, 2000), chapter 2; see also John Campbell, *Past, Space, and Self: Representation and Mind* (Cambridge, Massachusetts: MIT Press, 1994).

[18] Lynne Rudder Baker, *Persons and Bodies: A Constitution View* (Cambridge: Cambridge University Press, 2000), chapter 3; John Campbell, *Past, Space, and Self: Representation and Mind* (Cambridge, Massachusetts: MIT Press, 1994).

[19] Cf. Robert Kane, *The Significance of Free Will* (Oxford: Oxford University Press, 1998).

[20] Hence the position we are proposing is an incompatibilist view of free choice. Having alternate possibilities, that is, the ability to will otherwise, is essential to free choice and moral responsibility. It seems to us that the Frankfurt alleged counterexamples (proposed to disprove the principle of alternate possibilities) are not genuine counterexamples. In these alleged counterexamples there is a first agent who deliberates and decides, but there is a second, more powerful agent who in some way monitors the first agent and is ready and able to cause the first agent to do the act desired by the second agent if the first agent begins to will or perform otherwise than the desired outcome. It turns out, however (on the imagined scenario), that the first agent decides on his own to do the act that the second agent was ready to compel him to do. So, according to advocates of the Frankfurt examples, the first agent acted freely, was morally responsible, and yet could not have willed or acted otherwise. See Harry Frankfurt, "Alternate Possibilities and Moral Responsibilities," *Journal of Philosophy* 66 (1969): 829-839. For a recent defense of this approach, see John Martin Fischer and Mark Ravizza, *Responsibility and Control: A Theory of Moral Responsibility* (Cambridge: Cambridge University Press, 1998). The problem is that the monitoring device, however it is imagined, will be unable to alert the second agent that the first agent is about to, or has begun to, act otherwise than the second agent plans. The act of willing is not determinate prior to its occurrence and so cannot be known before it occurs. And once it has occurred, it is too late to prevent it. (This was the ground for Aquinas's position that not even God can know a future contingent precisely as future, that is, as it exists in its causes, but he can know it only as it is in act—yet, since God is not in time, what is future with respect to us is not future with respect to God. See St. Thomas Aquinas, *Summa Theologiae*, Pt. I, q. 14, a. 13.) The second agent could prevent the physical, external action carrying out the choice, but the act of will is free and undetermined even if the external behavior executing the choice is prevented. Although his argument against the Frankfurt examples is not precisely the one presented here, an article that overlaps somewhat with this argument is: Paul A. Woodward, "Why Frankfurt Examples Beg the Question," *Journal of Social Philosophy* 33 (2002): 540-547.

[21] A more extended argument can be found in Joseph M. Boyle, Jr., Germain Grisez, and Olaf Tollefsen, *Free Choice: A Self-Referential Argument* (Notre Dame, Indiana: University of Notre Dame Press, 1976); see also Peter van Inwagen, *An Essay on Free Will* (Oxford: Oxford University Press, 1986); and Peter van Inwagen, "Free Will Remains a Mystery," in *The Oxford Handbook of Free Will*, ed. Robert

Kane (Oxford: Oxford University Press, 2002), pp. 158-170.

[22] The argument here is indebted to Thomas Aquinas. See, e.g., *Summa Theologiae*, I-II, q. 10, aa. 1-2.

[23] This claim is derived from Thomas Aquinas and has been developed by Thomists and Aristotelians of various types. It is not necessary here to assume one particular development of that view against others. We need only the point that the basic principles of practical reason come from an insight—which may be interpreted in various ways—that what is to be pursued, what is worth pursuing, is what is fulfilling or perfective of me and others like me. For more on this see: Germain Grisez, Joseph Boyle, and John Finnis, "Practical Principles, Moral Truth and Ultimate Ends," *American Journal of Jurisprudence* 33 (1988): 99-151; John Finnis, Joseph M. Boyle, Jr., Germain Grisez, *Nuclear Deterrence, Morality and Realism* (Oxford: Oxford University Press, 1987), chapters 9-11; John Finnis, *Fundamentals of Ethics* (Washington, D.C.: Georgetown University Press, 1983); John Finnis, *Aquinas: Moral, Political, and Legal Theory* (Oxford: Oxford University Press, 1998); Timothy D. J. Chappell, *Understanding Human Goods: A Theory of Ethics* (Edinburgh: Edinburgh University Press, 1998); David S. Oderberg, *Moral Theory: A Non-Consequentialist Approach* (Oxford: Blackwell Publishers, 2000); Ralph McInerny, *Aquinas on Human Action: A Theory of Practice* (Washington, D.C.: Catholic University of America Press, 1992) and Mark C. Murphy, *Natural Law and Practical Rationality* (New York: Cambridge University Press, 2002).

[24] The argument presented here is similar to the approaches found in the following authors: Louis G. Lombardi, op. cit.; Michael Goldman, "A Transcendental Defense of Speciesism," *Journal of Value Inquiry* 35 (2001): 59-69; and William J. Zanardi, "Why Believe in the Intrinsic Dignity and Equality of Persons?" *Southwest Philosophy Review* 14 (1998): 151-168.

[25] The position that the criterion for full moral worth cannot be an accidental attribute, but is the rational *nature*, that is, being a specific type of substance, is defended in Patrick Lee, "The Pro-Life Argument from Substantial Identity: A Defense," *Bioethics* 18 (2004): 249-263. See also Dean Stretton, "Essential Properties and the Right to Life: A Response to Lee," *Bioethics* (18) 2004: 264-282, and Patrick Lee, "Substantial Identity and the Right to Life: A Rejoinder to Dean Stretton," in *Bioethics* 21 (2007): 93-97.

[26] Dean Stretton, op. cit.

# 17

# Two Arguments from Human Dignity

## Paul Weithman

Since World War II, it has been increasingly common for fundamental international and European documents to begin with ascriptions of human dignity.[1] In some of these documents, human dignity is said to be *concomitant* with important human entitlements, such as rights. Thus Article One of the *Universal Declaration of Human Rights* says that "All human beings are born free and equal in dignity and rights."[2]

Sometimes, however, these documents seem to make a stronger claim. They sometimes seem to imply that human dignity *entails* entitlements. For example, Article One of the *Charter of Fundamental Rights of the European Union* says that "Human dignity is inviolable. It must be respected and protected." The *Charter* proceeds immediately, in the subsequent articles, to enumerate rights and liberties that are to be accorded citizens of the member states.[3] The immediacy of the *Charter's* move from Article One's assertion of dignity to the enumeration of rights creates the clear impression that the dignity ascribed to human beings in Article One entails, or is the basis for asserting, the rights listed immediately afterwards. The *German Basic Law* says explicitly that the ascription of dignity is the basis for inferring rights-claims. The first clause of Article One in the *Basic Law*

435

says "Human dignity shall be inviolable. To respect and protect it shall be the duty of all state authority." The second clause of the Article says "The German people *therefore* [*darum*] acknowledge inviolable and inalienable human rights as the basis of every community, of peace and of justice in the world."[4]

I want to examine arguments of the kind that are presupposed by the EU's *Charter* and the *German Basic Law*, arguments *from* assertions of human dignity *to* claims about human entitlements. The entitlements I shall discuss will be entitlements to so-called "second-generation rights," such as welfare rights. I shall focus here on one especially popular and attractive argumentative strategy for establishing these rights, which I call the *via negativa*. Proponents of the *via negativa* try to show that they can move from the assertion that human beings have dignity to claims about entitlements by showing that the denial or withholding of those entitlements is inconsistent with or violative of human dignity. As I shall explain in section I, I want to show that even if these arguments succeed, they ultimately depend upon the conclusions of *other* arguments for basic entitlements—arguments to which the arguments from human dignity are often thought to be independent alternatives. Arguments from human dignity therefore do not provide the independent route to human entitlements that they are sometimes thought to promise.

The President's Council on Bioethics has frequently appealed to the value of human dignity in its published reports. I shall not discuss the arguments of the Council in any detail here, though I shall occasionally call attention to some of them. Though this attention is not concentrated or sustained, my analysis of arguments from human dignity underlines the importance of confronting some of the criticism the Council's work has received and of pursuing one of the questions that its work raises.

One objection can, I believe, be dispensed with quickly. It is sometimes assumed that the value of human dignity is an irreducibly theological value that, as such, ought not be given any weight in the formulation of public policy. The fact that dignity is sometimes said to depend upon our being images of God, and the frequent appeals to the value in Catholic moral thought, are sometimes taken to confirm this assumption. I believe that the assumption is mistaken, and that a careful reading of history would show the value of human

dignity to have a home in secular as well as in religious thinking.\*
So the allegation that human dignity is a theological value cannot
sustain an objection to the Council's use of it.

Ruth Macklin has famously criticized the Council's appeal to
dignity by arguing that, while dignity is frequently appealed to in
human rights documents and in Catholic social teaching, it is a "useless" and therefore dispensable concept. She concludes that it is a
dispensable concept because, she says, dignity "means no more than
respect for persons and their autonomy."[5] I do not contend that the
concept of human dignity is dispensable. On the contrary, I believe
that the concept of dignity can very helpfully be used to call attention to the fact that we human beings have features in virtue of which
we are worthy of great respect. Furthermore, the fact that the notion of human dignity is at home in a number of moral traditions
makes it an especially useful "second-level concept"—a concept for
expressing moral agreement among those who may differ about what
first-order ethical vocabulary best explains *why* human beings merit
respect. It is therefore just the concept one would expect to find in
public documents (such as international charters and the reports of
Presidential commissions) in which signatories from diverse traditions and schools of thought express such agreement.

But the conclusion advanced here about the dependence of dignity arguments on other arguments raises what should be a troubling
question for those who rely on arguments from dignity: the question
of how much of the work thought to be done by arguments from
dignity is in fact done by the prior arguments on which dignity arguments depend. If the conclusion advanced here is right, then the
Council needs either to take up this question or to distinguish its dignity arguments from dignity arguments of the sort considered here.
Furthermore, as we shall see at the end of this paper, the argument I
offer for my conclusion suggests that the Council needs to give considerably more attention to questions on which it has touched all too
briefly, questions about the bases and the equality of human dignity.

---

\* For a splendid and concise discussion of the historical sources of the notion of
human dignity, see Adam Schulman's introduction to this volume.

## I. Why Argue from Dignity?

I said that I shall focus on arguments for basic entitlements that follow the *via negativa*. I believe that arguments of the sort I take up have considerable intuitive appeal. The claim that human beings are possessed of a dignity unique to our kind has long exercised a powerful hold on secular and religious moral consciousness, at least in the West. That claim may therefore seem a natural starting point for arguments about what human beings are owed as such. Furthermore, offenses and conditions that strike us as denials or violations of dignity are all too familiar in the contemporary world. They run a lamentable gamut that includes religious coercion, human trafficking, the torture and degradation of prisoners, and the squalor of urban slums in which human beings are condemned to live without minimal sanitation or modesty. What has gone wrong in such cases, we may think, is that those in power have not honored the entitlements of those whose dignity is denied or violated. And it may be appealing to think that we can argue *to* those entitlements *from* the claim that human beings have a dignity that is denied or violated in cases such as these.

Arguments from human dignity to human entitlements have proven especially appealing to some of those who are dissatisfied with social contract arguments. The critics I have in mind object to these arguments because they think that the conception with which these arguments begin—the conception of the individual contractor—is an illegitimate abstraction. This objection takes at least two forms.

Some thinkers in the Aristotelian-Thomist tradition have argued that social contract theorists can begin with apolitical or pre-political individuals, and ask what kind of society they would choose to live in, only by abstracting away from the embeddedness or sociality of human beings. Since sociability is essential to us, the philosopher who idealizes it away in order to set up the fundamental question of contract theory begins his argument for human entitlements in the wrong place. The basic entitlements at which he arrives from there are therefore inadequate to provide political guidance.[6] For some thinkers in the Aristotelian-Thomist tradition, our social nature is one of the grounds of our dignity. An argument that begins with ascriptions of human dignity promises to avoid the individualism that allegedly undermines contractualist arguments.[7]

According to other thinkers, including others in the Aristotelian tradition, the contract theorist's abstraction goes wrong in a different way. Social contract theorists, it is said, typically ascribe human powers within the normal range to all the contracting parties and to all those to whom the terms of the social contract apply. This ascription abstracts away from human variability. It therefore leads contracting parties to choose norms that are insufficiently sensitive to morally relevant differences in the use human beings can make of the resources distributed under the terms of the contract. For these critics, human dignity depends upon the fact that human beings can develop certain distinctively human capacities. Beginning an argument for human entitlements with an assertion of dignity so understood makes it possible, they believe, to arrive at norms which are sufficiently sensitive to morally significant human differences.[8]

Thus those who offer either form of criticism treat arguments from human dignity as desirable alternatives to contractualist arguments. The first form of criticism is of considerable interest. As we shall see, the second form now enjoys some currency in the philosophical literature. Partisans of contract theory should eventually confront both. Here I shall concentrate on the second.

I want to show that arguments from human dignity understood in the second way—as grounded in our potential for distinctively human capacities—are not really alternatives to social contract arguments after all. Rather, they presuppose contract arguments of some form in order to sustain their conclusions about entitlements. This is because—to put it crudely—the grounds of human dignity include capacities that are properly respected only by consulting those who have those capacities about their own basic entitlements.

I shall defend these conclusions in section V, where I assess what I call the *Aristotelian Argument from Dignity*. The *Aristotelian Argument* depends upon considerations that are complex and sophisticated, and it has considerable force. The strength of the argument is best appreciated by looking in some detail at how the *Aristotelian Argument* improves on other arguments from dignity that have some initial appeal.

## II. The Fittingness Argument: Initial Statement and Clarification

The entitlements supported by the arguments in which I am interested are, as I said, so-called "second-generation rights," though for my purposes I do not believe anything essential turns on whether the rights at issue are first- or second-generation. Consider what I shall call the *Simple Argument from Dignity* for such rights:

(1) Human beings have dignity.
(2) A human being who lives in conditions of gross material deprivation is living a life that, for that reason, is lacking in human dignity.

But it seems obvious to some people that if human beings have dignity, then they should not have to live lives which lack dignity. Since they do have dignity by (1),

(3) Human beings should not have to live lives that are lacking in human dignity.

From these claims, a claim about basic entitlement follows, since (2) and (3) seem to support the conclusion that:

C: Human beings are entitled to access to material conditions that are not conditions of gross material deprivation.

If we assume that national governments are obliged to guarantee that people live in a dignified way, then national governments are obliged to guarantee that people do not live in conditions of gross material deprivation.

If the assumption about national governments is sound and if the *Simple Argument* is a good argument, we can see why fundamental documents—laying out the claims people can make on their governments—should move from claims about human dignity to conclusions second-generation rights. But is the *Simple Argument* a good one?

I believe that the *Simple Argument* is often taken to be a good one. Although the argument may not often be laid out explicitly, premises (1) and (2) express claims that are frequently heard in discussions of human rights. These claims are taken to support a conclusion like C. Presumably they are thought to support that conclusion by way of a premise like (3).

Yet on its face, the juxtaposition of (1) and (2) is bound to cause some puzzlement. How can a human life be lacking in dignity, as (2) alleges, if dignity is something every human being has, as (1) says? The juxtaposition is especially puzzling if dignity is something human beings have inherently. For if human beings have the dignity asserted in (1) inherently, then it is not immediately clear how they can lack it. That it can be absent from the lives they lead, as (2) says it can be, requires some explanation.

Similar puzzlement can be engendered by juxtaposing various claims from the reports of the President's Council. The Council has asserted in some places that all human beings have dignity[9] equally[10] and inherently[11], and that "every human life" has dignity "from start to finish."[12] Yet the Council has also said that human dignity can be "violated,"[13] "threatened,"[14] and "encroach[ed] upon."[15] One of the reports suggests that dignity can be traded off or sold in return for athletic achievement.[16] But how can a quality which human beings have inherently and at all stages of their lives regardless of their condition also be one of which they could be deprived or one which they can alienate in these ways?

The various claims that the President's Council makes may all have some ground in our moral experience. Perhaps our moral experience of dignity raises all the puzzles raised by the juxtaposition of these claims. Even so, the derivation of normative conclusions from claims about dignity requires working through these puzzles to formulate a notion of human dignity that is clear and consistent. My own view is that the puzzles show the need to distinguish dignity as a quality of persons from dignity as a quality of the way they live their lives. That is, they show the need to distinguish "dignity" understood *adjectivally*—as applied to persons—from "dignity" understood *prepositionally*—as describing either a quality with which persons live their lives or a condition in which the living is done.

Having drawn this distinction, I want to return to the *Simple*

*Argument from Dignity* and modify the steps. The modifications yield an argument from dignity that avoids the puzzles raised by the *Simple Argument* and that says more clearly than the *Simple Argument* does just how lives can lack dignity. The argument that results from these modifications is the *Fittingness Argument from Human Dignity*.

Premise (1) of the *Simple Argument* said "Human beings have dignity." I shall follow the OED in taking "dignity" to mean "worthiness," "worth," and "excellence." Let's therefore reinterpret (1) to say that (1f) "Human beings have worth." Though this may sound a bit awkward, what needs to be borne in mind is that—because of the OED's equation of "worth" and "excellence"—what is really being ascribed is *relative worth*. What is being asserted is that human beings have a worth or value that is high relative to the worth or the value of the things that human beings excel or surpass.

What is characteristic of the *Fittingness Argument* are the way it interprets premise (2) and the way it moves from there to the entitlement alleged in the conclusion. The *Fittingness Argument* relies on the intuitively appealing idea that if something has worth or excellence or worthiness, then there are some things—including some conditions—that it is worthy of and some things that are not worthy of it. According to the *Fittingness Argument*, a life is lacking in dignity—or is an undignified life—just in case it is a life that is not worthy of human beings or, as I shall say, is a life that "does not befit their worth." One of the things that can make a life one that does not befit human worth is the condition under which it is lived. So premise (2) of the *Simple Argument* can be reinterpreted to say that (2f) "A human being who lives in conditions of gross material deprivation is living a life that, for that reason, does not befit human worth."

The *Fittingness Argument* moves from (1f) and (2f) to an entitlement to relief from conditions of gross deprivation via the claim that human beings are entitled to live as befits their worth. So what I am calling the *Fittingness Argument* can initially be stated as follows:

(1f)   Human beings have worth.
(2f)   A human being who lives in conditions of gross material deprivation is living a life that, for that reason, does not befit human worth.

Assume that if human beings have worth, then they should not have to live lives which do not befit their worth. Since human beings do have worth by (1f):

> (3f)  Human beings should not have to live lives that do not befit their worth.

From (3f) and (2f) we get the claim that human beings should not have to live in conditions of gross material deprivation. And so the *Fittingness Argument* concludes:

> C:  Human beings are entitled to access to material conditions that are not conditions of gross material deprivation.

And if we assume—as I did when I laid out the *Simple Argument*—that national governments are obliged to guarantee that people do not have to live in ways that do not befit their worth, then the argument shows why national governments are obliged to guarantee that people do not have to live in conditions of gross material deprivation. The *Fittingness Argument* thus purports to show how fundamental documents could move from claims about human dignity to second-generation rights.

Like the *Simple Argument*, the *Fittingness Argument* may not often be laid out explicitly. Like the *Simple Argument*, it raises questions. Among the most pressing of these are questions about premise (1f), questions about human worth and its grounds. These questions will eventually have to be confronted, but I want to put them off for now. For looking at the rest of the argument enables us to appreciate its appeal.

To begin to see that appeal, note that there is an immediately apparent difference between the *Simple Argument* and the *Fittingness Argument*. If we modify premise (2) of the *Simple Argument* in the way that the *Fittingness Argument* does, then the conjunction of (1f) and (2f) does not raise the same puzzlement that the juxtaposition of (1) and (2) did. That juxtaposition was puzzling because (2) seemed to suggest that humans could lack the dignity that (1) said they have. By contrast, it does not seem nearly so problematic to say, as (1f) does, that human beings have dignity or worth but that they can live lives that lack dignity, understood in the sense of (2f) as "lives which do not befit their worth."

The advantage the *Fittingness Argument* enjoys over the *Simple Argument* may seem, however, to come at a considerable price. For premises (2f) and (3f) rely on the notion of "fittingness" or "befittingness." This notion itself raises a number of questions. What, we might wonder, *is* befittingness? Why should we think that some lives befit human worth but others don't, as (2f) implies? And even if some lives do befit human worth and others don't, why is it that human beings should not have to live lives which do not befit their worth, as (3f) says?

To answer these questions and to see the appeal of the *Fittingness Argument*, it helps to recall something that is sometimes said by those who appeal to human dignity to ground entitlements. A society in which someone is able to live a life that is not lacking in human dignity is sometimes said to be one in which he can live "a life *commensurate* with human dignity." Martha Nussbaum, for example, uses this locution in her recent work on human entitlements and human dignity.[17] The phrase was also used by Pope John Paul II, who frequently appealed to human dignity, when he spoke of the need for a world order "commensurate with human dignity."[18] Talk of commensuration, taken literally, suggests that there are measures of human dignity and of human lives, and that some correlation between the measures is possible.

I believe that if we take talk of commensuration literally, and press on it very hard, we get a picture with the following elements:

- Items in the world, including human beings, have worth.
- The worth of these items can be measured.
- The measure of worth is scalar.
- Human beings can be located on the scale of values with some precision.*

---

* Note that, for purposes of understanding the *Fittingness Argument*, it does not matter whether the scale of values has many or few gradations. The scale could be a finely graded "Great Chain of Being" or it could be a two-value scale which simply distinguishes—as Kant did—between items that have dignity and items that have fancy price.

- Living conditions can be located on a scale which, because it is commensurable with the scale of worth, can be correlated with it.

If we suppose that the proponent of the *Fittingness Argument from Human Dignity* is operating with this picture in the background, then we can read premise (2f) as asserting a "mismatch" between conditions of gross material deprivation and the place of human beings on the scale of worth. And we can read premise (3f) as asserting that human beings must have access to conditions that match their worth.

But why think that anyone who offers arguments from human dignity accepts this picture? Why think that any of them believe that worth is scalar? And why think that they believe there can be matches and mismatches of the sort asserted by (2f)? In sum, why think anyone endorses these critical assumptions of the *Fittingness Argument*?

Note first that it is common enough to speak as if we can locate human beings somewhere on a scale of value, as if we should be placed higher on the scale than some other things because we excel those things, and as if our placement on such a scale is a matter of our dignity or worth. For example, Leon Kass, the former chairman of the President's Council, has said:

> Although the term "human dignity" has a lofty ring, its content is quite difficult to define. To be more precise, different authors and traditions define it differently, as the readings in this chapter make abundantly clear. Yet all are struggling to reveal that elusive core of our humanity, *those special qualities that make us more than beasts yet less than gods.*[19]

Furthermore, conditions of deprivation are often described as "beneath human dignity" or as "subhuman." This description may initially seem metaphorical. But if someone operates with the picture I have sketched, then he can give what looked like spatial metaphors a more straightforward reference. So the description of conditions of deprivation as "subhuman" and "beneath human dignity," taken in conjunction with the scalar picture suggested by talk of "commensurability" and seemingly endorsed by Kass, suggests that some people may indeed accept (2f). This suggestion gets some support from the way we may be inclined to give voice to the instinctive revulsion we feel when we see pictures of human beings living in squalor. In my case, the revulsion is accompanied by the thought that "Human beings do not belong there," or "That is no place for something as great as a human being."

That some conditions are a "match" and others a "mismatch" for human value is also suggested by a different metaphor that is used to describe human value in western religious and philosophical traditions, and in contemporary discussions of human rights. In the *King James Version*, God speaks of righteous human beings as "jewels" (*Malachi* 3:17). In Section One of the *Groundwork*, Kant echoes this description by famously describing the good will as a "jewel." And one contemporary scholar says of the *German Basic Law*, "Article 1 is the Basic Law's crown. The concept of human dignity is this crown's jewel."[20] The use of the "jewel" metaphor in three such different sources at least suggests that the metaphor expresses a widely held way of thinking about human worth. If we think that the value of human beings is aptly likened to the value of a jewel, then we might think that some settings are appropriate for it but other settings are not. There are some settings, we might think, that naturally suit an item of such value, while others are incongruous with it.

Suppose, then, that familiar ways of speaking suggest the picture whose elements are laid out above, and that we can use that picture to make (2f) clear and acceptable. Even so—and despite the fact that the *Fittingness Argument* provides an interesting and perhaps a surprisingly rigorous elaboration of familiar ways of thinking about human worth—the real interest of the *Fittingness Argument* lies in where it goes wrong. For by seeing where the argument goes wrong, we can bring to light conditions that any argument from human dignity must meet.

To see where the *Fittingness Argument* goes wrong, we need to look more closely at how the argument moves from the lack of fittingness or the incongruity alleged in (2f) to the entitlement alleged in the conclusion. In the *Fittingness Argument* as laid out so far, that move depends upon (3f), the claim that human beings should not have to live in conditions that do not befit their worth. But why shouldn't they? Why should the lack of fittingness asserted in (2f) matter? And even if it matters, why should the lack of fittingness ground a basic entitlement to conditions that befit us or befit us better?

The proponent of the *Fittingness Argument* clearly thinks that a state of affairs in which human beings must live in conditions that do not befit their worth is bad. As I originally laid out the *Fittingness Argument*, its proponent asserts:

(3f)   Human beings should not have to live lives that do not befit their worth.

But now we can see that part of what he means by (3f) is:

(3f.1)   That humans should have to live lives which do not befit their worth is bad.

This claim, when taken together with (2f), implies that it is bad for human beings to have to live in conditions of gross material deprivation.

But how does this ground an entitlement to access to better conditions? Perhaps the idea is that, if human beings have worth, then the lack of "fit" alleged in (2f) and in (3f.1)—the incongruity of someone's having to live in a setting that does not befit his or her worth—is a bad state of affairs that must be averted. If this hermeneutical suggestion is correct, then when the proponent of the *Fittingness Argument* asserts (3f) he also means to say:

(3f.2)   The bad of a human being's having to live in conditions of gross material deprivation must be averted.

Reading (3f) as the conjunction of (3f.1) and (3f.2) seems to get us from (2f) to the conclusion of the *Fittingness Argument*.

Reading (3f) this way is, however, misleading. Note first that the entitlement to live as befits one, the entitlement asserted in the conclusion of the *Fittingness Argument*, is an entitlement held with respect to someone else. It is an entitlement in virtue of which other agents have duties toward the person whose entitlement it is—in this case, duties to avert the bad alleged in (3f.1). The *Fittingness Argument* as I have now elaborated it moves from the bad to that entitlement by alleging an imperative—a "must"—in (3f.2).

This way of reading the argument, with the impersonal "must," seems to suggest that the agents on whom the duty falls must avert the bad alleged in (3f.1) *because* by (3f.2) that bad must be averted. But this is surely a mistake. The badness of a state of affairs does not generate a free-floating imperative which explains why agents are obliged to avert it. Rather, if some bad state of affairs must be averted, it is surely because some agent or agents—maybe even all agents—have a duty to avert it. So to see whether the move from (3f.1) to the entitlement is justified, we need to see whose duty that is and where the duty comes from.

Because I began by talking about the EU *Charter* and the UN *Declaration* (which are signed by governments) and the *German Basic Law* (which establishes a government), I shall assume that the agents on whom the duty falls are governments. It falls to governments to avert the bad in question. Moreover, the proponent of the *Fittingness Argument* thinks it falls to government to avert that bad because government is supposed to be appropriately responsive to or respectful of the worth of human beings. So when the proponent of that argument asserts (3f), I believe that what he means is not (3f.1) and (3f.2), but rather (3f.1) together with:

(3f.2.1) The bad of a human being's having to live in conditions of gross material deprivation is one that government must avert if it is to be appropriately respectful of human worth.

(3f.2.2) Government must be appropriately respectful of human worth.

(3f.2.3) So the bad of a human being's having to live in conditions of gross material deprivation is one that government must avert.

With this elaboration of (3f) in hand, it is possible to elaborate the initial statement of the *Fittingness Argument*.

## III. The Fittingness Argument: A Fuller Statement and Assessment

As we saw, the *Fittingness Argument* begins with the assumptions that:

(1f)   Human beings have worth.

and that

(2f)   A human being who lives in conditions of gross material deprivation is living a life that, for that reason, does not befit human worth.

As we also saw, it assumes that if human beings have worth, then it is bad that they should have to live lives which do not befit that worth. This assumption, together with (1f), implies:

(3f.1)   That humans should have to live lives which do not befit their worth is bad.

The *Fittingness Argument* also assumes that, if having to live as does not befit one's worth is bad, then that bad is one that government must avert if it is to be appropriately respectful of human worth. It follows from this assumption, together with (2f) and (3f.1) that:

(3f.2.1)   The bad of a human being's having to live in conditions of gross material deprivation is one that government must avert if it is to be appropriately respectful of human worth.

The proponent of the argument takes for granted that:

(3f.2.2)   Government must be appropriately respectful of human worth.

So it follows from (3f.2.1) that:

(3f.2.3) The bad of a human being's having to live in conditions of gross material deprivation is one that government must avert.

From (3f.2.3), it seems to follow that human beings have a basic entitlement against their governments:

C: Human beings are entitled to access to material conditions that are not conditions of gross material deprivation, and that entitlement is one their government must honor.

Is the *Fittingness Argument* thus elaborated a good argument? I have already discussed (1f) and (2f), so I shall concentrate on (3f.1), (3f.2.1), (3f.2.2) and (3f.2.3).

(3f.2.2) says that government is bound to be appropriately respectful of human worth. This claim certainly seems to be right. But whether this gets us to (3f.2.3) and to C depends upon the forms of respect for human worth that government is bound to show. It depends, therefore, on whether (3f.2.1) is true.

To see whether (3f.2.1) is true, let's recall what the "bad" in question is. By (3f.1), the bad is an incongruity or lack of "fit" between human worth or human value and its setting, a lack of "fit" which I have supposed can be made clear by pressing on the language of "incommensurate." The guiding idea of the *Fittingness Argument* thus seems to be that, when human beings live in conditions of gross material deprivation, there is a lack of due proportion or correlation in the world that needs to be averted. And (3f.2.3) claims that government must avert it.

The problem with this idea is that it is hard to see that a bad of this kind is one it falls to government to avert. If we are to move from claims about human worth to claims about human entitlements, *via* the claim that government must respect human worth, the argument must plausibly connect human entitlements with forms of respect that government is supposed to show. But (3f.1) fails to draw such a connection because the bad it asserts—the bad that government is to address by (3f.2.1)—does not have the right kind of connection with the interests of citizens.

This may seem a surprising claim. For it is certainly contrary to the interests of citizens to have to live in conditions of gross deprivation. But the fact that having to live in such conditions is contrary to the interests of citizens is not the reason the *Fittingness Argument* provides for the government action required by C. Rather, the reason for government's action is the incongruity or lack of "fit" asserted in (3f.1). In this case, government's failure to take citizens' interests as its reason for action is a failure to be appropriately respectful of human worth. For if government acknowledges that living in gross deprivation is bad, but alleviates that bad in order to correct a cosmic imbalance,* then it is not showing appropriate respect to the citizens who would otherwise have to endure those conditions. When government is moved by the incongruity or lack of fit caused by poverty, rather than by the fact that poverty is bad for the people who suffer it, government at best treats its citizens as valued *objects*. It does not treat them as human *agents*, as beings capable of action and liable to suffering. But since a government that treats its citizens as objects (even as valued objects) rather than as agents is not showing respect for human dignity, the *Fittingness Argument* fails. It fails because, given what is meant by "befit" in (3f.1), (3f.2.1) is false.

## IV. The Aristotelian Argument: Initial Statement and Clarification

The argument from human dignity that I now want to explore promises to avoid the difficulty of the *Fittingness Argument* by showing that respect for human dignity requires government to advance certain identifiable human interests. It is an argument with some currency

---

* Joel Feinberg has suggested that ideas about injustice to the cosmos—consisting in acts and states of affairs which throw the cosmos "out of kilter"—persist in modern moral consciousness. Feinberg associates these ideas with what he calls "Platonic justice"; see his "Non-Comparative Justice," *The Philosophical Review* 83 (1974): 297-338, pp. 307*ff*. My own opinion is that what Feinberg calls "Platonic justice" is one member of a larger family of "Fittingness Views of Justice"; see the footnote on Nussbaum on pp. 458-459 below. I do not mean to deny Feinberg's suggestion about modern moral consciousness. Indeed, I believe my discussion of commensuration confirms it. But I do question—as I believe Feinberg would—whether putting the cosmos back in "kilter" is a proper aim of liberal democratic government.

in the philosophical literature. I believe it is roughly the argument recently put forward by Martha Nussbaum, though I shall not be primarily concerned with tying the argument I consider to the texts of any particular author. For reasons that shall become clear, I refer to it as the *Aristotelian Argument*.

How does the *Aristotelian Argument* go?

Like the *Simple Argument from Dignity*, the *Aristotelian Argument* begins with the claim that "Human beings have dignity." Like the *Fittingness Argument* it interprets that claim as:

(1a) Human beings have worth.

And like the *Fittingness Argument*, the *Aristotelian Argument* tries to support entitlements by exploiting the claim that having to live in certain conditions is unworthy of human beings. What is distinctive of the *Aristotelian Argument* is the way it supports that claim.

The proponent of the argument starts with the Aristotelian observations that there are some activities that are exclusively human, such as the discursive exercise of theoretical and practical reason, and that even those activities that are part of our animal life, such as eating, procreating and associating with others, are activities that human beings perform in a characteristic way. When human beings engage in the characteristically human activities, and when we perform activities in a characteristically human way, we act from affective and intellective habits, and exercise a repertoire of skills. We may choose not to engage in various of these activities—we might, for example, choose a friendless life. But if engaging in these activities is to be a live option for us, then we must have the developed capacities on which these activities draw, at least to some minimum degree. We must have, as I shall say, certain *threshold capacities*. And so, the proponent of the *Aristotelian Argument* observes, a life without the threshold capacities would be a life in which we cannot behave in ways that are characteristically human.

The proponent of the *Aristotelian Argument* then claims that the life of a person who cannot conduct herself in a characteristically human way—the life of someone who cannot associate with others, eat in a human way, converse, and so on—is not a life that is worthy of human beings. These considerations support the second premise of the *Aristotelian Argument*:

(2a)  A life in which someone lacks the threshold capacities is not a life worthy of human beings.

Thus a life in which someone lacks the ability to play or to be sociable, for example, is not a life worthy of a human being.

Like the *Simple Argument from Dignity* and the *Fittingness Argument*, the *Aristotelian Argument* assumes that if human beings have worth, they should not have to live lives that are not worthy of them. Since human beings have worth by (1a), it follows that:

(3a)  But human beings should not have to live lives that are not worthy of them.

And from (3a) and (2a), it follows that human beings should not have to live lives in which they lack the threshold capacities. And so it would seem to follow that:

C:  Human beings are entitled to develop the threshold capacities.

If living in conditions that are not conditions of gross material deprivation is necessary for the development of their threshold capacities, then human beings are entitled to access to living conditions that are not conditions of gross material deprivation. And if we assume—as we did when considering the *Fittingness Argument*—that national governments are obliged to guarantee that people can live in ways that befit their worth, then national governments are obliged to guarantee that people do not live in conditions of gross material deprivation. And so, proponents of the *Aristotelian Argument* conclude, we can see why fundamental documents, laying out the claims people can make on their governments, should include second-generation rights.

I said that the *Aristotelian Argument* I want to look at is of interest in part because it resembles a line of argument pursued by Martha Nussbaum in her recent work. The assertion of resemblance gains some confirmation from Nussbaum's emphasis on developing the basic capabilities and from her explicit endorsement of what I have called premise (2a).[21] It gains further support from her remarks on her own methodology. The *Aristotelian Argument* as I have laid it out follows what I called the *via negativa*, which Nussbaum follows as well. Thus after listing the capacities that she says people are entitled to develop to a minimum degree Nussbaum writes, "The basic idea is that with regard to each of these, we can argue, by imagining a life without the capability in question, that such a life is not a life worthy of human dignity."[22] Even aside from its intrinsic interest, then, this currency gives the *Aristotelian Argument* some claim on our attention.

The *Aristotelian Argument* attempts to support the same basic entitlements as the *Fittingness Argument*, while eschewing the reliance on "fittingness" or "incongruity" that ultimately undermined that argument. Does the *Aristotelian Argument* succeed where the *Fittingness Argument* failed?

Like the *Fittingness Argument*, the *Aristotelian Argument* enjoys one clear advantage over the *Simple Argument from Human Dignity*: the conjunction of its first and second premises does not raise the puzzles raised by the juxtaposition of the first and second premises of the *Simple Argument*. For the conjunction of these premises does not imply or suggest that people can have dignity while their lives lack it. Instead, the two premises say that people have worth but can, under some circumstances, live lives that are not worthy of human beings.

The first premise of the *Aristotelian Argument*—(1a) "Human beings have worth."—clearly raises a number of questions, just as did the first premise of the *Fittingness Argument*. Is the worth of human beings different from the worth possessed by valuable objects that have intrinsic worth, say? If so, is the difference a difference in kind? How is that difference to be understood? What are the properties of human beings in virtue of which they have it? But when I looked at the *Fittingness Argument*, I put these questions aside. Since I am trying to determine whether the *Aristotelian Argument* is more successful than that argument, I shall put them aside here as well, though I shall return to them later. The considerations supporting (2a), the distinctively Aristotelian premise of the argument, seem to me to be very powerful. I am inclined to grant (2a) for the sake of argument. I therefore want to focus attention on the move from (2a) to basic entitlements.

In the previous two sections, we saw that the third premise of the *Fittingness Argument* as initially stated—(3f) "Human beings should not have to live lives which do not befit their human worth."—had to be interpreted as conjoining a number of claims to support the move from the first and second premises to the conclusion. The same is true of the *Aristotelian Argument*. The third premise of that argument is:

(3a)   But human beings should not have to live lives that are not worthy of them.

But without some further argument, it is not clear why this is so. The critical move in the *Aristotelian Argument* is, I believe, like the critical move in the *Fittingness Argument*: both appeal to the need to avoid some bad state of affairs. So I take it that part of what the proponent of the Aristotelian argument has in mind in asserting (3a) is:

(3a.1)   That human beings should have to live lives that are not worthy of them is bad.

It may be tempting to move from (1a), (2a) and (3a.1) to basic entitlements by appealing to:

(3a.2)   The bad of someone's having to live a life in which she lacks the threshold capacities must be averted.

But in the discussion of the *Fittingness Argument*, we saw how misleading such a premise can be. It can suggest that the badness of a state of affairs generates what I called a "free-floating" imperative that explains or grounds the duties of those against whom the entitlement asserted in C is held. It can suggest, that is, that the badness of a state of affairs generates two imperatives, one immediately and the other mediately: (i) a free-floating and impersonal imperative that the bad is to be averted and (ii) a duty to honor the entitlement which is binding on some or all agents and which follows from the free-floating imperative. But at best this gets things the wrong way 'round. If the badness of someone's having to live without the threshold capacities is to be averted, that is surely a consequence of—and not the reason for—the obligation some agent or agents are under to avert it. The obligation of these agents is what is grounded immediately on the badness of the state of affairs. Since the entitlement in question is held against government, it must be that the bad is one that government is under an obligation to avert. And, the proponent of the *Aristotelian Argument* must think, it is a bad that government is obligated to avert if it is to be properly respectful of human dignity.*

Instead of supposing that the proponent of the Aristotelian Argument relies on (3a.2), I shall therefore suppose that he would move from (1a), (2a) and (3a.1) to basic entitlements by appealing to claims that are, in relevant respects, like those on which the *Fittingness Argument* relies:

(3a.2.1) The bad of a human being's having to live a life in which she lacks the threshold capacities is one that government must avert if it is to be appropriately respectful of human worth.

(3a.2.2) Government must be appropriately respectful of human worth.

and

(3a.2.3) The bad of a human being's having to live a life in which she lacks the threshold capacities is one that government must avert.

## V. The Aristotelian Argument: A Fuller Statement and Assessment

Let me recapitulate the *Aristotelian Argument* so that all the steps are before us. The argument begins, as we saw, with the claims that:

---

* Writing of her "capabilities approach" to justice, Martha Nussbaum says: "The aim of the project as a whole is to provide the philosophical underpinning for an account of basic constitutional principles that should be respected and implemented by the governments of all nations, as a bare minimum of what respect for human dignity requires." See her *Women and Human Development* (Cambridge: Cambridge University Press, 2000), p. 5.

(1a)   Human beings have worth.

and that

(2a)   A life in which someone lacks the threshold capacities is not a life worthy of human beings.

It assumes further that, if human beings have worth, then it is bad that they should have to live lives that are unworthy of them. Since (1a) says that people have worth, then (1a) together with this assumption implies that:

(3a.1)   That human beings should have to live lives that are not worthy of them is bad.

The *Aristotelian Argument* also assumes that if someone's having to live a life that is not worthy of her is bad, then—if government is to be appropriately respectful of human worth—that bad is one that government must avert. This assumption, when conjoined with (2a) and (3a.1), implies that

(3a.2.1)   The bad of a human being's having to live a life in which she lacks the threshold capacities is one that government must avert if it is to be appropriately respectful of human worth.

The proponent of the argument takes for granted that:

(3a.2.2)   Government must be appropriately respectful of human worth.

So it follows from (3a.2.1) that

(3a.2.3)   The bad of a human being's having to live a life in which she lacks the threshold capacities is one that government must avert.

(3a.2.3) seems to imply the conclusion of the *Aristotelian Argument*, now stated so as to make explicit that the entitlement in question is one that citizens can press against their government:

C: Human beings are entitled to develop the threshold capacities, and that entitlement is one their government must honor.

I do not want to linger over what it is to "honor" an entitlement. One natural way to take C is as providing the basis for at least some second-generation rights. For if living in gross material deprivation makes development of the threshold capacities impossible, then it seems to follow from C that human beings have a right against their government to access to living conditions that are not conditions of gross material deprivation.

Recall that the *Fittingness Argument* came to grief because the bad that it said needed to be averted—the bad asserted in (3f.1)—was the bad of an "incongruity" or lack of "fit" between human worth and conditions of gross material deprivation. I argued that because this bad is not appropriately connected to human interests, it was hard to see why a government that is supposed to be appropriately respectful of human dignity is bound to avert it.

What is the bad on which the *Aristotelian Argument* turns? The bad asserted in (3a.1) is that of having to live a life in which one lacks the threshold capacities—the capacities needed to conduct oneself in a characteristically human way, developed to a minimum degree. Since this is truly bad, (3a.1) is correct. Moreover—unlike the bad asserted in (3f.1)—the bad asserted in (3a.1) is bad *for the human beings who have to live that way.*\* It is this bad that (3a.2.1) says govern-

---

\* Nussbaum clearly accepts (3a.1). Of course, one could accept (3a.1) but insist—along with the proponent of the *Fittingness Argument*—that what is bad about someone's having to live without the threshold capacities is that it throws the universe "out of kilter." Indeed, according to what Feinberg calls "Platonic justice," "when functions…are not performed by the thing or person best fitted by its (his) own nature to perform them, there is injustice done, at least from a cosmic point of view"; see Feinberg, "Non-comparative Justice," p. 308. Nussbaum does not, however, defend Platonic justice, and she avoids the difficulties I have associated with it and other versions of the *Fittingness Argument*. That she thinks the bad (3a.1) asserts is bad for the persons who lack the threshold capacities is vividly confirmed by the fact that she likens having to live without those capacities to "a

ment must avert if is to be appropriately respectful of human worth. Since the bad the *Aristotelian Argument* says government must avert is connected with human interests, the *Aristotelian Argument* seems to avoid the problem that undid the *Fittingness Argument*, at least if (3a.2.1) is true.

Is (3a.2.1) true?

(3a.2.1) is a claim about what government must do if it is to be "appropriately respectful" of human worth. Human beings are agents—that is, we are purposive beings who can exercise practical reason to plan and lead our lives. In doing so, we draw on the skills and qualities that I have labeled the "threshold capacities." That we can live in a distinctively human way and are capable of distinctively human excellences seems to be—or to be an important part of—what gives us our dignity or worth. And so it seems that if any agent—including our government—is to be appropriately respectful of our dignity or worth, that agent must respect and treat us *as* agents who can live in this way. How such respect is to be shown may vary depending upon who is showing the respect. But it seems plausible that one of the ways that government—with the resources, responsibility and authority to serve the interests of its citizens—should show respect is by averting the bad state of affairs that occurs when its citizens have to live without the threshold capacities. Since this is just what (3a.2.1) says, (3a.2.1) may seem to be true.

The introduction of (3a.2.1) is clearly the critical move in the *Aristotelian Argument*. According to the line of reasoning just offered, that move depends crucially upon a claim about what a government must do if it is to respect and treat its citizens as agents. The requirement that government treat its citizens as agents is one that the proponent of the *Fittingness Argument* overlooks, since the *Fittingness Argument* came undone precisely because its crucial premise—(3f.2.1)—was compatible with a government's treating citizens merely as valued

---

kind of premature death"; see Nussbaum, *Frontiers of Justice*, p. 347. Nussbaum's endorsement of (3a.1) and her remark about premature death are what incline me to think that her argument for the right to develop threshold capacities follows the line plotted in the text; see also pp. 228-229 of her "Human Functioning and Social Justice," *Political Theory* 20 (1992): 202-246. The passage at the top of p. 169 of her "Nature, Function, and Capability: Aristotle on Political Distribution," *Oxford Studies in Ancient Philosophy,* Supplementary Volume (1988): 145-184, is harder to interpret and may lay out a different line of argument.

objects, somewhat like jewels, and not as agents. But what exactly is it to respect and treat citizens as agents who can develop and exercise the threshold capacities? Which capacities are relevant?

Among the capacities most human beings can exercise with proper nurture and training are the capacity to develop, articulate and exchange ideas about how they should live and about the material conditions under which they pursue their ends, and the capacity to live with others on mutually acceptable terms. More specifically, we can reason together about whether we are conducting ourselves justly, about what our own basic entitlements are, and about whether the conditions under which we live are just. We are, we might say, capable of developing and exercising a sense of justice.[23] Because human beings can develop and exercise a sense of justice, we can reflect on their own dignity or worth, and we can develop, articulate and exchange ideas about what conditions are and are not worthy of us.

This capacity for a sense of justice is a characteristically human capacity, hence a capacity for living in a distinctively human way. A life in which someone lacks the ability to reason about justice is a life lacking in human dignity, at least to that extent. This point is one that proponents of the *Aristotelian Argument* are well-positioned to appreciate, since it is a point that Aristotle pretty clearly implies in the first book of the *Politics* (1253a17). If government is to respect human worth, it must respond appropriately to the fact that people can develop and exercise a sense of justice. How is it to do that?

I suggest that if human beings can reason well about their own basic entitlements, then—if government is to respect its citizens as beings who can develop this capacity—it must foster the development of the capacity. This in itself is a significant conclusion, one which does not seem to have been reached by all proponents of the *Aristotelian Argument*.* But government must also do something more. If it is to be appropriately respectful of human worth, it must take as normative the conclusions its citizens would reach about their own basic entitlements when they reason well about them.

The requirement that government take those conclusions as

---

* It is difficult to see where the capacity for a sense of justice is included on Martha Nussbaum's list of basic capabilities; it is not included on her list as such. For Nussbaum's list, see the Appendix to her essay in this volume, as well as *Frontiers of Justice*, pp. 76ff.

normative is vague. One way to take those conclusions as normative would be to take them as dispositive. Taking the requirement this way implies that government must take the conclusions citizens would reach about basic entitlements as defining those entitlements. Another way to take them as normative would be to hold that, while the agreement they would reach does not automatically define basic entitlements, there is a rebuttable presumption that it defines them. There are other, still weaker ways we can imagine of taking the conclusions as normative. For my purposes, I do not need to be specific. I shall simply say that in arriving at what government must do if it is to be appropriately respectful of human worth, the conclusions human beings would reach about their own basic entitlements must be taken into account. This is a very weak requirement, but it is as strong as I need for the points about human dignity arguments that I wish to make.

What do I mean by "the conclusions citizens would reach about their own basic entitlements"? First of all, as I said above, I mean the conclusions citizens would reach when reasoning *well* together about their own entitlements. Determining what those conclusions are may require a fair amount of idealization and abstraction, since we do not always reason well about such matters in ordinary life. The conclusion to which my suggestion refers is therefore a hypothetical rather than an actual conclusion, as the word "would" in the suggestion implies. Various works in the social contract tradition offer different ways of modeling good reasoning about human entitlements and so offer different ways of determining what the content of the hypothetical conclusion would be. I shall not try to adjudicate among them. I simply note that some contractualist argument is needed to give substance to the idea of "conclusions citizens would reach."

My suggestion therefore comes to this. If human beings are capable of a sense of justice, then—if their government is to respect them as beings who can develop and exercise that capability—what states of affairs government must avert to show respect cannot be determined without taking into account the conclusions citizens would reach when reasoning well about their own basic entitlements.

Why accept the suggestion?

If human beings have the potential for a sense of justice, that is a very important fact about us. A government that is bound to be appropriately respectful of human worth must therefore respect human beings as beings who can develop and exercise this capacity. It is bound, that is, to respect us as beings who can arrive at conclusions about our own basic entitlements. Now suppose that a government determined how it was bound to show respect—and what, if any, basic entitlements it was bound to honor—without taking any account at all of what conclusions human beings would reach about their own entitlements. Then it is hard to see how it could be respecting its citizens as beings capable of reaching such conclusions. For to respect persons as beings who are capable of reaching conclusions is surely to take some account of the conclusions they would reach. If government is to respect its citizens as such beings, it must therefore take the object of their hypothetical consensus into account.

What does this suggestion imply about the structure of the *Aristotelian Argument*?

(3a.2.1) is the premise of the argument that says, "The bad of a human being's having to live a life in which she lacks the threshold capacities is one that government must avert if it is to be appropriately respectful of human worth." I sketched a defense of that premise that turned on a claim about what a government must do if it is to respect and treat its citizens as agents. If the suggestion I have just argued for is correct, then one of the things it must do to treat them as the kind of agents they are is to take account of the conclusions they would reach about their basic entitlements and about what they are due from their government. (3a.2.1) must therefore be the last step of an argument, one of the premises of which is a claim about the conclusion that would be reached when human beings capable of a sense of justice reason well together about their basic entitlements.

What the other premises are depends upon what we make of hypothetical reasoning, and upon what it means to take the conclusions of that hypothetical reasoning into account. I shall not pursue those questions here. What matters for my purposes is this: (3a.2.1) depends upon the content of a hypothetical consensus among citizens, and the conclusion of the *Aristotelian Argument* depends upon the truth of (3a.2.1). So—if human beings can develop and exercise a sense of justice—the basic human entitlements which the *Aristotelian Argument* is said to support cannot ultimately be determined without a hypothetical consensus about basic entitlements reached by those whose entitlements they are.

## Conclusion

As I noted in section I, arguments from human dignity are often presented as alternatives to arguments that rely upon a social contract. Even when arguments from dignity support the same entitlements as contractualist arguments, arguments from dignity are often thought to provide an independent route to those entitlements. Sometimes, as we saw, arguments from human dignity are said to be not just independent of contractualist arguments, but preferable to them. They are said to provide a justification for basic entitlements that does not suffer from the various defects that are alleged to afflict social contract theory.

I have examined two arguments that appeal to human dignity to ground basic entitlements. One, the *Fittingness Argument*, fails because it requires government to avert a bad that is not properly connected with the human interests government is supposed to advance. The argument therefore misconstrues the ways in which government must respect human worth. The *Aristotelian Argument* avoids the difficulties that undermine the *Fittingness Argument*. But if the arguments of the previous section are correct, then—if human beings can develop and exercise a sense of justice—the conclusions of the *Aristotelian Argument* need to be reached *via* conclusions about the content of a hypothetical agreement. In that case, the *Aristotelian Argument* depends upon a contractualist argument to support the basic entitlements asserted in its conclusion. This suggests that, if human beings can develop and exercise a sense of justice, then the contrast between contractualist arguments and the *Aristotelian Argument from Human Dignity* is a false contrast. The claim that the *Aristotelian Argument* can avoid the defects of contractualist arguments because it is independent of those arguments is mistaken.

I have not argued that the value of human dignity is dispensable or that it does not play an essential role in arguments from human dignity. Indeed, I have granted here that government must respect those features of human beings that are thought to ground human dignity. I said at the outset that I think the concept of human dignity can be used to draw attention to those features and to express agreement about their moral significance. "Dignity" is, I said, a useful second-level concept. And I have assumed that the duty to respect those features of human beings entails the duty to respect human beings as capable of a sense of justice when the ability to develop a sense of justice is present.

What I have been concerned to show here is that it is this latter duty which leads to the dependence of human dignity arguments on contractualist ones. Thus government's duty to respect human dignity or human worth is what, as it were, gets arguments for basic entitlements off the ground. But what that duty entails must be spelled out by reference to people's hypothetical reasoning about what their basic entitlements are. In defending this conclusion I am, of course, merely defending a claim that social contract theorists themselves have recognized.*

Note, finally, that the conclusion for which I have argued is conditional. I have argued that *if* human beings can develop and exercise a sense of justice, *then* their basic entitlements against government can be identified only by taking account of a hypothetical agreement among them.

I have assumed that most human beings can develop and exercise a sense of justice. If *all* human beings can do so, then *everyone's* basic human entitlements against government must be identified in this way. But what if there are some human beings of whom the antecedent of the conditional does not hold? What if there are some who cannot develop and exercise a sense of justice, or some of whom it makes no sense to suppose that they enter into a hypothetical agreement—perhaps because of severe handicaps? Do such persons, if such there be, have basic entitlements? If so, what are the grounds of those entitlements and how are those grounds connected to human dignity?

As I noted earlier, the President's Council appeals frequently to the value of human dignity. In one passage, the language of the Council raises the possibility that human beings may have different kinds

---

* See John Rawls's discussion of human dignity at *A Theory of Justice*, p. 513; that discussion concludes with the remark, "There is no way to avoid the complications of the original position, or of some similar construction, if our notions of respect and the natural basis of equality are to be systematically presented." See also Ronald Dworkin's very interesting interpretation of Rawls's view as a natural rights view in "Justice and Rights," in his *Taking Rights Seriously* (Cambridge, Massachusetts: Harvard University Press, 1977), pp. 150-83, especially pp. 180*ff*.

of dignity, depending upon their stage of development.[24] Other passages seem to foreclose this possibility by asserting that all human beings have dignity equally.[25] In one critical place, at which the Council tries to draw normative conclusions from ascriptions of dignity, the argument for those conclusions seems to depend, not just upon the claim that all have dignity equally, but also on the claim that the basis of human dignity is the same for all.[26]

It does not follow from anything I have said that human beings who are incapable of a sense of justice do not have basic entitlements, or that they do not have the same entitlements as those who can develop and exercise a sense of justice. But if they cannot develop and exercise a sense of justice, then it is hard to see how their government's respect for their dignity or worth requires it to respect them as beings who can develop and exercise that capacity. And it is hard to see how government could be bound to show respect for their worth by taking account of hypothetical reasoning into which they could or would enter. The grounds for the entitlements held by those who can and those who cannot develop a sense of justice would therefore seem to be different, even if the entitlements enjoyed by both groups turn out to be the same. If this is so then, while dignity may be a useful second-level concept, the hope that some unitary account of human dignity can provide a single foundation for the basic entitlements of all human beings would seem to be misplaced.

## Notes

[1] I am grateful to Elizabeth Anderson and Robert Audi for helpful comments on an earlier draft.
[2] See www.un.org/Overview/rights.html.
[3] The *Charter* is available via a link at www.europarl.europa.eu/charter/default_en.htm.
[4] Emphasis added; for an English translation of the Basic Law, see www.iuscomp.org/gla/statutes/GG.htm.
[5] Ruth Macklin, "Dignity is a Useless Concept," *British Medical Journal* 327 (2003): 1419-1420.
[6] See, for example, Louis Dupré and William O'Neill, SJ, "Social Structures and Structural Ethics," *The Review of Politics* 51 (1989): 327-344, especially pp. 336 and 342.
[7] See Jacques Maritain, *The Person and the Common Good* (Notre Dame, Indiana: University of Notre Dame Press, 1966), trans. John J. Fitzgerald, p. 13: "Our desire is to make clear the personalism rooted in the doctrine of St. Thomas and to separate, at the very outset, a social philosophy centered in the dignity of the human person from every social philosophy centered in the primacy of the individual and the private good."
[8] This paragraph summarizes a line of criticism pursued in detail in Martha Nussbaum, *Frontiers of Justice* (Cambridge, Massachusetts: Harvard University Press, 2006).
[9] The President's Council on Bioethics, *Human Cloning and Human Dignity: An Ethical Inquiry* (Washington, D.C.: Government Printing Office, 2002), p. 89; *Taking Care: Ethical Caregiving in Our Aging Society* (Washington, D.C.: Government Printing Office, 2005), p. 104.
[10] See *Taking Care*, pp. 103, 126, 127, 129.
[11] The President's Council on Bioethics, *Being Human: Readings from the President's Council on Bioethics* (Washington D.C.: Government Printing Office, 2003), introduction to chapter 10.
[12] See *Taking Care*, p. x.
[13] *Human Cloning and Human Dignity*, p. 87; The President's Council on Bioethics, *Monitoring Stem Cell Research* (Washington, D.C.: Government Printing Office, 2004), p. 92.
[14] The President's Council on Bioethics, *Alternative Sources of Human Pluripotent Stem Cells: A White Paper* (Washington, D.C.: Government Printing Office, 2005), p. 43; *Human Cloning and Human Dignity*, p. ix.
[15] *Human Cloning and Human Dignity*, p. 14.
[16] The President's Council on Bioethics, *Beyond Therapy: Biotechnology and the Pursuit of Happiness* (Washington, D.C.: Government Printing Office, 2003), p. 103.
[17] Martha Nussbaum, *Frontiers of Justice*, p. 44 (emphasis added). I hasten to add that, as will be apparent in the next section, I do not take Nussbaum to be a proponent of the *Fittingness Argument*. The quotation here is simply a prominent and

readily accessible example of a popular locution.

[18] See, for example, his "The Church and the State Are Not Rivals but Partners," Papal Address to New Turkish Ambassador to Holy See, February 23, 2004, available online at www.zenit.org/english/visualizza.phtml?sid=49511.

[19] Leon R. Kass, "Reflections on Public Bioethics: A View from the Trenches," *Kennedy Institute of Ethics Journal* 15 (2005): 221-250, p. 240 (emphasis added).

[20] Craig Smith, "More Disagreement Over Human Dignity: Federal Constitutional Court's Most Recent Benetton Advertising Decision," *German Law Journal*, vol. 4, no. 6, 1 June 2003.

[21] Cf. Nussbaum, *Frontiers of Justice*, pp. 82, 155, 161.

[22] Ibid., p. 78.

[23] The phrase "sense of justice" is, of course, taken from Rawls; see John Rawls, *A Theory of Justice* (Cambridge, Massachusetts: Harvard University Press, 1999), p. 41.

[24] See the enigmatic remark about "primordial dignity" in the introduction to chapter 10 of *Being Human*.

[25] See *Taking Care*, p. 103.

[26] See the argument against cloning in *Human Cloning and Human Dignity*, pp. 105*ff.*

# 18
# Dignity and Bioethics: History, Theory, and Selected Applications

Daniel P. Sulmasy, O.F.M.

The word "dignity" has become something of a slogan in bioethics, often invoked by both sides of debates about a variety of scientific and clinical issues, supporting contradictory conclusions. For instance, in arguments about assisted suicide, those who favor the legalization of the practice base their conclusion on a moral imperative to provide "death with dignity," while those who oppose legalization do so because they see intentionally rendering a human being dead, even out of mercy, as a direct assault on human dignity.[1] Certainly this suggests that dignity is a concept in need of clarification.

Ruth Macklin has noted this lack of conceptual clarity surrounding the use of the word "dignity" in the bioethics literature and has concluded that dignity is a "useless concept," reducible to respect for autonomy, and adds nothing to the conversation.[2] This hasty conclusion, casting aside thousands of years of philosophical writing, ignoring the contemporary bioethical discourse of continental Europeans, and sweeping away a whole body of international law, can be justified only by begging the question. If one defines a word completely in terms of another concept more to one's liking, it will always follow that the word in question adds nothing to the concept one already endorses. While shrouded in rhetoric, this is precisely the structure of Macklin's argument. Premise: dignity means nothing more than respect for autonomy. Conclusion: therefore dignity means nothing more than respect for autonomy and (Corollary) therefore dignity adds nothing to bioethical discourse.

A more careful treatment of the topic is in order. In this essay I will, first, describe three ways the word "dignity" has been used in moral discourse, both in the history of Western thought and in contemporary bioethics. I call these the attributed, the intrinsic, and the inflorescent uses of the word.

Second, I will argue that, while all three senses have moral relevance, the intrinsic sense of dignity is the most fundamental from a moral perspective. I will advance this argument in two ways. I will call the first the Axiological Argument and the second the Argument from Consistency.

Third, I will outline some of the general norms that follow from accepting the moral primacy of the intrinsic sense of human dignity.

Finally, I will show how this vigorous understanding of dignity helps to give shape to arguments in bioethics. As examples, I will show (briefly) how it applies to questions about justice and access to health care resources, the care of the disabled, embryonic stem cell research, cloning, euthanasia, and the care of patients in the so-called permanent vegetative state.

I will conclude that a notion robust enough to supply answers to all of these questions is not useless.

## Three Senses of Dignity

Throughout Western history and in contemporary debates, the word dignity has played a prominent role in ethical discussions. It may be surprising to both religious and non-religious persons to know, however, that dignity is not a word that entered the Western moral vocabulary through the Judeo-Christian heritage. Dignity is not an important word in either the Hebrew or Christian scriptures. For almost two millennia, it was not an important theological term. Until very recently, dignity was almost never invoked by moral theologians in making arguments about abortion, euthanasia, or economic justice.[3]

Neither was dignity an important concept for all Western moral philosophers. For instance, dignity was not an important word for Plato or Aristotle. The first Western philosophers for whom dignity was an important philosophical term were the Roman Stoics. Cicero and Seneca, especially, used the word to designate important concepts in their moral philosophies.

Cicero defined dignity as "the honorable authority of a person, which merits attention and honor and worthy respect" (*dignitas est alicuius honesta et cultu et honore et verecundia digna auctoritas*).[4] He used the word dignitas frequently in his writings. As one translator put it, the meaning of dignitas in Cicero's use is literally "worthiness," but he often used it (as did others in his day) to refer to a person's standing, reputation, or even office in the civitas.[5] Importantly, in Cicero's account, this dignitas is not so much dependent on the subjective evaluation of others as it is on the ability of everyone to recognize an instance of true human excellence. For example, in *De Officiis,* Cicero writes,

> If we wish to reflect on the excellence and dignity of our nature, we shall realize how dishonorable it is to sink into luxury and to live a dainty and soft lifestyle, but how honorable to live thriftily, strictly, with self-restraint, and soberly.
>
> *Atque etiam, si considerare volumus, quae sit in natura excellentia et dignitas, intellegemus, quam sit turpe diffluere luxuria et delicate ac molliter vivere, quamque honestum parce, continenter, severe, sobrie.*[6]

In other words, for Cicero, one's standing in the community ought to be based on one's true excellence. For him, to have dignity was to have a merited degree of respect from others because of one's excellence as a human being.

The Stoic use of the term, however, is not the only historical conception of dignity. Hobbes, for instance, defined dignity in a very different way. He eliminated any necessary connection to true human excellence and took the meaning of dignity to depend solely upon the inter-subjective judgments of the market. In the *Leviathan* he writes:

> The Value or WORTH of a man, is, as of other things, his price; that is to say, so much as would be given for the use of his Power; and therefore it is not absolute; but a thing dependent on the need and judgment of another.... The publique worth of a man, which is the Value set on him by the Commonwealth, is that which men commonly call DIGNITY.[7]

Hobbes writes clearly and bluntly. Dignity is the value one has to the Commonwealth regardless of whether one actually merits this based on one's true excellence as a human being or on one's nature as a human being.

Kant never explicitly cites Hobbes, but in presenting yet a third view of dignity, he seems to be writing in direct reaction to Hobbes. The Kantian view of dignity (*Würde*) continues to exert a powerful influence to the present day. Kant wrote,

> The respect I bear others or which another can claim from me (*osservantia aliis praestanda*) is the acknowledgement of the dignity (*dignitas*) of another man, i.e., a worth which has no price, no equivalent for which the object of valuation (*aestimii*) could be exchanged.[8]

Kant connected dignity with his idea that human beings should never be treated as pure instruments of another's will. In the *Grundlagen,* he writes, "...[T]hat which constitutes the condition under which alone something can be an end in itself has not merely a relative worth, i.e., a price, but has intrinsic worth, i.e., dignity."[9] More simply, he states elsewhere, "Humanity itself is a dignity."[10]

Thus, the Kantian view of dignity is neither based on one's value to others, nor on the esteem they ought to show based on one's degree of human excellence, but rather on one's humanity itself.[11] The Kantian view of dignity is powerful, influential, and substantially different from the notions that preceded it. The Kantian notion of *Würde* may be one of his greatest contributions to moral philosophy.

These three historical uses of the word "dignity" are illustrative of three senses of the word that are still active in philosophical discourse and in ordinary language today. These three general senses of dignity can be understood according to the following names and descriptions.

By attributed dignity, I mean that worth or value that human beings confer upon others by acts of attribution. The act of conferring this worth or value may be accomplished individually or communally, but it always involves a choice. Attributed dignity is, in a sense, created. It constitutes a conventional form of value. Thus, we attribute worth or value to those we consider to be dignitaries, those we admire, those who carry themselves in a particular way, or those who have certain talents, skills, or powers. We can even attribute worth or value to ourselves using this word. The Hobbesian notion of dignity is attributed.

By intrinsic dignity, I mean that worth or value that people have simply because they are human, not by virtue of any social standing, ability to evoke admiration, or any particular set of talents, skills, or powers. Intrinsic dignity is the value that human beings have simply by virtue of the fact that they are human beings. Thus we say that racism is an offense against human dignity. Used this way, dignity designates a value not conferred or created by human choices, individual or collective, but is prior to human attribution. Kant's notion of dignity is intrinsic.

By inflorescent dignity, I mean the way people use the word to describe the value of a process that is conducive to human excellence or the value of a state of affairs by which an individual expresses human excellence. In other words, inflorescent dignity is used to refer to individuals who are flourishing as human beings—living lives that are consistent with and expressive of the intrinsic dignity of the human.[12] Thus, dignity is sometimes used to refer to a state of virtue—a state of affairs in which a human being habitually acts in ways that expresses the intrinsic value of the human. We say, for instance, that so-and-so faced a particularly trying situation with dignity. This use of the word is not purely attributed, since it depends upon some objective conception of human excellence. Nonetheless, the value to which this use of the word refers is not intrinsic, since it depends upon a prior understanding of the intrinsic value of the human. The

Stoic use of the word, while it sometimes borders on an attributed sense, is generally an inflorescent sense of dignity.

These conceptions of human dignity are by no means mutually exclusive. Attributed, intrinsic, and inflorescent conceptions of dignity are often at play in the same situation. Yet each has been taken as the central basis for particular moral claims in bioethics.

Does it matter which of these senses of dignity one invokes in ethical discourse? The short answer would seem to be "yes." At the very least it seems important to keep these senses straight. For example, those who claim that death with dignity requires that euthanasia be permissible seem to be using the word "dignity" in an attributed sense,[13] while those who claim that euthanasia is a direct offense against human dignity appear to be using the word in an intrinsic sense.[14] Still others who oppose euthanasia appear to argue from an inflorescent sense of dignity, suggesting that the practice represents less than the most noble and excellent response a human being can make in the face of death.[15] Merely noticing these distinctions can help us clarify arguments and understand points of disagreement.

But more than this, is there anything that can be said about the relationship between these senses of dignity? Is there an order or moral priority? If there is a conflict between moral claims based on differing senses of dignity, does one count more than the other?

I will argue that the intrinsic notion of dignity is foundational from a moral point of view. I will advance two arguments to support this claim. I call these the Axiological Argument and the Argument from Consistency.

## The Axiological Argument

The axiological argument depends on the theory of value or axiology.[16] By understanding what values are, how values get into the world, what sorts of values there are, and how they are related, it will be argued that one can arrive at the conclusion that the intrinsic sense of dignity is the fundamental sense.

Classically, axiology distinguishes between intrinsic and instrumental values. Instrumental values, however, are best characterized as a subclass of attributed values. I have argued that the primary distinction in axiology is between intrinsic values and attributed values.[17]

Intrinsic value is the value something has of itself—the value it has by virtue of its being the kind of thing that it is. It is valuable independent of any valuer's purposes, beliefs, desires, interests, or expectations. Truly intrinsic values, according to environmental ethicist Holmes Rolston III, "are objectively there—discovered, not generated by the valuer."[18]

Attributed values are those conveyed by a valuer. Attributed values depend completely on the purposes, beliefs, desires, interests, or expectations of a valuer or group of valuers. That is why I argue that instrumental values are a class of attributed values. An instrumental value is one that is attributed to some entity because it serves a purpose for a valuer. The instrumental value of the entity consists in its serving as a means by which the valuer achieves some purpose. But there can be non-instrumental attributed values as well. For example, the value of humor may serve no clear instrumental purpose.

Attributed values play important roles in human life. The authority of government, for instance, is attributed. The value of money is attributed. The value of technology is attributed. Importantly, some attributed values are morally flawed, such as attributing value to human skin color or attributing too much value to the opinions of other persons.

Intrinsic values and attributed values are asymmetrically related. Intrinsic values, as intrinsic and objective, must be recognized by an intelligent valuer. Recognition, of course, requires attribution, and thus an intelligent valuer must attribute intrinsic value to whatever does have intrinsic value in order to be correct in his or her evaluation. It would be incorrect for the valuer to attribute no value to what has value intrinsically. This is not to suggest that the act of evaluation confers the value, but that the value must be attributed to whatever has intrinsic value in order for the act of evaluation to be correct. By contrast, the mere fact that value has been attributed to an entity has no logical implications with respect to intrinsic value. One may freely attribute value to things on the basis of individual preferences, social customs, or instrumental needs. One may also recognize (i.e., correctly attribute value to) an entity that has intrinsic value. The bare fact that value has been attributed does not allow us to conclude whether the value at stake is attributed or intrinsic.

I have suggested that there is yet a third category of values, inflorescent values. Certain processes or states of affairs in an intrinsically valuable entity are considered especially valuable. This is the case because these processes or states of affairs either are conducive to or instantiate the flourishing of an intrinsically valuable thing as the kind of thing that it is. The flourishing of a member of a natural kind is a good state of affairs, but that goodness depends upon something about the kind of thing that is flourishing. Thus, the value of that state of affairs is, in a sense, derivative. One might be tempted to say that flourishing is intrinsically good, but the goodness of flourishing is always dependent upon the kind of thing that is said to be flourishing, and thus that state of affairs is not, strictly speaking, intrinsically valuable. Rather, it is the thing that is flourishing that is intrinsically valuable, and its flourishing can only be understood in terms of the intrinsic value of that thing.

On this view, human virtues, such as courage, are not, in a technical sense, intrinsically valuable. We seek virtue not for its own sake, but for the sake of our humanity. For instance, since the virtue of courage is a state of affairs of an individual member of the human natural kind, the value of courage is dependent upon knowledge of what kind of thing a human being is and upon the value of being human. Human virtues are good because they instantiate aspects of the flourishing of the human natural kind in virtuous individuals.

What relationship does this discussion have to dignity? "Intrinsic dignity" is just the name we give to the special type of intrinsic value that belongs to members of natural kinds that have kind-specific capacities for language, rationality, love, free will, moral agency, creativity, aesthetic sensibility, and an ability to grasp the finite and the infinite. The phase "attributed dignities" refers to several non-instrumental values that are attributed to members of any natural kind that has intrinsic dignity. The phrase "inflorescent dignity" refers to a variety of states of affairs in which a member of a natural kind that has intrinsic dignity is flourishing as the kind of thing that it is. By definition, then, intrinsic dignity is the fundamental notion of dignity. One defines attributed and inflorescent dignity in terms of intrinsic dignity.

The next step in the argument is to note that, if there are intrinsic values in the world, the recognition of the intrinsic value of something depends upon one's ability to discern what kind of thing it is. This brings me to the notion of natural kinds, a relatively new concept in analytic philosophy.[19] The fundamental idea behind natural kinds is that to pick something out from the rest of the universe, one must pick it out as a something. This, in turn, leads to what its proponents call a "modest essentialism"—that the essence of something is that by which one picks it out from the rest of reality as anything at all—its being a member of a kind. The alternative seems inconceivable—that reality is actually completely undifferentiated and that human beings merely carve up an amorphous, homogeneous universe for their own purposes. Reality is not homogenous but "lumpy." It comes differentiated into kinds of things. It seems bizarre to suggest that there really are no actual kinds of things in the world independent of human classification—no such things, de re, as stars, slugs, or human beings.

Intrinsic value, to repeat, is the value something has by virtue of its being the kind of thing that it is. Thus, the intrinsic value of a natural entity—the value it has by virtue of being the kind of thing that it is—depends upon one's ability to pick that entity out as a member of a natural kind. Intrinsic dignity, then, is the intrinsic value of entities that are members of a natural kind that is, as a kind, capable of language, rationality, love, free will, moral agency, creativity, aesthetic sensibility, and an ability to grasp the finite and the infinite.

One should note that this definition is decidedly anti-speciesist. If there are other kinds of entities in the universe besides human beings that have, as a kind, these capacities, they would also have intrinsic dignity—whether angels, extra-terrestrials, or (arguably) other known animal kinds.

Importantly, the logic of natural kinds suggests that one picks individuals out as members of the kind not because they express all the necessary and sufficient predicates to be classified as a member of a species, but, rather, by virtue of their inclusion under the extension of a natural kind that, as a kind, has those capacities. The logic of natural kinds is extensional, not intensional. As Wiggins puts it,

> [The] determination of a natural kind stands or falls with the existence of law-like principles that will collect together the

actual extension of the kind around an arbitrary good specimen of it; and these law-like principles will also determine the characteristic development and typical history of members of this extension.[20]

For example, very few bananas in the bin in the supermarket express all the necessary and sufficient conditions for being classified as fruits of the species *Musa sapientum*. We define a banana as a yellow fruit. Yet some specimens in the bin are yellow, some are green, some are spotted, some are brown, and some are even a bit black. Nonetheless, they are all bananas. They fall under the extension that gathers them around an arbitrary good specimen (or two) of a banana.

Health care depends profoundly upon this logic. It is not the expression of rationality that makes us human, but our belonging to a kind that is capable of rationality that makes us human. When a human being is comatose or mentally ill, we first pick the individual out as a human being, then we note the disparity between the characteristics of the afflicted individual and the paradigmatic features and typical development and history of members of the human natural kind. This is how we come to the judgment that the individual is sick, and make the diagnosis of a disease.

So, if there is such a thing as intrinsic value in the world, then intrinsic dignity is the name we give to the value of all the individual members of any and all kinds that, as kinds, share the properties we think essential to the special value we recognize in the human. Thus, because a sick individual is a member of the human natural kind, we recognize that this individual has the intrinsic value we call dignity. It is in recognition of that worth that we have established the healing professions as our moral response to those of our kind who are suffering from disease and injury. The plight of the sick has little instrumental value, rarely serving the purposes, beliefs, desires, interests, or expectations of any of us as individuals. Rather, it is because of the intrinsic value of the sick that health care professionals serve them. Thus I would argue that intrinsic human dignity is the foundation of health care.

## The Argument from Consistency

The argument from consistency is an alternative means of reaching the conclusion that intrinsic dignity is the primary moral sense of dignity. The argument is simple in its form. Consistency is at least a necessary condition of a valid moral argument, even if one would quickly add that consistency is not sufficient.[21] In discussions about its fundamental moral meaning, the word "dignity" can be defined as the value or worth that a human being has either: (a) in terms of some property that some entities have and some do not, or (b) in terms of simply being human.* But I will show that defining the fundamental moral meaning of dignity as the value certain entities have by virtue of their possession of any particular candidate property leads to gross inconsistencies in our universally shared, settled moral positions if applied to all human beings. Therefore, one is led to the alternative: that dignity, in its fundamental moral sense, is defined in terms of simply being human—i.e., as an intrinsic value. This kind of argument depends on the exhaustiveness of the list of candidate properties and is not decisive. But at least it puts the burden of proof on those who oppose assigning moral priority to the intrinsic sense of dignity to come up with an alternative property (such as age, size, strength, brainwaves, or skin color) to define what gives an entity the fundamental worth or value we call dignity.

## What Sorts of Candidate Human Properties Might Be Proposed?

First, some have argued that human dignity, in its most fundamental moral sense, depends upon the amount of pleasure and pain in a human life. Hedonism certainly has its adherents, whether egoistic or utilitarian. But even hedonists might not want to promote the pleasure/pain calculus as a theory of human dignity. Certainly, most of us are able to tell stories about the extraordinary lessons in human dignity we have learned from persons whose lives have been racked

---

* There is a third logical possibility that I will not discuss, although some nihilists accept it—namely, that human beings have no dignity.

by pain, and most of us also know undignified human beings who have spent their whole lives in the pursuit of pleasure. Basing morality squarely on a balance between pleasure and pain has seemed, since the time of Aristotle, to be an anemic account of morality and human dignity, and one that most people would reject.[22]

Second, some might think that Hobbes was right—that human dignity depends upon one's market price. But there are problems with such a conception of human dignity. The unemployed, the severely handicapped, the mentally ill, and all others who cannot contribute to the economic well-being of society would then have no dignity. Yet our society has gone to great lengths to recognize the dignity of such persons. If we did not believe that human dignity remains even if people are disabled and lose their economic value to society, then we would not be making access ramps for them. This Hobbesian conception of dignity seems inconsistent with some of our most basic moral and social views.

Third, some might think that human dignity depends upon the active exercise of freedom. Dignity, on this view, is the value we give to entities that actively express a capacity for rational choice. But this view is also hard to sustain consistently. One would have to hold that those who have lost control of certain human functions, or have lost or never had the freedom to make choices, have lost or have never had dignity. This would mean that infants, the retarded, the severely mentally ill, prisoners, the comatose, and perhaps even the sleeping would have no human dignity. This seems obviously wrong.

Now some might suggest that these are "straw man" arguments. What counts, they would aver, is the possibility of exercising control and freedom, not the actual exercise of control and freedom. One might suggest that some individuals without full control and freedom nevertheless deserve to be treated with dignity either because they have a potential for exercising such a capacity (so that children, for instance, come to be regarded as placeholders for actual persons with dignity), or they have a history of having exercised such a capacity (so that the demented, for instance, come to be regarded as remnants of persons with dignity).[23] But these arguments are quite tenuous. Who would feel dignified and secure as a placeholder or a remnant? Further, these arguments still cannot answer why those who never could and never will make free, rational choices (such as the severely mentally retarded) are worthy of being treated in accord with human dignity.

Certain advocates of the position that dignity means the capacity to exercise rational choice (at least above a certain threshold level) do not believe their argument is thus refuted. They fail to see how arguments that would lead to the moral legitimization of practices such as infanticide[24] and experimentation upon permanently unresponsive patients without their consent[25] need to be regarded as *reductio ad absurdum* refutations of their position. Rather, these philosophers fancy themselves heroes, bravely embracing these stark conclusions as the moral consequences of a new and enlightened form of thinking, finally free from the prejudices that weigh the rest of us down.

To argue against this position, one must move the argument one step logically prior to the argument about dignity. One must investigate the underlying theory of the good that drives some philosophers to cling so tenaciously to the idea that dignity means the active exercise of free choice, that they are willing to become champions of infanticide rather than give up the idea of dignity as freedom. One must ask, are things good merely because we choose them? Although space limitations preclude a fuller discussion, simply put, is it not the case, rather, that we choose what we think is good, aware that we can be mistaken in our choices? The meaning of the human good is not exhausted by the exercise of free choice. It is metaphysically impossible to choose one's biological parents. It is metaphysically impossible to choose to come into existence. It is impossible to choose to be loved by someone. In the instant that the choice is one's own rather the free choice of one's lover, what one receives ceases to be love. And it is impossible to choose not to die. Thus, defining the most fundamental human good as the exercise of free choice results in a moral system that simply cannot account for the great human questions, among them: existence, biological relationship, love, and death. The human good must be far deeper than the freedom to choose. The most fundamental meaning of human dignity is not human freedom and control.

Fourth, and finally, some might think that human dignity is something individuals are free to define as they choose, according to their own inner lights. But this view also leads to major moral inconsistencies. First, the concept of a moral term implies that it has universal meaning, a position acknowledged both by Kant[26] and by utilitarians such as R. M. Hare.[27] Second, to say that human dignity is subjective is to claim that one person can never reliably recognize the dignity of another person, because one can never know exactly what the other thinks dignity means at any given moment. This explains why empirical projects designed to understand dignity by asking each in a collection of individuals to describe "what dignity means to me," while well-intended, are profoundly misguided.[28] Morality seems to depend upon our mutual commitment to knowing that each of us has dignity before we open our mouths and explain our notions of dignity to each other. Human dignity cannot be a purely subjective concept.

Thus, the argument from consistency claims that fundamental human dignity must be something each of us has simply because we are human. It is the notion of dignity that drove the U.S. civil rights movement. It is the notion the Rev. Dr. Martin Luther King, Jr., says he learned from his grandmother, who told him, "Martin, don't let anyone ever tell you that you're not a somebody."[29] No matter what value others may attribute to persons because of properties such as skin color, or how free they are to do as they would like, they have dignity because they are somebodies—human beings. Being somebody, being a human being, is the foundation of the notion of human dignity. The argument from consistency says that, if this is what dignity means in civil rights, this is what dignity must mean in bioethics.

## Norms Derivable from Intrinsic Dignity

The conclusion that intrinsic dignity is the fundamental sense of dignity has significant moral implications. The notion of intrinsic dignity entails both self-regarding and other-regarding moral duties for beings that have intrinsic dignity. One of the primary features distinguishing the intrinsic value of a natural kind that has intrinsic dignity from other natural kinds is a kind-typical capacity for moral agency. All members of a natural kind that has intrinsic dignity (and are individually capable of exercising the moral agency that is distinctive of their natural kind) have moral obligations to themselves, to any other entities that have intrinsic dignity, and to the rest of what exists. The following list describes some of these duties. Space limitations preclude a full discussion of how these principles follow from this theory of dignity, but many will appear quite plausible on their face. This list is also not meant to exhaust the fundamental principles of ethics. It is limited to those fundamental principles that are most directly connected to the theme of dignity. But these duties should be taken as sufficiently fundamental and general to be considered true principles. All members of a natural kind that has intrinsic dignity and are, as individual members of that natural kind, capable of exercising the moral agency that in part constitutes their intrinsic dignity, have the following duties:

P-I. A duty of perfect obligation to respect all members of natural kinds that have intrinsic dignity.

P-II. A duty of perfect obligation to respect the capacities that confer intrinsic dignity upon a natural kind, in themselves and in others.

P-III. A duty to comport themselves in a manner that is consistent with their own intrinsic dignity.

P-IV. A duty to build up, to the extent possible, the inflorescent dignity of members of natural kinds that have intrinsic dignity.

P-V. A duty to be respectful of the intrinsic value of all other natural kinds.

P-VI. A duty of perfect obligation, in carrying out PP-I-V, never to act in such a way as directly to undermine the intrinsic dignity that gives the other duties their binding force.

While the language of these principles might seem unfamiliar to bioethicists, the concepts are quite familiar. The second formulation of Kant's categorical imperative might be considered a corollary of P-I. Together, P-I, P-II, P-III, and P-VI elaborate the meaning of Respect for Persons; P-III sounds as if it comes directly from a Stoic discourse on dignity; P-IV and P-VI are related to Beneficence and Non-Maleficence; P-V is the clarion call of environmental ethics. Justice arises from the need to balance the requirements of PP-I-V.

It is also important to note that the duty to build up the

inflorescent dignity of any human being depends logically on the intrinsic dignity of human beings. The primary duty is to recognize and respect that intrinsic dignity. The duty of building up the inflorescent dignity of human beings is a way of concretizing the fundamental duty of respect for intrinsic dignity. If one is to show respect for a dynamic, developing, living natural kind as an intrinsically valuable thing, then it follows that one ought to show that respect by concrete actions that help to establish the conditions by which that thing can flourish as the kind of thing that it is. Thus, one waters a rosemary bush and assures that it has proper sunlight. One feeds a human child and teaches him or her to read.

It is the intrinsic value of the human that grounds our moral duties towards our fellow human beings and gives these duties their special moral valence. It is a minor indiscretion to go on vacation and forget to arrange for someone to water one's rosemary bush. It is an unspeakably immoral evil to neglect to feed or educate one's child. Human beings have a special intrinsic value, and it is this value that commands that we act towards our fellow human beings in a special way. The ground of our duties towards our fellow human beings is not merely that they have interests. Rodents also have interests. As David Velleman has argued, from an ethical point of view, there must be something more fundamental to ethics than interests—i.e., a reason to respect a fellow human being's interests in the first place. The question can be asked, for example, why should I care that this person has lost a degree of independence that I have the capacity to restore through the medical arts? Velleman's answer is that we seek to protect and promote a fellow human being's interests because we first respect the human being whose interests they are.[30] This fundamental respect is for intrinsic dignity—the "interest-independent" value of a human being. Without this primary respect, there is no basis for interpersonal morality.

## Consequences of This View for Bioethics

This conception of dignity has important implications for addressing f issues in bioethics.

## Justice and Access to Health Care

Access to health care and the just distribution of health care resources are pressing questions both within individual nations and between the nations that constitute our globalized world community. Human dignity is often invoked in such discussions, but without much clarity or rigor.

Intrinsic dignity, as elaborated in this essay, can be understood as the foundation of all human rights. We respect the rights of an individual because we first recognize his or her intrinsic dignity. We do not bestow dignity because we first bestow rights. Human beings have rights that must be respected because of the value they have by virtue of being the kinds of things that they are.

Intrinsic dignity is at the core of all our beliefs about moral obligation. Of particular relevance to discussions of access to health care resources are principles P-I and P-IV.

Absolute rights (also called negative rights or natural rights) are based on P-I, the duty to respect all members of natural kinds that bear dignity. These include, for example, the rights not to be killed, not to be treated disrespectfully, and not to be experimented upon without one's consent. These rights can and should be respected by all persons and all societies regardless of their ecological, historical, physical, social, or economic circumstances. In Kantian terminology, these rights entail duties of perfect obligation.

I have argued that health care is not an absolute right or a natural right in this sense of the word.[31] To assert a right to health care is to assert a positive right—a right to goods and services that must, of necessity, vary according to the ecological, historical, physical, social, and economic circumstances of individual persons and societies. In Kantian terminology, these rights entail duties of imperfect obligation. They apply to the degree that they can be instituted in various circumstances. Such so-called positive rights are based on P-IV, the duty to build up the inflorescent dignity of individuals belonging to a natural kind that has, as a kind, intrinsic dignity.

Health is critical for the flourishing of any member of any living natural kind. This is no less true for members of the human natural kind. Diseases diminish health. Accordingly, the concept of disease necessarily includes reference to the adverse effects of the condi on the flourishing of the affected individual. As I have defined it elsewhere, "A disease is a class of states of affairs of individual members of a living natural kind X, that: (1) disturbs the internal biological relations (law-like principles) that determine the characteristic development and typical history of members of the kind, X,...(4) and at least some individuals of whom (or which) this class of states of affairs can be predicated are, by virtue of that state, inhibited from flourishing as Xs."[32] Thus, an anatomical variation such as an anomalous branch in the brachial artery going around the median nerve may violate the law-like generalizations and characteristic development of human beings, but such a variation has no adverse effect on the flourishing of any human being and is not a disease. By contrast, a condition such as rheumatoid arthritis inhibits one's ability to walk, to care for oneself, to open a jar, or to hold a spoon. It causes such pain that one may lose the ability to concentrate on other aspects of life. It is a real disease. Rheumatoid arthritis inhibits one who bears the stamp of intrinsic dignity from flourishing as a human being, either directly or by virtue of the fact that health is required for so many other forms of human flourishing—family life, friendship, work, art, politics, scholarship, and more. Respect for an afflicted individual requires, in recognition of this dignity, a concrete response. Medicine is one of the major forms of human response to such affliction, capable at times of restoring the flourishing of the individual, and at other times limiting the degree to which the disease or injury detracts from human flourishing. In terms of concrete medical practice this can mean either cure, or assistance with the activities of daily living, or amelioration of pain or other symptoms if this is possible. The duty to provide such care follows from P-IV. A society that fails to provide for health care has violated P-IV.

Health is also a fundamental condition for attributions of value, either reflexively by an individual, or by the attribution of others. To see this, one need only reflect on the ways in which illness and injury assault the attributed dignity of human beings. Those who are ill are robbed of their stations in life. They lose valued independence. They often become disfigured. They lose their social productivity. They lose esteem in the eyes of others and may even begin to question their own value. If there are any duties to build up the attributed dignities of human beings, surely health care is one of the primary means of doing so.

As argued above, however, the fundamental reason one provides health care is out of respect for intrinsic dignity. And intrinsic dignity inheres in the human with a radical equality. In its intrinsic sense, dignity is inalienable and does not admit of degrees. Thus, a duty to build up the inflorescent dignity of human beings through health care, founded upon respect for intrinsic human dignity, applies equally to all. So, while there might not be a natural right to health care, a just society has a moral obligation, founded upon human dignity, to provide equal access to health care, to the extent possible in its particular ecological, historical, physical, social, and economic circumstances.

Thus the conception of dignity presented here provides a normative basis for determining what it means for a society to distribute health care resources justly. This would seem to make dignity a useful concept.

## Euthanasia

As I discussed earlier, understanding the three senses of dignity presented in this essay helps to explain three very different ways the word has been invoked in debates about euthanasia and physician-assisted suicide. This, in itself, seems a significant contribution to bioethics. Proponents of euthanasia and assisted suicide argue that the practice ought to be permitted because the assaults that illness and injury mount upon the attributed dignities of human beings can be so overwhelming that some patients might be led to attribute no more worth or value to themselves, thus making euthanasia a reasonable option. Opponents of euthanasia make two dignity-based arguments: one based on an inflorescent sense of dignity and the other based on an intrinsic sense of dignity. Neither argument denies the assault that illness and injury can mount against the attributed dignity of a human being. The argument from inflorescent dignity suggests, however, that the value of the human is expressed most fully (i.e., flourishes) in the ability to stand up to such assaults with courage, humble acceptance of the finitude of the human, not even love. To kill oneself in the face of death or to ask to on this view, is precisely the opposite of what it means to face death with dignity.

The argument from intrinsic dignity suggests that the fundamental basis for the duty to build up the inflorescent dignity of sick human beings—the root of any motivation to attribute dignity to them—is the intrinsic value of the human, the value human beings have by virtue of being the kinds of things that they are. As argued above, no circumstances can eliminate that intrinsic dignity. As Duty P-VI states, there is a duty of perfect obligation, in carrying out PP-I-V, never to act in such a way as directly to undermine the intrinsic dignity that gives the other duties their binding force. Thus, while one might, out of human sympathy, suggest that a duty to build up attributed dignity legitimizes euthanasia, the conception of dignity presented in this essay would argue that this cannot be permitted because it undermines the fundamental basis of morality itself—respect for intrinsic dignity.

A conception of dignity with the explanatory power to understand the basis for arguments on both sides of the debate about euthanasia as well as the normative power to settle that argument in favor of prohibiting the practice seems much more than a "useless" concept.

## The Care of the Disabled

The proper treatment of persons with disabilities has become a matter of great controversy in bioethics, with significant implications for our society. A famous philosopher has even argued with a disability rights activist about these issues in the pages of the *New York Times Sunday Magazine*.[33] Could the conception of dignity presented here illuminate these debates?

First, it is clear that disability does not transform a human being into another natural kind. One classifies a person as disabled because one has first picked that individual out as a member of the human natural kind, noting the kind-typical features that the individual does not express. The disabled therefore have intrinsic dignity. Respect for intrinsic dignity would dictate, as argued above, that one recognize the radically equal intrinsic dignity of a severely mentally retarded adult and of a philosophy professor at an Ivy League university. No matter how severe the disability, there are no gradations in intrinsic dignity. It is the value one has by virtue of being the kind of thing that one is—a member of the human natural kind.

Second, respect for intrinsic dignity would prohibit, as described above, euthanizing disabled human beings of any age on the basis of their disability. As discussed, in violation of P-VI, this practice would undermine the most fundamental basis of any human morality.

Third, as discussed above, the duty to build up the inflorescent dignity of human beings—a duty based on respect for intrinsic dignity—carries with it a notion of the radical equality of the intrinsic dignity of all human beings. Just as skin color, income, education, and social worth ought not be the basis for differential access to health care, likewise disability ought not be invoked as a basis for justifying unequal access to health care.

Yet, as a duty of imperfect obligation based on P-IV, the duty to provide health care to the disabled will have limits even in the wealthiest society. A disabled person cannot be euthanized, but there will be limits to how far one goes in sustaining the life of a disabled person, just as there will be limits to how far one must go in sustaining the life of any person. These limits include the physical, psychological, social, spiritual, and economic resources of the individual in his or her particular circumstances as well as the limits of a society's resources. It is critically important to add, however, that any criterion for deciding upon limits must not be based on the disability in itself, since this would constitute a judgment regarding the worth of the person and violate the principle of equal respect for intrinsic dignity. Rather, such judgments must be based on the same criteria one would use for deciding on the limits of care for any individual, whether disabled or not. That is, based on the inefficacy of the intervention, on absolute scarcity, or on the individual's own judgments about burdens and benefits. Limits based on judgments of social worth, whether made by physicians or third parties, are inconsistent with the meaning of respect for intrinsic dignity.

Thus, the conception of dignity presented here is in full harmony with the traditional distinction between killing and allowing to die, converging on that distinction by noting differences in the types of dignity and the moral duties associated with each. The conception of dignity presented here provides a strong basis for preventing discrimination against the disabled and for supporting claims of equality of access to health care for the disabled. Such a conception of dignity would appear quite useful to bioethics.

## Embryonic Stem Cell Research

A currently vexatious issue facing biomedical science is the morality of using human embryonic stem cells for research. Arguments opposing this practice on the basis of respect for human dignity have been vigorously attacked in the bioethics literature as vacuous. Does the conception of human dignity presented in this essay shed any light on these arguments?

If there is such a thing as intrinsic value, then, as I have argued, it is the value something has by virtue of its being the kind of thing that it is. Intrinsic value inheres in natural kinds, since artifacts have only attributed, and not intrinsic, value. I defined intrinsic dignity as the intrinsic value of natural kinds that have, as natural kinds, the capacity for language, rationality, love, free will, moral agency, creativity, aesthetic sensibility, and an ability to grasp the finite and the infinite. These are characteristic features of the human natural kind. Thus, the human natural kind (at least) has intrinsic dignity.

As I have argued, this value is not based on the active expression by an individual of any one (or even several) of the particular characteristics that confer intrinsic dignity on the natural kind as a whole. I made this argument in two ways. First, I explained that the extensional logic of natural kinds dictates that one first pick out an individual as a member of a kind by including it under the extension provided by one or two representative samples of the kind, backed by a full understanding of the typical history, the development, and the law-like generalizations that characterize members of that kind. The very notion of natural kinds entails acceptance of this "modest" essentialism. The presence or absence of no single specifiable characteristic or set of characteristics is sufficient to determine this "essence," in all of its modesty. Second, I showed that each of the candidate characteristics one might suggest, by intensional logic, as the dignity-conferring characteristic, leads to gross inconsistencies when applied universally, clashing with our most deeply held moral views. One is therefore led, by a process of elimination, to accept that dignity is the worth all human beings have simply by being human.

On the basis of all that I have explained about dignity thus far, it follows that if a human embryo is a member of the human natural kind, then it has all the intrinsic dignity of the human natural kind. And if that is true, then it cannot be killed, even to do good for others, without violating the fundamental moral duties that flow from recognizing intrinsic dignity. Thus, the fundamental question with respect to whether a human embryo has intrinsic dignity is whether that embryo is an individual member of the human natural kind.

What else is a human embryo, however, but an individual member of the human natural kind at the earliest stages of its development? This is what a human embryo is, biologically and ontologically. It is not a different kind of thing (say a slug or a porpoise). It is what every human being is (or was) at 0-28 days of development.

Judith Thompson has argued that "a fetus is no more a human being than an acorn is an oak tree."[34] Thompson is precisely correct in her analogy, but precisely wrong in the biological, ontological, and moral conclusions she draws from it. Despite her rhetorical fervor, Thompson has it backwards. A fetus (or an embryo) is a member of the human natural kind at the earliest stages of development, just as an acorn is a member of the oak tree natural kind at the earliest stages of its development. Every human being's history can be traced back, as a continuous existent, to its own embryonic stage. Every oak tree's history can be traced back, as a continuous existent, to its own acorn stage.[35] In fact, the continuity is clearer in the case of human development. The concept of natural kinds has been introduced into philosophy to do just this: to account for the continuity and change of individuals over time. "Embryo" and "acorn" are not terms used to sort different natural kinds. Rather, these words are used to distinguish phases within the development of two distinct biological natural kinds. "Embryo" is a phase-sortal term for animals and "acorn" is a phase-sortal term for oaks.[36] If intrinsic value inheres in individuals as members of kinds, then it inheres in them throughout their natural histories as members of that kind undergoing the development that typifies the kind. Thus the intrinsic dignity of the human inheres in embryonic members of the human natural kind every bit a as it does in adult members of the human natural kind.

Space limitations preclude a full discussion of long-standing arguments about the distinction between persons and members of the human natural kind. Suffice it to say that "person" is not a phase-sortal, like "fetus" or "adolescent." Even if "person" were a phase-sortal, one could not make personhood the basis for intrinsic dignity without completely subverting the notion of intrinsic value, which must, by definition, inhere in each individual by virtue of its being the kind of thing it is, and not by virtue of the phase it is in during its development as a member of that kind.

Some have argued that the fact that an early human embryo can split into two, forming twins, means that there is no individual until after 14 days of development, so that any developing entity younger than 14 days is not an individual human being and therefore has no dignity. As Germain Grisez[37] and Robert P. George[38] have pointed out, however, this argument is totally specious. The fact that one amoeba can split into two amoebas is not an argument that what was there before the split was not an amoeba. It is among the law-like generalizations and is typical of the natural history and features of individual members of the human natural kind that they can split before 14 days of development and form identical twins. This is hardly an argument that human embryos younger than 14 days are not individual members of the human natural kind in whom intrinsic dignity inheres.

Finally, some have argued that the fact that some human zygotes will develop into tumors known as hydatidiform moles means that one need not regard the developing entity as human, since it could be a mole.[39] For simplicity's sake I will consider only the case of a complete hydatidiform mole. It is uncertain whether this "mole" objection is intended as an ontological argument or an epistemological argument. Interpreted as an ontological argument, it is tainted with genetic reductionism, presuming (falsely) that whatever has a 46 XX or XY set of chromosomes is a human being. But a hydatidiform mole is neither a human being nor a human embryo. A mole is not even an organism. Its chromosomes are only of paternal origin, and these are abnormally imprinted, even if the DNA sequence is totally human. No actual embryo ever develops, only abnormal trophoblastic tissue. From its origin, a mole is a different kind of thing, even though it has human genes. As a different kind of thing, a mole does not have intrinsic dignity. Therefore, the possibility of mole formation is not an argument that a human embryo in the Petri dish does not have intrinsic dignity. If what is in the dish is a human embryo, then it has intrinsic dignity. If what is in the dish is a mole, then it does not.

Interpreted as an epistemological argument, however, this line of reasoning suggests that, because one might not be able to determine until later in development whether what is growing in the uterus or the Petri dish is a mole, one therefore cannot speak meaningfully of the intrinsic dignity of a five-day old blastocyst. It is true that, *in vivo,* given current technology, there is no good way to tell an embryo from a mole at 5 days of developmental age. *In vitro,* by contrast, it has been demonstrated that even at the 2-cell stage one can detect characteristic abnormalities in hydatidiform moles.[40] However, prescinding from the question of whether one has epistemic access to the true (if modest) essence of the thing undergoing development, as a practical matter this possibility does not seem morally decisive. Moles are rare. If there is a 99.9% chance that what I see stirring in the woods is a fellow hunter, and a 0.1% chance that it might be a deer, prudence suggests not shooting. And any epistemic doubts I might have about what stirs—in the woods, the womb, or the Petri dish—do not suffice to change the ontological status of the thing that stirs. There is a correct answer to the question, is this a mole or an embryo? If what is in the dish is an individual member of the human natural kind in the embryonic stage of development, then it has intrinsic dignity. My uncertainty does not change the kind of thing that it is, nor does my uncertainty change its intrinsic value.

A theory of dignity that can provide such explanations and guidance in moral decision-making about the treatment of human embryos would not seem useless.

# Cloning to Bring Babies to Birth

All of the arguments I raised above about why it is a violation of intrinsic human dignity to destroy already existing human embryos for research purposes apply *a fortiori* to creating human embryos expressly in order to destroy them for research purposes. However, a different set of considerations arises in examining the morality of cloning to bring babies to birth.

Curiously, cloning to bring babies to birth has met with widespread opposition by persons of many different philosophical and theological orientations. Most subscribe to the notion that this practice would deeply offend human dignity. There has yet to be, however, an entirely compelling explanation of exactly why this might be so. Does the conception of dignity offered in this essay shed any light on this bioethical issue?

The intuitions of many observers may be captured by attempting to understand how the difference between an artifact and a natural kind is related to the conception of dignity that I have presented. Artifacts have no intrinsic value. The value of an artifact is purely attributed—conferred on the artifact by its artificer. Typically, this attributed value is instrumental. I make a knife in order to cut things because cutting them is useful to me. I manufacture a mobile telephone because telephones have an instrumental value to me that is enhanced by making that instrumental value portable. The very notion of the intrinsic value of biological entities, as I have discussed, entails the notion of natural kinds—the value things have by virtue of being the kinds of things that they are. Intrinsic dignity is the name we give to the intrinsic value of members of the human natural kind. This value is discovered, not made. It is decidedly noninstrumental.

The introduction of various reproductive technologies into clinical medicine has worried many observers for many years, but few have articulated these worries carefully. The possibility of cloning for reproductive purposes seems to have led many observers to agree that these long-standing worries have had genuine moral substance. The President's Council on Bioethics has expressed this unease as the difference between begetting and manufacture.[41] A child born of the normal course of affairs is begotten. A child brought to birth after having been cloned seems manufactured. The conception of dignity expressed in this essay perhaps gives a more fundamental basis for explaining the worry captured by the pithy distinction between begetting and manufacture. Cloning blurs the line between the value one discovers in the human as a natural kind (i.e., intrinsic dignity) and the value that is merely conferred upon artifacts by human attribution.

In one very serious sense, a human clone would be an artifact. As such, it would have value only to the extent that value would be conferred upon it by its artificers. If the clone were created and then destroyed for research purposes, perhaps one could convince oneself that what one had destroyed was not a member of the human natural kind and therefore had no dignity. But if that clone were brought to birth, one could not avoid confronting the artifact vs. natural kind question. The scientist would stare the clone in the eye and say, "I have created you." The value of the clone would be artifactual, not already given, commanding recognition and respect. An artifact's value is purely instrumental and attributed. Thus, the very notion of intrinsic human dignity would be radically threatened. And with it, our whole system of morality, founded upon respect for intrinsic dignity, would be threatened.

In another sense, of course, a cloned human being brought to birth would have intrinsic dignity. While born out of the natural course, perhaps suffering from genetic disorders associated with that manner of coming into being, the clone would still be a member of the human natural kind. Clones are not created from scratch—from a soup of nucleotides and DNA polymerase. Somatic cell nuclear transfer depends on the pre-existence of members of the human natural kind from which the clones would be derived. A human clone brought to birth would be picked out as falling under the extension of the human natural kind. While quite likely to be genetically defective, such an individual would still have a developmental history traceable back to a human embryo. Such an individual would still obey most of the law-like generalizations that characterize the human natural kind. Thus, such an individual would be a member of the human natural kind and would still have intrinsic dignity.

Given the way in which the individual came into being, however, the real and acute worry would be that this individual's intrinsic dignity would be open to question, because the individual might be considered an artifact and not a member of a natural kind, and might therefore be considered to have only attributed and not intrinsic value. And when the intrinsic value (the intrinsic dignity) of any member of the human natural kind is threatened, the moral system that characterizes us as a kind is threatened.

A theory of dignity that explains the common intuition that the bringing to birth of a cloned human being would be a transgression against dignity is a robust theory of dignity. This suggests that the concept of dignity is not irrelevant to bioethics but, rather, extremely important.

## The Care of Persons Suffering from Post-coma Unresponsiveness

The proper care of persons suffering from the Permanent Vegetative State and related neurological conditions has become a highly contentious bioethical topic in the Western world. Even the name of the condition has become a matter of controversy. Although a good biologist or philosopher who has studied Aristotle knows that the term "vegetative" is purely descriptive and not pejorative, many persons, sadly, have abused the term and have called patients who suffer from the condition "vegetables." Because of this, the Australian term, "post-coma unresponsiveness" may be the most descriptive name one can use for this condition and may also be the least liable to misinterpretation.[42] Accordingly, "post-coma unresponsiveness" is the term I will use to describe the condition of persons who initially become comatose after anoxic or traumatic brain injury, but gradually develop into a state in which they are able to open their eyes, have intact brain stem functions and are able to breathe and exhibit sleep-wake cycles, but never recover signs of cognitive awareness or conscious interaction with their environments.

One line of argument in bioethics suggests that such individuals have lost all dignity and therefore should either be euthanized, experimented on, or denied access to life-prolonging therapies. The conception of dignity presented in this essay provides a basis for understanding that this line of argument cannot be sustained. That is because such arguments are based solely on an attributed sense of dignity.

Human beings suffering from post-coma unresponsiveness (PCU) have not undergone an ontological change. Such patients have not become some other kind of thing. We pick them out as members of the human natural kind as a precondition for our judgment that they are severely ill. Even an argument, for example, for euthanizing such patients, based on their profound loss of attributed dignity, presumes, as I have argued, that they are members of the human natural kind and still have intrinsic dignity. All duties to build up or to create conditions conducive to a patient's possibilities for inflorescent dignity depend upon respect for intrinsic dignity. Likewise, any perceived duty to build up diminished attributed dignity also depends upon respect for intrinsic dignity. Respect begins with recognition, and recognition does require an act of attribution, yet this attribution does not create the value. Rather, recognition is best described as an act of attributing correctly, an acknowledgement of the intrinsic dignity of the patient that cannot be eliminated even should it go unrecognized. The dignity here acknowledged is an objective value that presents itself as worthy of respect. Before we can attribute any additional values to human beings, whether sick or well, and call those values "dignities," we must first recognize and respect them as bearers of intrinsic dignity. Those suffering from PCU may represent a limiting case. They have severely diminished attributed dignity, and extremely limited possibilities for inflorescent dignity. Yet it is only by virtue of having first picked them out as members of the human natural kind and having recognized their intrinsic value that we concerned about either their attributed or their inflorescent value. Those who strive to build up the attributed dignity of patients suffering from PCU have already conceded that there is such a thing as intrinsic dignity by the very fact that they show concern for these patients. While extraordinarily impaired, these individuals still have intrinsic dignity by virtue of being the kinds of things that they are—members of the human natural kind. Therefore, according to the moral duties that follow from a fundamental duty to respect intrinsic dignity, someone suffering from PCU cannot be euthanized or experimented upon without consent (P-VI).

Such individuals have an intrinsic dignity that also demands equality of treatment. Accordingly, such individuals cannot be denied access to care that other ill human beings would be afforded merely on the basis of their medical conditions. Treatment might be refused, but treatment must be offered. Comfort, care, and respect must never be abandoned. As discussed above, this duty to provide care is limited by the individual's physical, psychological, social, spiritual, and economic resources in his or her particular circumstances as well as the availability of a given society's resources. The diagnosis of PCU itself, however, must never be the basis for unilaterally withholding or withdrawing care that would be rendered to others.

It is undeniably true that such individuals are extremely restricted in their ability to flourish as the kinds of things that they are. They are incapable of expressing courage, or honor, or even understanding their predicaments. Thus, their capacities for inflorescent dignity are profoundly restricted. No one wishes to be in such a state. Therefore, respect for equal intrinsic dignity also ought to assure such persons the same rights as others to withhold or withdraw life-sustaining treatments that are futile, or more burdensome than beneficial.

The conception of dignity presented in this essay thus also has concrete implications for understanding how to care for individuals suffering from post-coma unresponsiveness. This gives further evidence of the critical importance of a serious consideration of dignity in debates about pressing issues in bioethics.

## Conclusion

In this essay, I outlined three ways the word "dignity" has been understood in the history of Western thought and explained how these three senses of dignity—the attributed, the intrinsic, and the inflorescent—are still at play in contemporary bioethical debates. I offered two arguments about why the intrinsic sense of dignity is the most foundational—the Axiological Argument and the Argument from Consistency. In so doing, I stressed the importance of the conception of natural kinds to all three senses of dignity. I then outlined several general moral norms that specify what it means to respect dignity. Finally, I applied this theory of dignity and its associated moral norms to a variety of pressing ethical questions in contemporary bioethics, showing how this conception of dignity is extraordinarily powerful in helping us to understand how we ought to proceed in answering these questions. Space has precluded a fuller explication of this theory or a full consideration of counter-arguments. However, it seems clear that if this is what dignity means, then dignity is anything but a useless concept.

# Notes

[1] Daniel P. Sulmasy, "Death, Dignity, and the Theory of Value," *Ethical Perspectives* 9 (2002): 103-118, reprinted in *Euthanasia and Palliative Care in the Low Countries*, ed. Paul Schotsmans and Tom Meulenbergs (Leuven, Belgium: Peeters, 2005), pp. 95-119.
[2] Ruth Macklin, "Dignity is a Useless Concept," *BMJ* 327 (2003): 1419-1420.
[3] Charles Trinkaus, "The Renaissance Idea of the Dignity of Man," in *Dictionary of the History of Ideas*, vol. 4, ed. Philip P. Weiner (New York: Charles Scribner's Sons, 1973), pp. 136-147; Daniel P. Sulmasy, "Death with Dignity: What Does it Mean?" *Josephinum Journal of Theology* 4 (1997): 13-24.
[4] Cicero, *De Inventione* I.166.
[5] Miriam T. Griffin and E. Margaret Atkins, "Notes on Translation," in *Cicero: On Duties* (New York: Cambridge University Press, 1991), pp. xlvi-xlvii.
[6] Cicero, *De Officiis* I.106, trans. Walter Miller (New York: Macmillan, 1913), pp. 106-109.
[7] Thomas Hobbes, *Leviathan*, chapter 10, ed. Richard Tuck (Cambridge: Cambridge University Press, 1991), pp. 63-64.
[8] Immanuel Kant, "The Metaphysics of Morals, Part II: The Metaphysical Principles of Virtue," Ak419-420, in Kant, *Ethical Philosophy*, trans. James W. Ellington (Indianapolis, Indiana: Hackett, 1983), pp. 80-81.
[9] Immanuel Kant, *Grounding for the Metaphysics of Morals*, Ak 434, trans. James W. Ellington (Indianapolis, Indiana: Hackett, 1981), p. 40.
[10] Ibid.
[11] Thomas E. Hill, Jr., *Dignity and Practical Reason in Kant's Moral Theory* (Ithaca, New York: Cornell University Press, 1992), p. 43.
[12] In my essay, "Dignity and the Human as a Natural Kind," included in *Health and Human Flourishing*, ed. Carol R. Taylor and Roberto Dell'Oro (Washington, D.C.: Georgetown University Press, 2006), pp. 71-87, I called this the "derivative" sense of dignity. However, some commentators, especially those who would be counted as using the word this way, have worried that "derivative" sounds less "dignified" than is appropriate.
[13] Timothy E. Quill, "Death and Dignity: A Case of Individualized Decision Making," *New England Journal of Medicine* 324 (1991): 691-694.
[14] Dónal P. O'Mathúna, "Human Dignity in the Nazi era: Implications for Contemporary Bioethics," *BMC Medical Ethics* 7 (2006): E2.
[15] Leon R. Kass, *Life, Liberty and the Defense of Dignity: The Challenge for Bioethics* (San Francisco, California: Encounter Books, 2002), pp. 231-256.
[16] See Noah M. Lemos, "Value Theory," in *Cambridge Dictionary of Philosophy*, ed. Robert Audi (New York: Cambridge University Press, 1995), pp. 830-831; also Michael J. Zimmerman, "Intrinsic vs. Extrinsic Value," *Stanford Encyclopedia of Philosophy* (2004 edition), ed. Edward N. Zalta, available online at http://plato.stanford.edu/entries/value-intrinsic-extrinsic/. The standard views either distinguish intrinsic from instrumental values, or intrinsic from extrinsic values.

The theory of intrinsic value outlined in this essay, however, following Holmes Rolston III, *Environmental Ethics* (Philadelphia: Temple University Press, 1988), aligns with the views of Kant, Brentano, Broad, Ross, and others, that whatever is intrinsically good is worthy of being valued in itself.

[17] See Sulmasy, "Death, Dignity, and the Theory of Value."

[18] Rolston, *Environmental Ethics*, p. 116.

[19] Credit for initiation of the discussion of natural kinds is usually given to Saul Kripke, in his two essays, "Identity and Necessity," in *Identity and Individuation* ed. Milton K. Munitz (New York: New York University Press, 1971), pp. 135-164, and "Naming and Necessity," in *Semantics of Natural Language*, ed. Gilbert Harman and Donald Davidson (Dordrecht, Netherlands: Reidel, 1972), pp. 253-355. For a good contemporary approach to the concept of natural kinds, see David Wiggins, *Sameness and Substance* (Cambridge, Massachusetts: Harvard University Press, 1980), pp. 77-101, and his *Sameness and Substance Renewed* (Cambridge: Cambridge University Press, 2001).

[20] Wiggins, *Sameness and Substance*, p. 169.

[21] Tom L. Beauchamp, *Philosophical Ethics* (New York: McGraw-Hill, 1982), pp. 5-21.

[22] Aristotle, *Nicomachean Ethics* 1095b, trans. Terence Irwin (Indianapolis, Indiana: Hackett, 1985), p. 7.

[23] H. Tristram Englehardt, Jr., *The Foundations of Bioethics* (New York: Oxford University Press, 1986), p. 213.

[24] Michael Tooley, *Abortion and Infanticide* (Oxford: Oxford University Press, 1983).

[25] Raymond G. Frey, "Pain, Vivisection, and the Value of Life," *Journal of Medical Ethics* 31 (2005): 202-204.

[26] Kant, *Grounding for the Metaphysics of Morals*, Ak 421, p. 30.

[27] Richard M. Hare, *Moral Thinking: Its Levels, Methods, and Point* (New York: Oxford University Press, 1981), pp. 107-116.

[28] Thomas F. Hack, et al., "Defining Dignity in Terminally Ill Cancer Patients: A Factor-analytic Approach," *Psychooncology* 13 (2004): 700-708.

[29] Garth Baker-Fletcher, *Somebodyness: Martin Luther King, Jr. and the Theory of Dignity*, Harvard Dissertations in Divinity, No. 31 (Minneapolis, Minnesota: Fortress Press, 1993), p. 23.

[30] J. David Velleman, "A Right to Self-Termination?" *Ethics* 109 (1999): 605-628.

[31] Daniel P. Sulmasy, "Dignity, Rights, Health Care, and Human Flourishing," in *Human Rights and Health Care*, ed. G. Diaz Pintos and David N. Weisstub (Dordrecht, Netherlands: Springer, in press 2007).

[32] Daniel P. Sulmasy, "Diseases and Natural Kinds," *Theoretical Medicine and Bioethics* 26 (2005): 487-513.

[33] Harriet McBryde Johnson, "Unspeakable Conversations," *New York Times Sunday Magazine*, February 16, 2003, p. 50. The philosopher was Peter Singer.

[34] Judith Jarvis Thompson, "A Defense of Abortion," *Philosophy and Public Affairs* 1 (1971): 47-66.

[35] Robert P. George and Patrick Lee, "Acorns and Embryos," *The New Atlantis* 7 (Fall 2004/Winter 2005): 90-100.
[36] Alfonso Gómez-Lobo, "Does Respect for Embryos Entail Respect for Gametes?" *Theoretical Medicine and Bioethics* 25 (2004): 199-208.
[37] Germain G. Grisez, "When Do People Begin?" *Proceedings of the American Catholic Philosophical Association* 63 (1990): 27-47.
[38] Robert P. George, "Human Cloning and Embryo Research," *Theoretical Medicine and Bioethics* 25 (2004): 3-20.
[39] Carlos A. Bedate and Robert C. Cefalo, "The Zygote: To Be or Not Be a Person," *Journal of Medicine and Philosophy* 14 (1989): 641-645; Thomas J. Bole, III, "Metaphysical Accounts of the Zygote as a Person and the Veto Power of Facts," *Journal of Medicine and Philosophy* 14 (1989): 647-653.
[40] Nicanor Austriaco, O.P., "Are Teratomas Embryos or Non-embryos?" *National Catholic Bioethics Quarterly* 5 (2005): 697-706.
[41] The President's Council on Bioethics, *Human Cloning and Human Dignity: An Ethical Inquiry* (Washington, D.C.: Government Printing Office, 2002), pp. 104-107.
[42] National Health and Medical Research Council of Australia, "Post-Coma Unresponsiveness (Vegetative State): A Clinical Framework for Diagnosis," December 18, 2003, available online at http://www.nhmrc.gov.au/publications/synopses/_files/hpr23.pdf.

# Part VI.
# Human Dignity and the Practice of Medicine

# 19

# Human Dignity and the Seriously Ill Patient

## Rebecca Dresser

Respecting human dignity is a central moral and social aim when it comes to either health policy or everyday medical care. Yet like other important concepts, such as "happiness"[1] and "fairness," the meaning of dignity can be difficult to pinpoint.

At the same time, one attraction of the dignity concept is that it lacks a settled interpretation. Elasticity in the definition of dignity creates the possibility for rich and diverse scholarship about the concept, such as the essays in this volume. As the essays illustrate, writers may examine the meaning of dignity from a variety of vantage points. They may explore the concept from a broad, comprehensive perspective, or consider dignity in a single context. They may approach the concept from a historical, religious, biological, or humanistic vantage point. They may consider dignity at the abstract level, or apply it to individual cases. They may describe dignity, defend it, or criticize it.

Many of the writers in this volume consider questions related to the proper subjects of human dignity. Should we extend dignity to humans in the early stages of development? Should we extend it to potential future beings with enhanced, "superhuman" features? Should we extend it to certain nonhuman animals or intelligent machines? And how can we defend the idea that humans are owed dignity, when contemporary science and theory seem to undercut the traditional religious justifications for this idea?

My question is different. If human dignity applies to anyone, it applies to people experiencing serious illness. Every author in this volume would agree that human patients should be treated with human dignity.* But what does this mean today? What constitutes dignified treatment for patients receiving care in the context of contemporary medicine?

In this essay, I examine dignity from the bottom up. I consider how the concept of dignity bears on the treatment of patients with serious illness. I argue that dignity merits more scholarly attention in bioethics, that it is no less problematic than other bioethics concepts, and that it is a central concern for patients and caregivers in the clinical setting. My analysis draws on scholarly work and on my personal experience as a cancer patient.

## The Bioethics Critique

For many years, certain bioethics scholars, medical professionals, and policy officials have embraced preservation of human dignity as a clinical and policy goal. Securing a "Death with Dignity" for patients was an early preoccupation of the bioethics field.[2] The need to preserve human dignity has also been recognized in work on the new reproductive technologies, genetics, medical training, and research on human subjects.[3]

Yet the concept of dignity has recently come under attack. The sharpest critique comes from philosopher and bioethicist Ruth Macklin, who claims that "appeals to dignity are either vague restatements of other, more precise, notions or mere slogans that add nothing to an understanding of the topic." In the worst case, she argues, dignity acts as a slogan to substitute for substantive argument favoring a particular position. In other cases, Macklin sees appeals to dignity as redundant, adding nothing to the analysis. For example, in the end-

---

* As the contributions by Gelernter, Meilaender, and Sulmasy suggest, however, there may be disagreement over what constitutes dignified treatment for permanently unconscious individuals like Theresa Schiavo or for advanced dementia patients.

of-life context, she contends that appeals to dignity are actually appeals to promote patient autonomy in decisions about life-sustaining treatment. Appeals to dignity may also stand in for other principles, such as respect for persons, confidentiality in the doctor-patient relationship, or bans on "discriminatory and abusive practices." Macklin concludes that dignity "is a useless concept in medical ethics and can be eliminated without any loss of content."[4]

Macklin's provocative challenge has generated many responses and in that sense has served as a useful trigger to further examination of the dignity concept. Although some writers share Macklin's disdain for the concept, others see human dignity as a distinct ideal, one that is both morally and practically significant. I am part of the second group. Like any other moral arguments, appeals to dignity may be inappropriate or superficial, or they may mask inadequately supported claims. But it does not follow from this that bioethics should abandon appeals to dignity.

Macklin's argument that we should eliminate dignity from bioethics analysis is unpersuasive for at least three reasons. First, the claim that the concept of dignity is too vague to be useful implies that other bioethics concepts are free of this problem.[5] Yet many bioethics concepts are imprecise. Examples are the concepts of justice, fairness, and rights.[6] All of these concepts are defined and applied in a variety of ways by different groups and individuals. Indeed, the proper meaning of the concepts Macklin prefers, such as autonomy, respect for persons, discrimination, and abuse, are sufficiently imprecise to generate extensive scholarly debate over how they should be defined and applied. Macklin sets up a double standard in demanding a clear and widely accepted definition of dignity.

Second, Macklin's critique is premature. It is true that individuals and groups invoking dignity in bioethics do not always supply a clear account of its meaning. And bioethics scholars have not devoted much effort to discussing the concept.[7] Yet these are not reasons to abandon dignity. Rather, they are reasons to pay more attention to it. The shortcomings of the existing literature should attract more scholarly work and policy debates over the proper meaning and applications of human dignity.

Other writers make similar arguments. While acknowledging that dignity can mean different things to different people, Ann Gallagher contends that Macklin's argument "urges us...not to throw dignity out but rather to reclaim it, embrace it, draw on and develop existing theoretical and empirical work...."[8] Timothy Caulfield and Audrey Chapman conclude that "a pronouncement that something infringes human dignity should be viewed as an opportunity to debate the values at play and the cultural underpinnings of the concern."[9] What is needed, then, is more work on the dignity concept. It is too early to consign dignity to the scrapheap.

A third shortcoming in Macklin's claim is its lack of respect for the individuals and groups that see dignity as a significant bioethical concern. As Gallagher puts it, "In response to Professor Macklin's question, 'Why, then, do so many articles and reports appeal to human dignity, as if it means something over and above respect for persons or for their autonomy?' it might be asserted 'Because it does mean something over and above respect for persons and autonomy.'"[10] A belief's popularity is not necessarily evidence of its validity, of course. But widespread popularity is a reason for critics to consider that belief carefully, instead of dismissing it outright.

## Dignity from the Patient's Perspective

There are many ways that we could learn more about the meaning of human dignity. The concept deserves further theoretical and empirical investigation from a variety of vantage points. One possibility would be to conduct surveys of different individuals and groups to elicit their views on the matter. Such surveys might identify similarities that suggest empirical agreement on the meaning of dignity in various settings.

In the remainder of this essay, I adopt a form of this approach. I present my own and other writers' views of how dignity concerns arise in medical care. Human dignity is implicated when patients and families face decisions about ending life, but it also is implicated before that, when patients are undergoing treatment for serious illness. During this time, the patient's dignity can be honored or compromised in numerous ways. Here, I describe how privacy, communication, personal knowledge, and dependence connect to dignity for people facing serious illness.

The concerns I describe are separate from the bioethics concepts Macklin invokes. As Miles Bore observes, "While [patients] might voluntarily agree to a medical procedure, be well informed of the procedure, have their records of the procedure kept in strict confidence, be unharmed by the procedure and actually benefit from the procedure, they might still incur and feel a loss of dignity."[11]

Dignity concerns arise in connection with the broader area of personal privacy, but contrary to Macklin, they go beyond protecting the confidentiality of medical communications. Patients enter a world of forced and one-sided intimacy with strangers. Besides the physical exposure that goes along with clinical care, there can be unwanted exposure to members of the public.

Patients feel a loss of dignity when care intrudes into areas raising particular privacy concerns. Having to wear "flimsy and revealing hospital gowns" and being gossiped about by staff are some of the violations that can occur.[12] Other examples include being bathed, using a bedpan, and receiving an enema.[13] Being wheeled through the halls in a wheelchair or on a gurney feels undignified too, especially when the halls are public places with visitors and others who cannot resist staring at the sight. Having medical students and residents troop into a hospital room to make one an object of study can also be experienced as an indignity. Having to open one's bedroom to home care professionals is yet another example of the forced intimacy patients endure.

Although some personal invasions are probably unavoidable, clinical care should minimize them as much as possible. The ordinary norms governing physical privacy should be observed unless there are good medical reasons to deviate from them. Clinicians and students entering the examining room, hospital room, or home should acknowledge the intrusion and undertake compensatory efforts to preserve the patient's dignity. As I discuss below, communication, respect for personal knowledge, and responses to dependency can reduce the indignities accompanying the loss of privacy that illness brings.

Communication can have a lot to do with preserving patients' dignity. The outward signs of illness create a heightened need to be treated in a dignified manner. Hair loss, severe weight loss, and other unwelcome changes make patients sensitive about appearing in public. Small actions, such as making eye contact with a skinny, bald cancer patient, are ways to confer dignity on such patients. Other methods of reaching out, in person or in writing, can make a huge difference in how a patient experiences the burdens of illness.

It is all too tempting to look away from people who are obviously ill, in part because they are reminders of human frailty and mortality. But the person inside still needs to be recognized, to be honored and valued. If dignity is "a psychospiritual connection...that involves empathy, presence, and compassion,"[14] sincere efforts to communicate are essential to establishing this connection.

Another dimension of dignity is respect for the patient's personal knowledge. Being diagnosed with a life-threatening illness is life-altering. Priorities, relationships, and social roles undergo drastic change. Patients face mortality in ways that healthy people cannot imagine. In this sense, patients know more than the relatives, friends, and clinicians around them. Many patients suffer through chemotherapy, radiation, surgery, and other burdensome interventions, and this demands a kind of strength never before required. Dignity is promoted when others honor the patient's ordeal and look up to the person enduring the assaults of illness and treatment.

Serious illness also brings a new kind of dependence, and being dependent feels undignified to many people. Sometimes clinicians respond to a patient's desire for independence by giving her too much responsibility for decisions she is unequipped to make. Telling a patient that it is up to her to decide whether her symptoms merit hospitalization is inappropriate when the patient lacks the medical expertise needed to make such a choice. Expecting patients on high doses of pain medication to exercise full autonomy is inappropriate, too. On the other hand, pressuring patients to accept beneficial treatments they are resisting can be appropriate.

Clinicians and informal caregivers respect human dignity when they attend to patients' needs for help in navigating the complicated course of a serious illness. Thoughtless invocations of autonomy can conflict with patients' dignity interests. Patients are persons deserving of high-quality care, and sometimes this requires others to assume or share with them the authority for making difficult medical

## Conclusion

Patients may have the freedom to decide about treatment, yet still feel subjected to indignities. Patients' interests in confidentiality and being protected from abuse and discrimination may be adequately addressed, but they may still experience care as impersonal and demeaning. Many dignity violations occur when patients feel they are regarded as objects, rather than as persons worthy of equal respect. In this situation, it would be dangerous to tell clinicians (and bioethicists) that they need not worry about the dignity of seriously ill patients.

The bioethics field has existed for several decades, but many people still feel devalued when they receive medical treatment or are hospitalized. This is the case even though patient autonomy is much more respected than it used to be. One could argue that bioethicists' failure to emphasize protection of dignity has hindered efforts to improve the medical experience for patients. In support of this view, Hilda Bastian argues that dignity's place in medical ethics must be recognized: "Maybe when there's no indignity possible in illness or medical procedures, when all caregivers, policymakers and members of ethics committees are superhumans incapable of having lapses in empathy, then retiring this notion from active duty could be considered."*

The good news is that many clinicians do treat patients with dignity. The doctors and nurses in this group would be horrified by the notion that dignity no longer matters. For them, treating patients with dignity seems to be part of their character, as well as their sense of professional integrity. People concerned with bioethics should join them in recognizing dignity as a crucial component of ethical patient care.

For patients, dignity is a precious possession. Serious illness threatens one's place in the human community. Ordinary activities fall by the wayside and relationships are no longer the same. How should the patient, clinicians, loved ones, and others respond to this

---

* Hilda Bastian, "An Offensive Slogan." Michael Marmot makes a similar point: "Having had experience of the way patients are treated in large public hospitals in different parts of the world, I have little doubt that human dignity is fragile and can be affected by the way one is treated." Michael Marmot, "Dignity and Inequality," *Lancet* 364 (2004): 1019-1021.

disruption, this new vulnerability? These matters are fertile ground for the inquiry into human dignity. They deserve a high priority in bioethics scholarship and teaching.

## Notes

[1] Miles R. Bore, "Dignity: Not Useless, Just a Concept in Need of Greater Understanding," *BMJ Rapid Responses*, February 17, 2004 (available online at http://bmj.bmjjournals.com/cgi/eletters/327/7429/1419).

[2] See Rebecca Dresser, "Precommitment: A Misguided Strategy for Securing Death with Dignity," *Texas Law Review* 81 (2003): 1823-1847.

[3] See Ruth Macklin, "Dignity is a Useless Concept," *BMJ* 327 (2003): 1419-1420, and Timothy Caulfield and Audrey Chapman, "Human Dignity as a Criterion for Science Policy," *PLoS Medicine* 2 (2005): 736-738 (available online at www.plosmedicine.org).

[4] Macklin, op. cit.

[5] Mary C. Beach, Patrick Duggan, and Gail Geller, "Don't Confuse Dignity with Respect," *BMJ Rapid Responses*, January 21, 2004 (available online at http://bmj.bmjjournals.com/cgi/eletters/327/7429/1419).

[6] Anthony Staines, "What is Dignity?" *BMJ Rapid Responses*, December 25, 2003 (available online at http://bmj.bmjjournals.com/cgi/eletters/327/7429/1419).

[7] Exceptions are Deryck Beyleveld and Roger Brownsword, *Human Dignity in Bioethics and Biolaw* (Oxford: Oxford University Press, 2001), and Leon R. Kass, *Life, Liberty and the Defense of Dignity: The Challenge for Bioethics* (San Francisco, California: Encounter Books, 2002). See also Richard E. Ashcroft, "Making Sense of Dignity," *Journal of Medical Ethics* 31 (2005): 679-82; Matti Häyry, "Another Look at Dignity," *Cambridge Quarterly of Healthcare Ethics* 13 (2004): 7-14; and "Dignity at the End of Life (Thematic Issue)," *Journal of Palliative Care* 20 (2004): 133-216.

[8] Ann Gallagher, "Defending Dignity," *BMJ Rapid Responses*, January 12, 2004 (available online at http://bmj.bmjjournals.com/cgi/eletters/327/7429/1419).

[9] Caulfield and Chapman, op. cit., p. 738. See also Häyry, op. cit, pp. 11-12.

[10] Gallagher, op. cit.

[11] Bore, op. cit.

[12] Alexander M. Capron, "Indignities, Respect for Persons, and the Vagueness of Human Dignity," *BMJ Rapid Responses*, December 31, 2003 (available online at http://bmj.bmjjournals.com/cgi/eletters/327/7429/1419).

[13] Hilda Bastian, "An Offensive Slogan," *BMJ Rapid Responses*, December 19, 2003 (available online at http://bmj.bmjjournals.com/cgi/eletters/327/7429/1419).

[14] Stanley M. Giannet, "Dignity Is a Moral Imperative," *BMJ Rapid Responses*, December 25, 2003 (available online at http://bmj.bmjjournals.com/cgi/eletters/327/7429/1419).

# 20

# The Lived Experience of Human Dignity

## Edmund D. Pellegrino

*The problem in question is that of understanding what happens to human dignity in the process of technicalization to which man today is delivered.*

—Gabriel Marcel[1]

Gabriel Marcel wrote these words in 1963 when biotechnology was a set of optimistic promissory notes, and bioethics had yet to be born. Humans then only dimly foresaw, usually in literary fancies, that technology could grow to overshadow its makers. They were still secure in the confidence they inherited from the Renaissance humanists that human beings were the only creatures endowed with reason and the freedom to use it to determine their own destiny.[2] That freedom, they thought, placed us firmly between the angels and the apes and endowed us with an inherent dignity that set us apart from both.

Today dignity has become problematic, and its future is questioned. Biotechnology has expanded beyond anything heretofore imagined so that its powers threaten to overshadow humanity itself. Bioethics has expanded beyond its medical confines to challenge humanity's claims to a unique dignity and to the moral entitlements such a status entails. Together biotechnology and bioethics are reshaping what it is to be human and what human being is.

As a result, among the intensive debates that roil contemporary culture, there are few that are not intimately related to Marcel's question. Even a cursory and incomplete survey of those debates, e.g., the controversies concerning embryonic stem cell research, preimplantation genetic diagnosis, enhancements of human physical or mental capabilities, the practice of regenerative medicine, the uses of nanotechnology, and re-engineering the human species, suffices to underscore this assertion. Some believe that we must explore every possibility these technologies offer; others think certain technologies should never be pursued. For some, the decisions must rest on traditional ethical analyses grounded in classical notions of human dignity; others see such ethical constraints as outmoded limitations on human freedom and progress.

Technology may exalt or imperil human dignity, depending on what we take human dignity to be. Is dignity simply a matter of the degree of biological complexity an animal possesses? Or is it a quality that can only be predicated of humans? Is it the imprint of a personal God on the beings He has created? Or is it simply the fortuitous outcome of the intersections of the laws of chance variation and natural selection? Is the whole notion of human dignity a useless remnant of the days before autonomy became the signal mark of our humanity? Is the idea of dignity too vague to have meaning or, worse, an illicit and covert intrusion of religion into bioethics, as Ruth Macklin would have it?[3]

Whatever one's perspective, the fact remains that biotechnology and bioethics converge whenever humans decide whether a given technological advance is good or bad for humans as humans. Most of the dissonance between and among bioethical systems today rests on how we see human dignity. In the end, the edifices of bioethical systems are grounded in some idea of the purposes and destiny of human life. This is, of course, the anthropological question: "What are human beings?" Our answers provide the templates for decisions we make about which technologies we believe contribute to, or detract from, our flourishing as the kind of being we are.[4]

To understand what happens to human dignity in Marcel's sense, we must understand human dignity not only abstractly as a concept and an idea, but also as an experience, a lived reality of human life. All too often, dignity, like many of the more precious but intangible phenomena of human life, is taken for granted. Only when it is threatened, demeaned, or wrenched forcibly from us do we understand how inseparable our dignity is from our humanity.

For many centuries, and especially the last, a multitude of humans have experienced the degradation of the human spirit that follows from the systematic deprivation of human dignity. To illustrate, one need only mention the Holocaust, slavery, genocide and ethnic cleansings, and the political murders of massive numbers of dissidents by the ideological tyrannies of Maoism, National Socialism, and Stalinism.[5] To the victims, the resulting indignities were the cause of horrific suffering. To the rest of us, their sufferings were so crushingly obvious that to ignore them would have undermined—and in some cases did undermine—our own dignity as well.

The *Universal Declaration of Human Rights* of the United Nations in 1948,[6] and the recent UNESCO *Declaration on Bioethics and Human Rights*,[7] gave clear voice to our moral revulsion. Both documents make human dignity the first principle and the inescapable grounding for all human rights. Remarkably, these declarations were agreed upon between and among nations of vastly different religions, cultures, metaphysical beliefs and historical backgrounds.[8]

It took the collective lived experience of the loss of human dignity to focus the world's attention on its full meaning. Only in this way could flesh be put on the abstract concept. However, without the abstract concept to stimulate critical reflection, the lived experience would have been without meaning for those who were, themselves, not deprived of dignity. But it was the lived experience that gave dignity its axiomatic credibility. As John Keats had so acutely observed:

> Axioms in philosophy are not axioms until they are proven on our pulses; we read fine things but never feel them fully until we have gone the same steps as their author.[9]

Keats's poetic insight connecting thought and experience was reinforced more than a century later when philosophers became more interested in the phenomena of human existence and experience.

One of these philosophers, Gabriel Marcel, linked philosophy with experience in this way:

[P]hilosophy…is experience transmuted into thought….*

and

Philosophy is…a certain way for experience to recognize itself.†

I will focus here on the lived experience of dignity. By a "lived experience" I mean the way human dignity is perceived by human beings as they respond to the valuations of their worth and worthiness by others or by themselves. From a philosophical perspective, a focus on experience re-embeds the concept in the complex daily life from which that concept was extracted. Neither the concept alone nor the experience alone can transmit the full meaning of the word. As a lived experience, dignity is the product of intra- and inter-subjectivity. The underlying conviction of this essay is that the intelligibility of so elusive a notion as dignity must be grounded in our lived experiences of dignity either personally or collectively or, as the rest of the world experienced the Holocaust and the other horrors of the last century, vicariously.

This will require an effort to philosophize about dignity as a concept arising from, and returning to, experience in the real world of everyday life. My aim is thereby to supplement the conceptual analyses so ably conducted in the majority of essays in this collection. I do not suggest that such phenomenological reflections can replace theory. But concepts do and must stand in a dialectical relationship to the lived experience of dignity. In this I proceed in parallel with Rebecca Dresser's reflections in this volume on the experiences of seriously ill

---

* Gabriel Marcel, *Du refus a l'invocation* (Paris, Gallimard, 1970 [1940]), p. 39: "Le point de départ d'une philosophie authentique—et j'entends par là une philosophie qui est l'expérience transmutée en pensée, c'est cependant la reconnaissance aussi lucide que possible de cette situation paradoxale qui non seulement est la mienne, mais *me fait moi.*"

† Gabriel Marcel, op. cit., p. 25: "La philosophie, c'est bien une certaine façon pour l'expérience de se reconnaître, de s'appréhender—mais à quelle niveau d'elle-même."

patients, including her own.* I also believe that the lived experience of dignity inevitably raises the thorniest questions about our place in the cosmos and our stance toward divinity. These questions have been probed with remarkable acuity and candor in a recent dialogue between Jürgen Habermas and Cardinal Joseph Ratzinger (now of course Pope Benedict XVI), and I offer some concluding reflections on the future of human dignity in the light of the conversation between these eminent thinkers.

## Thinking About the Experience of Dignity: Gabriel Marcel and John Newman

At the outset, it is essential to indicate my concurrence with the concept of intrinsic dignity set forth by Sulmasy† on the basis of the theory of natural kinds, by Lee and George on the basis of natural law,‡ and by Meilaender on the basis of man's special relation with his Creator.§ Each of these authors makes a clear distinction between intrinsic human dignity and attributed or imputed dignity. From their viewpoints, intrinsic human dignity is expressive of the inherent worth present in all humans simply by virtue of their being human. Intrinsic dignity cannot be gained or lost, expanded or diminished. It is independent of human opinions about a person's worth. It is the inherent grounding for the moral entitlements of every human to respect for one's person, one's rights, and one's equal treatment under the law in a just political order.

Extrinsic or imputed dignity, on the other hand, is the assessment of the worth or status humans assign to each other or to themselves.[10] It is based on external measures of worth or value as perceived in a person's behavior, social status, appearance, etc. It sums up certain perceived attributes judged admirable or condemnable by other persons, by culture, by political or social criteria, by fashion, or by membership in certain groups. Imputed dignity can be gained or lost simply by one's own self-judgment or by the judgment of others.

---

\* See Rebecca Dresser's essay in this volume.
† See Daniel P. Sulmasy's essay in this volume.
‡ See the essay by Patrick Lee and Robert P. George in this volume
§ See Gilbert Meilaender's essay in this volume.

It can be taken away or granted by law or social convention or by one's opinion of one's own worth in comparison with others.

All of us make imputed judgments of value or worth consciously and unconsciously. These judgments affect the way we respond to others and to our own inner selves. Together, these judgments and responses are the phenomena that make up our lived world of the experience of dignity. Imputations of dignity have no essential relationship to intrinsic dignity, from which they are ontologically distinct. To conflate intrinsic and extrinsic dignity is especially dangerous in bioethics, where what we think it is to be human is the basis of what we think ought and ought not to be done.

The intricacies of attempts both to define the concept and to characterize the experience of human dignity are amply demonstrated in a brilliant essay written some years ago by the philosopher Aurel Kolnai.[11] Kolnai sets out a dazzling array of metaphors and images evoked by the concepts and the experiences of both dignity and indignity. It would be an error to take Kolnai's exhaustive description of the richness of the "conceptual aura or halo" of details that "cluster round the phenomenon" as grounds for abandoning the project of clarifying the meaning of dignity.[12]

Instead, Kolnai provides us with a rich mosaic of lived experiences that underlie any abstract concept of human dignity. It becomes clear that neither the concept, nor the lived experiences from which the concept was abstracted, can by themselves yield the full meaning of the term. Thinking about dignity entails an oscillatory reflection between what can be deduced logically and deductively on the one hand and what must be existentially and concretely experienced on the other.

Two philosophers, in my opinion, have articulated well this oscillatory mode of cognition—on the one hand empirico-psychological, and on the other logico-deductive. I refer here to John Henry Newman with his notion of the "illative sense" and to Gabriel Marcel with his signature distinction between "mystery" and "problem." A brief excursus into their ways of thinking seems helpful in our project of understanding human dignity and its loss.

Human experiences of dignity and indignity are the deep wells from which the abstract conceptions of both inherent and attributed dignity are retrieved. But abstraction by its nature moves us away from the experience itself. A return to experience for an evaluation of the adequacy of our conception is in order so as to complete the meanings of the concept. This "reality check" is necessary to avoid an error that worried Marcel:

> I think the philosopher who first discovers certain truths and then sets out to expound them in their dialectical or systematic interconnections always runs the risk of profoundly altering the nature of the truths he has discovered.[13]

Marcel is admittedly an elusive thinker. I do not suggest that his critique of conventional philosophical modes of thinking is destructive of those modes. Rather, I think it invites us to look a little more fully into his attempt to understand the presence and absence of dignity in human experiences. To this end, we might look briefly at the hallmark distinction of Marcel's thought—his distinction between a "mystery" and a "problem."[14]

For Marcel a "problem" is a question that can be examined objectively. It is susceptible to the scientific method of observation, experiment, and deduction. He calls this method the examination of experience by "primary" reflection.

A "mystery" on the other hand, is a question not susceptible to purely objective analysis. It involves what is given and experienced but cannot be totally objectified. The word "mystery" does not mean an infused truth, a revelation in the religious sense, nor is it shorthand for the unknowable or a flight into total subjectivity. A mystery is examined, as it were, from "within," as the concrete experience of a person as person.[15] It is examined by secondary reflection, "… replunging into the ocean's immediacy from which its concepts are scooped up at the same time [it] re-establishes the primacy of the existential."[16] This contrasts with primary reflection, which makes concepts by abstraction from concrete details to arrive at ideas and essences. Abstraction done in this way tends to reify the concept. Secondary reflection uses the same instruments of thought as primary reflection. However, it orients them in a different direction—toward transcending experience in a way that recognizes the mystery enmeshed in the concrete details of experience. In this way primary and secondary reflection complement each other.

Marcel's insistence on concrete experience and the ways of thinking about it is analogous in some ways to John Henry Newman's thinking in his well known work on the "Grammar of Assent."[17] In that work, Newman recognizes two ways of arriving at truths and giving assent to them. The first is notional, belonging to the world of the intellect, depending on abstraction, syllogistic reasoning, and proofs. The other way is through individual experiences of individual things, acts, and feelings. Here assent to a truth is through the immediacy of our perceptions. It does not depend solely on the notional form of reasoning. Rather, assent arises from implicit inference which perceives the relations between things and ideas without formal syllogistic proof.

For Newman's non-notional way of thinking about experience we must use inferential thinking that involves our whole person. Newman ascribes this non-notional thinking to an illative sense.[18] This sense is an internal guide to inferential thinking. This he takes to be an acquired capacity to make non-syllogistic inferences that nonetheless reveal truths about the way things are in the world. Newman's illative sense is a guide to prudential reasoning and decision-making. Newman's way of philosophizing about experience is closer to clinical thinking with its emphasis on prudence. It is in Newman's insistence on remaining within the horizon of experience that he most resembles Marcel.

Marcel, Newman, and others who emphasize the lived experiences of human persons make us appreciate what Collins said of Marcel: "The full force of evidence is not realized until it is envisaged as being in the inquirer's life and conduct."[19] Or, to put it another way:

> One transcends experience by means of concepts which make experience possible and are only meaningful in relation to experience.[20]

To invoke the reflections of Marcel and Newman on experience is not to suggest that intuitive thinking can entirely replace abstract thinking. What is crucial is to recognize the bipolarity of human dignity between its concept and its lived experience and to respect the dynamic oscillation between the two. How to comport ourselves with respect to the dignity of any human being does not admit of a formulaic resolution. It is instead a prudential judgment, which is the focus of Marcel's and Newman's reflections. The distinction I outlined above between human dignity as inherent in what it means to be human and the way dignity is perceived and imputed to ourselves and others holds conceptually. But even then we must appreciate that inherent and perceived dignity will often overlap and can be confused partially or totally with each other. This will become especially apparent as we move next to the lived experience of dignity.

## Dignity and the Human Predicament of Illness

Against this background of Marcel's and Newman's ways of thinking about experience and Kolnai's reflections on the phenomenon, we can now turn to the experience of dignity and its real and apparent loss in the clinical encounter. I will draw on personal experience as I have observed the challenges to dignity in my patients in the midst of the realities of illness and healing. Such experience is to be examined, as Marcel suggests, by secondary reflection, which involves the subject. I will focus on the patients' perceptions of the experience of dignity.

As I indicated earlier, humans become most acutely aware of their own dignity and that of others when it is threatened by the acts and opinions of their fellow humans or by the circumstances of one's life, work, social, political or community life, or by the way one reacts to the exigencies of those encounters. What is most significant for our understanding of our own or another's dignity is that we experience them only in community with others. Assessment of my own dignity is disclosed in the personal encounter with another. The experience of dignity is inescapably a phenomenon of intersubjectivity. Only in the encounter with others do we gain knowledge of how we value each other and ourselves. The personal and intersubjective nature of the experience of dignity thus fits the idea of "mystery" as Marcel has conceived it. We cannot objectify our experience of our own dignity or another person's attributions, nor explain it fully, simply by classifying it or treating it as a problem to be "solved" psychologically or sociologically or by any other empirical or analytical methodology. We apprehend the reality of a particular experience of dignity by non-syllogistic inference in Newman's sense. In any case, as John Crosby has so aptly pointed out, it is not just the external qualities or behavior that carry worth or admirability but the particular human person who has them: "When we speak of the dignity of the human person we do not speak of a goodness for the human person but of a goodness human persons have in themselves."[21]

## Dignity and the Clinical Experience

Some of the more complex experiences of dignity are those most relevant for bioethics. They are epitomized in the clinical encounter. The central relationship is the one between patient and physician, though nurses and other health professionals also participate to varying degrees. The person in need, the being around whom the drama centers, is a patient, someone literally bearing a burden, suffering and in distress, anxious, frightened, and no longer able to cope without professional help.

The clinical encounter is a confrontation, a face-to-face encounter between someone who professes to heal and someone in need of healing. Its locus is the doctor-patient, or nurse-patient, relationship. It is a phenomenon of intersubjectivity, and it is in this sense that it is a locus for the experience of human dignity and its loss. The doctor-patient relationship is paradigmatic for other "healing" relationships, those that involve humans in states of need and vulnerability. The same perceptions of threats to or loss of dignity accompany those myriad encounters in which one person seeks the help of another. In all these relationships there are always the silent questions: How will my plight be perceived? Has my vulnerability diminished the respect I deserve as a fellow human being? Is my need for help perceived as a manifestation of a physiological or psychological weakness? Does that perception erode my dignity in the eyes of the one whose help I need?

It is especially as a petitioner that the person's dignity is "on the line." Consciously or unconsciously, merely admitting the need for help places a person in a state of vulnerability. The patient's perception of his or her independence and freedom are exposed, by necessity, to the full view of another person. How another person responds to our need can sustain or undermine our perception of our own dignity.

The patient is in a state of unusual vulnerability, a predicament that compels entry into a relationship of inequality in knowledge and power. This predicament must be confronted by submitting to the danger of loss of a patient's imputed dignity. Such disproportionate allotment of power is especially problematic in democratic societies. In those societies, personal autonomy is a cherished right, as is the right to privacy. Both can be threatened or endangered by the doctor's or the nurse's orders. However, our autonomy cannot exist apart from our humanity. Its moral force is rooted in our inherent dignity as humans. To experience a loss of autonomy is to experience a loss of only our imputed dignity. Although we are sometimes tempted to conflate our imputed with our inherent dignity, our inherent dignity as human beings cannot be lost. In times of suffering, disfigurement, or certainty of death, patients often lose their confidence in their own worth or dignity. The gravity of that experience obliges physicians, nurses, family and friends to reassure the patient that his intrinsic dignity is enduring and inviolable. For that assurance to be authentic the patient must be treated with dignity to the end.

Patients know that, in the end, they must take some doctor's advice. Before making that choice, they may diligently search the doctor's credentials, qualifications and practice record, but there is a moment of truth that patients cannot avoid. Whether one is president of the most powerful country in the world, or a peasant tilling the soil, one ultimately needs to accept, or refuse, another person's medical advice as authoritative. The patient's dignity as a rational being is preserved by others respecting his or her freedom to make that choice. But that dignity is endangered by having to do so in a human relationship of inequality.

The challenge to one's perceptions of one's own dignity is exacerbated by the guilt one may feel for being sick in the first place. Guilt leads to self-deprecation, to feelings of unworthiness, and even to the misperception of a loss of inherent dignity. Sickness exposes us to our mortality, the one unmovable boundary to our pride. In an age when the pursuit of health has become something of a cult, to become sick can suggest that we have failed at prevention somewhere— not enough dieting or exercise, "bad genes," or emotional instability.

Which, how many, and to what extent have I allowed those things to escape my control? Shouldn't I be ashamed of neglecting my health? This is a question often implied, even if not overtly asked.

Shame is another experience that adds to the distress of being ill, because illness weakens the safeguards that our sense of shame puts between the public and private perceptions of who we are.[22] It is this sense of the invasion of our protected, carefully controlled, private space that undermines our personal perceptions of dignity. The health care professional has become an observer whom we are forced to admit into the privacy of our bodies. Speaking of shame, Erwin Straus sees it as "….a protective against the public in all its forms."[23] It is, in Straus's terms, an original feature of human existence, while shamelessness is an acquired behavior.[24]

This sense of shame as a shield against loss of dignity is immediately challenged when we take on the status of patient. Usually, we must disrobe and expose our body to expert scrutiny with all its imperfections revealed. What we are and who we are is suppressed in the objectification of our person that a scientific appraisal of our physical state might demand. We may be infantilized, especially if we are elderly, but even if we are in our prime. The hospital routine, the order of procedures, and the vast array of "policies" may engulf us despite the best efforts of our care providers.

The experiences of threats to and loss of dignity are well-known to hospital patients. They begin with the haughty receptionist, continue with the admitting clerk and the interrogation about insurance, and are followed by lying on the gurney waiting in the hall for the x-ray technician. Being the "next case" does little to reassure us. There are subtle variations in the list of cumulative assaults on one's sense of dignity. I have heard the litany from my own patients, and know it from personal experience. It takes a stronger perception of one's inherent dignity than most of us possess not to feel humiliated. "Humiliation" is the word I hear most often from patients describing the experience of being ill and seeking help.

Most patients survive those routine humiliations, but there are many occasions when the experience entails deeper repercussions and, hence, much greater moral significance. Chronic illness, mental illness, dying, and death are occasions when the patient's perception of loss of his or her dignity is deep enough and persistent enough to be, itself, an additional source of suffering. This suffering is often more distressing than the pains, discomfort, or disability caused by the disease itself. Cumulative assaults on the dignity of the dying are often the reason for a desperate request for euthanasia or assisted suicide as well as for the prevalence of clinical depression among dying patients.

Perceptions of loss of dignity also contribute significantly to a person's assessment of the quality of his or her life and can dramatically shape their decisions to accept or reject even effective treatment. When patients have the capacity for decision-making, their assessment of the quality of their lives is dispositive. No one can ethically make quality of life decisions for an autonomous patient.

With those who have never had, or have lost, the capacity for decision-making—the retarded, the demented, those in states of serious brain dysfunction—surrogate decisions are necessary but perilous. They can overtly, or covertly, signify a devaluation of the "worth" of the patient with which the patient might, or might not, agree. In such cases, the temptation to treat the patient as one would treat oneself is strong but problematic.

In a sincere attempt to reassure a patient anxious about the loss of dignity in the impersonal milieu of modern medical care, a physician will sometimes promise to treat the patient "as he would his own mother." Ordinarily, such a well-intentioned promise is understood as such by the patient. In some situations, however, this kind intention can distort the application of the "Golden Rule." In fact, the doctor's values may not at all be those of his patient. Rather, the doctor is obliged to learn of the patient's wishes and adhere to them—unless they violate the physician's personal and professional moral integrity. When such an impasse occurs, the physician should make his position known so that either the patient can discharge him, or the doctor can ask to be relieved of his responsibility to provide care.

Caution must also be observed by physicians tempted to use a "best interests" standard as decided by "reasonable people." What is often hidden behind such notions, unintentionally one hopes, is a confusion of the intrinsic dignity of the patient with the dignity imputed by the physician or other observers.

Finally, all decisions about a "dignified death," or a "dignified life," or a "quality" life, are perilous when made by a surrogate and even when made by the patient himself. Sensitivity to the subtle differences between inherent and perceived dignity must be developed in physicians and all who minister to the sick or to persons in distress for any reason.

Ascertaining the patient's own quality-of-life choices does not entail an obligation on the part of physicians to suppress their moral beliefs in deference to the patient's wishes. This would violate the dignity inherent in each physician; how, ethically, to deal with such conflicts is a question for another occasion.

## Chronic Illness

Any serious illness is an assault on the whole person, one that challenges the image we have fashioned of ourselves over a lifetime. That image is pieced together carefully to form a synthesis of who we think we are, who we wish to be, and who we are in fact. Our aspirations are carefully molded to fit our physical, mental, or social limitations. Throughout life, we repair or adjust our image as it is challenged by the events in our lived world. Most of us reach some sort of equilibrium between our hoped-for worthiness and our worthiness as judged by others. We settle somewhere between the dignity we would prefer to have attributed to us and the dignity we possess in the eyes of the world we live in.

Serious illness shatters that equilibrium. It forces upon us a new image of ourselves, often drastically altered compared to our old self-image. The business mogul who suffers a massive heart attack, the truck driver who has had his first epileptic episode, the housewife and mother whose lymphoma is outpacing her chemotherapy—each suffers an ontological assault. The image they cherish of their own worth and the worth of their lives to others is forcibly shattered.

Some patients can renovate their self-images. Many cannot, or do not, do so. Too many lose all sense of personal worth and despair of regaining identifiable dignity. They often become depressed or suicidal. Others present heroic examples of recapturing a new sense of dignity and grow with the experience. Still others fear dying without dignity. The way each responds becomes a determinant of the dignity, or indignity, others impute to them.

As disease becomes chronic and unrelenting and progresses to foreseeable death, the experience of indignity becomes more insistent. It becomes ever harder to believe in one's underlying inherent dignity. It is difficult to controvert the ravages of a long illness—emaciation, loss of appetite, inability to care for one's most personal needs, overwhelming weakness and fatigue, and the deterioration of physiognomy and affect. Those realities powerfully force the conclusion of personal unworthiness on the patient.

None of these phenomena occurs in isolation. Health professionals, friends, family, and fellow patients are all participants. Seriously ill and dying patients are acutely sensitive to the way others in their presence react to them. The visitor's look of shock on entering the patient's room, the poorly disguised pity, the slight turning away of the eyes, the ever shorter visits, the struggle to say something meaningful, the mournful countenance, the recoil from bodily contact—those reactions all sustain the patient's conviction that she or he is no longer a respected, needed, or wanted member of their community or society. These phenomena feed the patient's perception of being a burden and even an embarrassment to his family, friends, and physicians.

Some patients may act "nobly" and "with dignity," while others may not. But in all, the experience of indignity is a reality for the patient and for those who witness the patient's experience of illness and dying. The way these witnesses respond to their experience of the decline of their patient, friend, or family member has serious consequences for that patient's perception of his worth. Those in the patient's presence are inevitably co-actors and participants in the unfolding drama. As such they incur certain ethical obligations to which I shall turn shortly. For the moment, it suffices to say that the observer's intended or unintended signals of body language, word, and countenance are all too often affirmations for the patient of his perceived loss of dignity.

Another facet of the experience of threat to or of a loss of a human being's dignity is the spiritual crisis that accompanies impending death. This crisis accompanies every serious illness and especially the approach of death. The term "spiritual" is used here in its broadest sense, extending from the religious and mystical to the acknowledgement of a transcendent reality of some sort beyond human cognition. That reality may be a personal God or some blind force of nature or simply a sense of identity with the mystery of the cosmos.

In the clinical confrontation with one's own finitude that dying or the threat of dying forces upon us, there is an unavoidable personal challenge to human dignity. What is the meaning of our personal existence? Is there any meaning? If there is a God, does God care at all? Have we been created and left alone in the universe? Is there anything after death? What is it? Religious believers, atheists, agnostics, materialists, cynics and skeptics, nihilists—all face those questions in some form. Each does so in a particular way. They are the same questions so poignantly addressed in that most poetic lament by Job—Why, oh Lord? Why me? Why now?[25]

## Ethical Obligation and the Experience of Dignity and Indignity

Our focus on the experiential dimensions of human dignity must not lead to the erroneous conclusion that dignity and indignity are irrelevant for those who cannot consciously experience them. Those in comatose states, in states of total or partial brain damage, those with various forms of dementia, the mentally retarded, as well as the infant and the very young child, all retain their inherent dignity. The concept of dignity to which I subscribe assigns an inalienable, inherent dignity to all human beings simply by virtue of being the kinds of beings they are. None of the patho-physiological mechanisms that impair the human capacity for conscious experience can alter dignity. Patho-physiological abnormalities of consciousness are in the realm of imputed or attributed dignity; they are not about intrinsic or inherent dignity.

Most of the essayists in this anthology have deduced certain ethical implications from the particular construal of human dignity they favor. That is wholly legitimate for the analysis of dignity as a problem in Marcel's sense of the term. But in addition, if we wish to probe dignity as a mystery in Marcel's sense, we must locate some of those obligations in concrete experience. This is not to disparage the deductive-conceptual model but to add to it the immediacy of a lived experience.

Karol Wojtyla (Pope John Paul II) saw the ethical experience this way:

> Every human action involves a particular lived experience that goes by the name of ethical experience. This whole lived experience has a thorough empirical character.[26]

Later on in his essay he goes directly to the core of ethical experience in the moral agent:

> ...[T]he only value that can be called an ethical value is a value that has the acting person as its efficient cause..., and this is also where the very core of ethical experience lies.[27]

The clinical encounter, because of its ubiquity and intensity, is a locus of the ethical experience to which Wojtyla refers. The "acting persons" in this case are the patient herself or himself, the physician, nurse, and other health professionals, and the non-professional observers—family, friends, and visitors. Again, the observation we make in the clinical encounter can analogously, if not precisely, relate to other situations such as those of the disabled person; the person without access to health care; the cultural or ethnic outcast; and those deprived in any way, physically or emotionally, by the mores of the society in which they live. Thus, loss or perceived loss of dignity is a common phenomenon in encounters between lawyer and client, priest and penitent, teacher and student. In each instance, dependent and vulnerable humans needing help must expose their fragile sense of self-worth to the gaze of others.

## Preserving Human Dignity, Preventing Indignity

Toward the end of his pointed indictment of the corrosive effects of modern mass society on human dignity, Marcel has this to say:

> It is within the scope of each of us within his own proper field, in his profession, to pursue an unrelaxing struggle for the dignity of man against everything that today threatens to annihilate man and his dignity.[28]

Marcel goes on to urge that this struggle be carried out in the field of law. But the struggle to which Marcel calls the professions is most acutely needed today in bioethics and medicine. In medicine, the concept and the experience of human dignity as the foundation for biomedical ethics is facing its most serious challenges. In law, the corrosion of human dignity weakens human rights; but in medicine, its corrosion weakens human beings' humanity itself—i.e., the foundations for both the rights and the obligations inherent in humans as humans. Medical practice and the clinical encounter are paradigm occasions where the defense of dignity must be pursued with diligence. Attention should also, of course, be given to encounters with other health professionals and with family, friends, and all who enter the patient's experience of illness, suffering, and dying.

The preservation of human dignity and the prevention of indignity are obligations built into the ends of medicine. The ends of medicine are focused on the good of the patient as a human person. Medicine's ends are ultimate, intermediate, and proximate. Ultimately, medicine aims to restore health; its intermediate aim is to cure, ameliorate, or prevent illness. Most proximately, it is to make a right and good healing decision, for a particular patient in a particular clinical encounter. Any behavior that frustrates those ends or causes suffering is a violation of the moral trust patients must place in physicians if they are to be helped. This is the trust physicians implicitly or explicitly promise to live up to when they offer to be of assistance. It is the source of physicians' obligation to be faithful to their promise to help.

To be faithful to that trust, the physician must avoid the vice of arrogance, one of the most frequent complaints I hear from patients. The inequality of power and knowledge between doctors and patients feeds the inordinate pride and self-importance that most physicians exhibit at one time or another. Self-importance is an intoxicant for the young physician and can become an addiction for the older ones. Self-importance tempts to certitude where only probabilities exist. It demeans the patient as well as fellow health professionals and adds to the indignity of the illness itself. It entraps the physician in the cage of pride, which breeds false pretensions of infallibility. It also endangers the healing relationship, since error or misstep can no longer be admitted. Ultimately, arrogance subverts and subordinates the good of the patient to the preservation of the physician's own self-image.

Physicians, instead, must be the unfailing advocates and defenders of patient dignity. They must be cognizant of those many times when the "system," the "team," or the "teaching hospital" may function to the detriment of the patient's self-esteem. Physicians are not guiltless if their staff and those around them in any way demean patients who lack education or financial means, or are elderly, or easily confused, or experience language barriers, etc. The therapeutic process begins when a patient in need calls the doctor's office and is greeted by the physician's receptionist or is admitted to the hospital. Some patients are robbed of their dignity right at the entry point by the attitude and tone of voice that greets them.

What patient has not, at one time or another, experienced the telephone rebuff, the refusal of personal contact with the doctor, or the supercilious interrogations of the person at "the front desk"? Some of this may be the result of a response to patient agitation and anxiety, to be sure, but frustration with a patient's personality is a weak excuse for treating patients with disrespect. Other weak excuses include being busy, wrestling with one's own problems, or simply being temperamentally unsuited to dealing with fellow human beings in distress.

Too many physicians distance themselves from the actions of those who act in their name on the basis of lack of time, difficulty in "getting good help," or simple insensitivity to anything not susceptible to resolution by a prescription or a procedure. More seriously, the behavior of his or her team may be a reflection of the physician's arrogance. Obviously, physicians cannot observe everything, but the devoted patient advocacy expected of the ethical physician dictates a higher degree of vigilance than is now common.

The physician is also obliged to respect the other professionals with whom she or he works for the good of the patient. The nurse, technician, social worker, chaplain, psychologist, etc., have justifiable pride in their expertise and recognize how essential they are to the patient's care. The day is happily past when physicians could discount the dignity of other health professionals with impunity. On the other hand, we cannot allow respect for our fellow workers to obscure those occasions when they may be incompetent, abusive, or insensitive to the dignity of those they treat. If we physicians do not move to correct the injurious behavior of health care workers who assault patient dignity, we ourselves are complicit in their misbehavior.

Physicians cannot ignore those many assaults on human dignity, intrinsic as well as attributed, that are taken for granted in the bureaucratic, commercialized, and impersonal places that hospitals have, all too often, become. Some of this is indeed unavoidable, given the complex nature of contemporary medical care. But physicians, administrators, and policy-makers must always ask, "What is the impact of our organization or 'system' on the care of the persons they were designed to help?" A more collective sense of shared responsibility for the "dehumanization," the "depersonalization," or the "alienation" that the sick feel in today's health and medical care institutions must fall on the physician. Physicians can exert enormous moral influence if they take their advocacy role seriously as part of their common professional ethic.

The physician plays a central role here: seeing the patient in his or her weakest moments, assessing the physical ravages of the disease, and prognosticating its severity and likely outcome. The physician decides when treatment has become futile, when the patient's private affairs must be put in order, and when care in a hospice is to be considered. At each step, the physician must try to bolster the patient against a sense of unworthiness and guilt. The physician must avoid false humor, unrealistic expectations, and the temptation to avoid the ultimate questions. Somehow, the physician must be truthful and realistic and, at the same time, try to mitigate the impact of the mounting evidence of the patient's decline. The patient must always feel worthy of the physician's time and attention.

In many ways, the most important doctoring occurs just when it becomes obvious that the patient's finitude must be confronted. How this is done while respecting the patient as a human person is the subject of much thought today. My aim here is not to provide a lexically ordered list of obligations. Rather, it is to establish a grounding for a serious ethical obligation to protect the patient against the loss of dignity that leads to despair and, often, to a desperate plea for relief by euthanasia or assisted suicide.[29]

A final, and often neglected, obligation of physicians is to help family and friends to understand that the ways they respond to the patient's plight and vulnerability are important determinants of the degree to which the patient will feel alienated from the human community. All who enter the patient's presence can become complicit in the patient's loss of self-worth.

In teaching institutions, students and residents will look to their clinical teachers for guidance in protecting patient dignity. Clinical teachers must be aware that arrogance, indifference, and ineptitude can lead patients to feel alienated and undignified, reduced to lesser members of the human community. All who enter the presence of the seriously ill person become accomplices if the patient feels a loss of dignity. Unconsciously, the members of the health care team thus can contribute to the patient's sense of unworthiness.

The need to sensitize physicians and other health professionals is an urgent one in today's mechanized experience of illness. All caregivers now rotate constantly. The patient must constantly re-establish identity relationships. The preservation of dignity becomes increasingly more difficult. Physicians must have the humility to recognize that other health professionals, family, and friends will often be more sensitive to this predicament.

This latter admonition is highly relevant in teaching institutions. Students and medical residents must be taught in settings in which human dignity is expressly addressed. Students will easily learn good and bad habits. Indifference, ineptitude, and arrogance are transmissible. Courses designed to teach compassion, intercultural competency, and the like may help. But, ultimately, students and residents model their attitudes about patient care on their clinical teachers' behavior. The same is true of the institutions within which they take their first steps as clinicians. The virtues of dignity-responsive care can only be learned in personal and institutional settings that sustain those virtues.

## Dignity in a Post-secular Society

This essay has focused primarily on only one common lived experience of dignity and indignity. That is because the clinical experience is, or will be, familiar to everyone either personally or in the lives of family and friends. Lived experiences of the same kind are encountered in other professional relationships, e.g., in law, ministry, and teaching. Even more universally, the experience of dignity is a reality in every conceivable kind of human relationship. Whatever concept of dignity one favors will, in the end, be abstracted from a concrete experience.

This account of human dignity has shown the untenability of two of the rash assertions in Ruth Macklin's diatribe against the idea of human dignity. First, can an experience so ubiquitous, and momentous, for all human beings be so summarily discounted? The question answers itself. And, second, can it be replaced by autonomy? Emphatically not. Humans possess autonomy because of their intrinsic dignity; they are not dignified because they are autonomous. Holocaust victims did not lose their dignity or the rights that it entailed because they were despoiled of their autonomy. Nor do infants, the comatose, or the brain-damaged lack dignity because they are not fully autonomous.

Macklin's third assault on dignity, her demand that it be banished from public discourse because it has religious overtones, is equally off the mark. Such a prohibition ignores the fact that religious faith is part of being human for millions. For them, as William James observed, "…religious experiences are absolutely authoritative over the individuals to whom they come."[30] These experiences will inevitably become public because they are elemental to the identities of the persons who hold them. That is why, as Stephen Carter has shown, "…religion has always been in the public square."[31]

Religious faith does in fact go beyond the canons of discourse that secularization would impose. But it cannot be ignored on that account. Secularists cannot deny the connection between moral belief and moral practice. The trajectory of modern culture is toward secularization, but the reality is that we now live, and will live, in a post-secular society. In that society, neither religion nor secularism will triumph over the other. They are almost certain to exist side-by-side for the foreseeable future, and their interrelations will be complex. As Jürgen Habermas has emphasized, a post-secular society will require "a complementary learning process" in which both sides "take seriously each other's contributions to controversial subjects in the public debate."[32]

Dignity, and the possibilities of its loss or erosion, are ineradicable phenomena of being human. The question for bioethics and contemporary culture is not how to eliminate dignity from public discourse but how to understand and acknowledge the variations in its meanings. The consequences for society, and for the way it meets the ethical challenges of biotechnology, are enormous.

Two contrary, but not necessarily contradictory, world views will dominate the discourse in our post-secular civilization. Two images of human dignity compete for moral authority. One is the scientific, the other the religious. Neither is likely to capitulate to the other. Is a productive dialogue and dialectic between these two world views possible, and how is it to be conducted?

Extremists on both sides, militant atheists and intransigent dogmatists, insist there can be no common ground. More responsible proponents of both views hope for a productive dialogue and appeal to the necessity of a common ground in the public arena, even while metaphysical foundations remain disputed. One hopeful sign is the recent dialogue between two of Europe's most eminent thinkers. One is the social philosopher and non-believer, Jürgen Habermas; the other is the Roman Catholic theologian and now Pope Benedict XVI, Joseph Ratzinger.[33]

Each thinker expresses genuine interest in the insights of the other. Each remains faithful to the metaphysical presuppositions of his own world. Both sincerely believe that each view can gain something from the other. Each recognizes the need for a "translation" of his ideas into the language of the other.

Interestingly, both use the concept of dignity as a subject for their "translational" methodology. The philosopher Habermas puts it this way:

> One such translation that salvages the substance of a term is the translation of the concept of "man in the image of God" into that of the identical dignity of all men that deserves unconditional respect. This goes beyond the borders of one particular religious fellowship and makes the substance of biblical concepts accessible to the general public who have other faiths and those who have none.[34]

Ratzinger puts the same thought this way:

> One final element of the natural law that claimed (at least in

the modern period) that it was ultimately a rational law has remained, namely, *human rights*. These are incomprehensible without the presupposition that man qua man, thanks simply to his membership in the "species" man, is the subject of rights and that his being bears within itself values and norms that must be discovered—but not invented. Today we ought perhaps amplify the doctrine of human rights with a doctrine of human obligations and human limitations.[35]

Throughout their dialogue, both participants are frank about some of the weaknesses and even the "pathologies" of their own positions. They deprecate the hubris that inhibits the kind of dialogue they seek, and they acknowledge the necessity to be open to each other without relinquishing their independence.

In another place, Habermas warns us against the hubris that makes a misinterpretation of human dignity an invitation to the latent illusion of humans that ultimately they will be their own deity. Speaking of genetic engineering, Habermas issues a warning with which Benedict XVI could agree:

> Would not the first human being to determine, *at his own discretion*, the natural essence of another human being at the same time destroy the equal freedoms that exist among persons of equal birth in order to ensure their difference?[36]

These are extraordinary men, neither of whom can be accused of eager compromise in the service of empty intellectual irenicism. They are acutely aware of the need to find a common ground and a common language—one that will recognize the perdurability of the concept of human dignity in an age of technology. Their willingness to seek practical truths of ethical action while holding to different world views should embolden all of us who hope to ease strife, indecision, and injustice in our use of biotechnology for human good.

That such a hope is not entirely fanciful is clear from the agreement in the declarations of the UN and UNESCO that both in the foundation of human rights and in bioethics, human dignity is the first principle. To arrive at this conclusion the participating nations did, indeed, use a translational methodology akin to that used by

Habermas and Ratzinger, even while each held to its own metaphysical beliefs.

Sadly, the world had to experience the massive deprivations of human dignity of World War II and the world scene following it to understand human dignity in a way no purely conceptual analysis could. To paraphrase John Keats, dignity became an axiom only when it was "proven" on the "pulses" of the whole world. Only when we all had gone some way on the "same steps" did we grasp how intimately our humanity was embedded in our inherent dignity. We then understood what happens to dignity when humanity is "delivered" to tyrannical regimes; let us hope we will not also have to learn what happens to human dignity when humanity is delivered to "the process of technicalization," the "problem" that troubled Marcel.

# Notes

[1] Gabriel Marcel, *The Existential Background of Human Dignity* (Cambridge, Massachusetts: Harvard University Press, 1963), p. 158.

[2] Paul Oskar Kristeller, *Renaissance Thought II, Papers on Humanism and the Arts* (New York: Harper and Row, 1965), pp. 108-109; Giovanni Pico Della Mirandola, *Oration on the Dignity of Man* (1486), trans. Robert Caponigri (Chicago: Henry Regnery, 1956); Eugenio Garin, "Italian Humanism," in *Philosophy and Civil Life in the Renaissance*, trans. Peter Munz (New York: Harper and Row, 1965), pp. 105-106.

[3] Ruth Macklin, "Dignity is a Useless Concept," *BMJ* 327 (2003): 1419-1420.

[4] Edmund D. Pellegrino, "Toward A Richer Bioethics," in *Health and Human Flourishing*, ed. Carol R. Taylor and Roberto Dell'Oro (Washington, D.C.: Georgetown University Press, 2006), pp. 247-269.

[5] On the lived experience of human dignity in the context of the Holocaust, see Victor Frankl, *Man's Search for Meaning* (Boston: Beacon Press, 2006 [1959]). On the relevance of that era for bioethics, see Dónal P. O'Mathúna, "Human Dignity in the Nazi Era: Implications for Contemporary Bioethics," *BMC Medical Ethics* 7 (2006): 2, available online at: www.pubmedcentral.nih.gov/articlerender.fcgi?artid=1484488.

[6] United Nations General Assembly, *Universal Declaration of Human Rights*, General Assembly Resolution 217 A (III), 10 December, 1948 (New York: United Nations General Assembly Official Records, 1948), available online at www.un.org/Overview/rights.html.

[7] *Universal Declaration on Bioethics and Human Rights*, adopted by acclamation at the 33rd session of the UNESCO General Conference, October 19, 2005; available online at www.unesco.org/ibc.

[8] See Jacques Maritain, *Man and the State* (Chicago: University of Chicago Press, 1951), p. 80.

[9] John Keats, "Letter 64 to J. H. Reynolds, 3 May 1818" as cited in *Oxford Dictionary of Quotations*, 2nd ed. (London: Oxford University Press, 1955), p. 289.

[10] Edmund D. Pellegrino, "The False Promise of Beneficent Killing," in *Regulating How We Die*, ed. Linda L. Emanuel (Cambridge, Massachusetts: Harvard University, 1998), pp. 71-91.

[11] Aurel Kolnai, "Dignity," *Philosophy* 51 (1976): 251-271.

[12] Ibid., p. 252.

[13] Gabriel Marcel, *The Mystery of Being, Volume 1: Reflection and Mystery* (*Gifford Lectures, 1949-50*) (South Bend, Indiana: St. Augustine's Press, 2001).

[14] Gabriel Marcel, *Being and Having: An Existentialist Diary*, trans. Katherine Farrer (New York: Harper and Row, 1965), pp. 100, 117, and 126 (first published in French as *Etre et avoir* in 1935); Kenneth T. Gallagher, *The Philosophy of Gabriel Marcel*, with a foreword by Gabriel Marcel (New York: Fordham University Press, 1975), Chapter 3.

[15] Sydney Rome and Beatrice Rome, "Interrogations of John Wild," in *Philosophical*

*Interrogations* (New York: Holt, Rinehart & Winston, 1964), p. 129.
[16] Gallagher, op. cit., p. 43.
[17] John Henry Newman, *An Essay in Aid of a Grammar of Assent* (Notre Dame, Indiana: University of Notre Dame Press, 2006), pp. 270-299 (first published in 1870 after a gestation of twenty years).
[18] Bernard Lonergan later used Newman's illative sense as a stimulus for his own in-depth explorations of the idea of "insight." See Bernard J. Lonergan, *Verbum: Word and Idea in Aquinas*, ed. David Burrell (Notre Dame, Indiana: University of Notre Dame Press, 1967), p. 47.
[19] James Collins, *The Existentialists* (Chicago: Henry Regnery, 1958), p. 150.
[20] Alexei Kukuljevic, "De Levze's Metaphysics and the Reality of the Virtual," *Philosophy Today* 49 (2005): 146.
[21] John F. Crosby, *The Selfhood of the Human Person* (Washington, D.C.: The Catholic University of America Press, 1996), p. 177. Crosby means here to distinguish relational goodness, that which is relative to one's own ends or to another's satisfaction, from the intrinsic goodness in itself that is the essence of human dignity.
[22] Erwin W. Straus, *Phenomenological Psychology*, trans. Erling Eng (New York: Basic Books, 1966), pp. 217-224.
[23] Ibid., p. 222.
[24] Ibid., p. 223.
[25] Edmund D. Pellegrino, "The Trials of Job: A Physician's Meditation," *Linacre Quarterly* 56 (1989): 76-88.
[26] Karol Wojtyla, *Person and Community—Selected Essays*, trans. Theresa Sandok, OSM (New York: Peter Lang, 1994), p. 5.
[27] Ibid., p. 38.
[28] Gabriel Marcel, *Man Against Mass Society*, trans. George F. Fraser, with a foreword by Donald McCinnon (Chicago: Henry Regnery, 1967), p. 244.
[29] Edmund D. Pellegrino, "The False Promise of Beneficent Killing," cited in note 10 above.
[30] William James, *Varieties of Religious Experience* (1902), reprinted in *Philosophy of Religion: Selected Readings*, 3rd edition, ed. Michael Peterson, William Hasker, Bruce Reichenbach, and David Basinger (Oxford: Oxford University Press, 2006), p. 16.
[31] Stephen Carter, *The Culture of Disbelief: How American Law and Politics Trivialize Religious Devotion* (New York: Doubleday, 1993), p. 100.
[32] See Habermas's contribution to Joseph Cardinal Ratzinger (Pope Benedict XVI) and Jürgen Habermas, *Dialectics of Secularization: On Reason and Religion*, ed. and with a foreword by Florian Schuller (San Francisco, California: Ignatius Press, 2006), pp. 46-47.
[33] Ibid.
[34] Jürgen Habermas, *The Future of Human Nature* (Cambridge: Polity Press, 2003), p. 41.
[35] Ratzinger and Habermas, *Dialectics of Secularization*, p. 71.
[36] Habermas, op. cit., p. 115.

# Contributors

- Adam Schulman is Tutor at St. John's College, Annapolis, and Senior Research Consultant at the President's Council on Bioethics.
- F. Daniel Davis is Senior Research Scholar at the Center for Clinical Bioethics at Georgetown University, and Executive Director at the President's Council on Bioethics.
- Daniel C. Dennett is Austin B. Fletcher Professor of Philosophy and Director of the Center for Cognitive Studies at Tufts University.
- Robert P. Kraynak is Professor of Political Science and Director of the Center for Freedom and Western Civilization at Colgate University.
- Alfonso Gómez-Lobo is Ryan Family Professor of Metaphysics and Moral Philosophy at Georgetown University, and a member of the President's Council on Bioethics.
- Patricia S. Churchland is University of California President's Professor and Chair of the Department of Philosophy at the University of California at San Diego.
- Gilbert Meilaender is Richard and Phyllis Duesenberg Professor of Christian Ethics at Valparaiso University, and a member of the President's Council on Bioethics.
- Holmes Rolston III is University Distinguished Professor of Philosophy at Colorado State University.

- Charles Rubin is Associate Professor of Political Science at Duquesne University.
- Nick Bostrom is Director of the Future of Humanity Institute at the University of Oxford and Fellow of St. Cross College.
- Richard John Neuhaus is founder and editor of *First Things*.
- Peter Augustine Lawler is Dana Professor and Chair of the Department of Government and International Studies at Berry College, and a member of the President's Council on Bioethics.
- Diana Schaub, a member of the President's Council on Bioethics, is Professor of Political Science at Loyola College in Maryland and a member of the Hoover Institution Task Force on the Virtues of a Free Society.
- Leon R. Kass is Addie Clark Harding Professor in the Committee on Social Thought and the College at the University of Chicago and Hertog Fellow in Social Thought at the American Enterprise Institute, and was a member of the President's Council on Bioethics until 2007. He was chairman of the Council from 2002 to 2005.
- Susan M. Shell is Professor and Chair of the Department of Political Science at Boston College.
- Martha Nussbaum is Ernst Freund Distinguished Service Professor of Law and Ethics at the University of Chicago.
- David Gelernter is a National Fellow at the American Enterprise Institute in Washington, D.C., and Professor of Computer Science at Yale University.
- Patrick Lee is Professor of Bioethics and Director of the Bioethics Institute at the Franciscan University of Steubenville.
- Robert P. George is McCormick Professor of Jurisprudence and Director of the James Madison Program in American Ideals and Institutions at Princeton University, and a member of the President's Council on Bioethics.
- Paul Weithman is Professor and Chair of the Department of Philosophy at the University of Notre Dame.
- Daniel P. Sulmasy, O.F.M., is Professor of Medicine and Director of the Bioethics Institute of New York Medical College and holds the Sisters of Charity Chair in Ethics at St. Vincent's Hospital, Manhattan.

- Rebecca Dresser is Daniel Noyes Kirby Professor of Law and Professor of Ethics in Medicine at Washington University in St. Louis, and a member of the President's Council on Bioethics.
- Edmund D. Pellegrino is Professor Emeritus of Medicine and Medical Ethics and Adjunct Professor of Philosophy at Georgetown University. He has been Chairman of the President's Council on Bioethics since 2005.

# Index

## A

abortion  220–221, 222, 373, 374, 430, 471
Adler, Mortimer  431
Ainslie, George
  *Breakdown of Will*  56
alcohol  *See* drugs and alcohol
Alzheimer's  4
American Founding  12, 15, 287, 292, 318, 360  *See also The Federalist Papers*
Anderson, Roland C.  144
Anderson, Stephen R.  136
anencephalic child  363, 385
animals  *See* dignity: of animals; *See* humans: as animals; *See* humans: as more than animals; *See* right(s): animal; *See* soul: animal
Aquinas  *See* Thomas Aquinas
Aristotle  45, 63, 72, 83, 84, 101, 102, 105, 106, 168, 175, 181, 219, 224, 356, 419, 420, 438, 471, 480, 496  *See also* dignity: Aristotelian Argument from; *See also* dignity: Aristotelian/Marxian account of; *See also* soul: Aristotelian account of
  and capabilities  357–362, 451–465
  *Nicomachean Ethics*  70, 219
  *On the Soul*  69–70
  *Politics*  219, 460
Arneson, Richard  415

Arnold, Matthew
  *Dover Beach*  144
assisted suicide  *See* death
Augustine  74, 218, 230–232, 247, 248, 250, 278
autonomy  5, 9, 10, 11, 14, 20, 24, 26–27, 31–32, 65, 66, 146, 192, 216, 222, 235–237, 242, 243, 244, 245, 246, 247, 270, 290, 300, 302, 312, 313, 333, 334, 336, 337, 339, 382, 384, 387, 388, 437, 469, 507, 508, 510, 511, 514, 523, 525, 534  *See also* dignity; *See also* dignity: as autonomy; *See also* humans: as autonomous chimps; *See also* Kant, Immanuel: as father of "autonomy"; *See also* patients: and autonomy

## B

Bacon, Francis  157, 217
Barrow, John D.  141
Barth, Karl  227
Bayes, Thomas  192, 209
Bear, Mark F.  143
Beauchamp and Childress
  *Principles of Biomedical Ethics*  270
Beauchamp, Tom L.  25
Beecher, Henry K.  22
beneficence  23, 24
Benny, Jack  41
Bentham, Jeremy  366, 374, 413

545

Berns, Walter 258
Beyleveld, Deryck 273–274, 275
Bible 10, 33, 62, 94, 181, 244, 282, 290, 342, 446 *See also* dignity: Biblical notion of; *See also* God: Biblical
*Colossians* 78
*Deuteronomy* 100
*Ecclesiasticus* 77
*Exodus* 100, 322
*Genesis* 8, 74–78, 81, 86–87, 135, 322–329, 396, 399
*Job* 109, 227, 528
*Leviticus* 392
*Micah* 389
*Philippians* 78
*Psalms* 16, 77, 168
*Romans* 78
*Wisdom* 77
biography *See* humans: as biographical
Birnbacher, Dieter 9
Blackburn, Simon 389
*The Blue Angel*, film 307
Boehm, Christopher 149
Boethius 412
Bostrom, Nick 161
  commentary on 207–212
Bowles, Samuel 104
Boyd, Robert 131
Brave New World 304, 313 *See also* Huxley, Aldous
Brecht, Bertolt 222
Brennan, William 258
Brownsword, Roger 273–274, 275
Bush, George W., President 57
  August 9, 2001, televised address 27–28
  Executive Order 13237 29
Byrne, Richard 132

# C

capabilities *See* Aristotle: and capabilities; *See* dignity: through capabilities or capacities; *See* Nussbaum, Martha: central human capabilities
capital punishment *See* death
Carter, Stephen 534
Cash, Johnny 241
Cat Man *See* enhancement: Cat Man
Chesterton, G. K. 207, 249
Childress, James F. 254 *See also* Beauchamp and Childress: *Principles of Biomedical Ethics*
chimeras
  animal-human 16, 17, 175
chimpanzees 103, 114, 131–133, 138, 142, 147, 149, 243, 364, 365, 366, 375 *See also* humans: as autonomous chimps
  and culture 131
  and justice 148
Christianity 8, 62, 73–79, 84, 207, 230–232, 247, 248, 263, 279–280, 284–290, 318, 373, 470 *See also* persons: Christian; *See also* virtue: Christian and classical
  Catholicism 124, 174, 224, 226
  evangelical 226
  fundamentalist 87
Churchill, Winston 53, 291–292, 421
Churchland, Patricia S.
  commentary on 122–125
Cicero 174, 188, 355, 471, 499
Clinton, William J., President: Executive Order 12975 28
cloning 8, 9, 12, 16, 17, 18, 40, 61, 80, 81, 175, 197, 205, 264, 269, 276, 277, 298, 305, 313, 375, 388, 393, 394, 396, 403–404, 470, 493–496
Collins, James 520
Confucius 102
Copernicus, Nicolaus 65
corpses *See* death

Crosby, John 522
culture 130, 131, 132, 133, 148, 149
  origin of 103–105

# D

Dalai Lama 105
Darwall, Stephen 199
Darwin, Charles 65, 66, 90, 91, 404
  *The Descent of Man* 116
Darwinism 66–67, 68, 84, 89, 90, 91, 92, 242, 243
  Social 67, 90, 91
Davies, Paul 54, 71–72, 73, 93, 94
  *Are We Alone?* 73
Deacon, Terrence W. 135
death
  assisted suicide 108, 305, 373, 469, 487, 525, 532
  capital punishment 40, 258, 418
  conquering 61, 80, 156, 299, 302, 375–377
  corpses 47, 48
  euthanasia 175, 297, 299, 305, 315, 390, 430, 471, 474, 487–488, 489, 525, 532
  fear of 17
  murder 75, 161, 169, 253, 288, 322–326, 391–392, 402, 411, 416, 426
  with dignity 217, 304, 305, 311, 326, 469, 488, 506, 525, 526
Declaration of Independence 10, 219, 221, 249, 261, 262, 266, 284, 286, 288, 289, 292, 316–318, 398
De Gaulle, Charles, cloned 80
DeLillo, Don
  *White Noise* 17
Delsol, Chantal 239, 246
Dennett, Daniel C. 66–67, 68
  commentary on 89–98, 278–283
  *Darwin's Dangerous Idea* 66, 91
  *Freedom Evolves* 45
dependence *See* patients: and dependence
Descartes, René 44, 46, 63, 96, 157 *See also* soul: Cartesian
  pop Cartesianism 246
Dewey, John 102, 106
Dickens, Charles
  *Bleak House* 169
dignity
  and enhancement 180–204
  Aristotelian Argument from 451–465
  Aristotelian/Marxian account of 352, 357–360, 365
  as accidentally comparative 310
  as a quality 175–178, 180–204, 207–208
  as a quality (defined) 175
  as aristocratic 14, 166, 259, 260, 284, 286, 309
  as autonomy 255, 273, 300, 437
  as constraint 273, 274
  as egalitarian 255, 257, 259, 261, 263, 264, 265, 268, 316, 320
  as humanity 4, 15–16, 17, 393–394
  as price 335
  as respect for persons 129, 313, 437
  as sanctity 14, 259, 322, 326, 333, 394–397, 400, 405
  Biblical notion of 10, 14
  classical notion of 6–8, 14
  etymology of 6, 134, 176, 260, 308
  from a patient's perspective 508–510
  intrinsic, attributed, and inflorescent defined 473–474
  Kantian notion of 10–11, 12, 14
  modern and American 247–251
  of animals 365–367
  of being "in-between" 168, 269, 270, 321–329, 445
  of human being and being

human  304, 306, 326
  of the "high" and the "low"  305, 313, 321, 325, 383
  of trees  134, 196, 198, 347, 353, 359
  Stoic account of  7–8, 10, 14, 33, 352–357, 362, 367, 471
  through asserting rights  318
  through capabilities or capacities  257, 320, 362–365
  through having a rational nature  425–429
  through natural kind membership  476–478, 482–484
  through species membership  319, 412
  transhumanist  157–167
  "Un-Dignity"  188, 194, 201, 202
disabilities  9, 363, 364, 366, 470, 480, 488–490  See also right(s): disability
  mental retardation  5, 363, 364, 385, 411, 481
Douglass, Frederick  289, 292
Dresser, Rebecca  516
drugs and alcohol  188, 371–372, 381
duties  See right(s): vs. duties
Dworkin, Andrea  340–341

### E

egalitarianism  6, 356  See also dignity: as egalitarian; See also equality; See also right(s): equal
embodiment  See humans: as embodied; See humans: as embodied souls; See soul: embodied rational
embryos  9, 11, 16, 40, 81, 98, 108, 124, 289, 298, 304, 305, 313, 345, 382, 384–386, 411, 430, 470, 490–493
  and Kant  345–347
enhancement  3, 5, 124, 155–172, 217, 272, 298, 300, 301, 303, 304, 305, 344, 345, 505, 514
  aesthetic  340
  and dignity  180–204
  Cat Man  164, 169, 208
  defined  179
  emotion modification  187–191
  in sports  7, 272, 372
  mood control  11, 16, 240–241
  performance  299, 313
Epictetus  7
equality  255, 298, 363  See also dignity: as egalitarian; See also egalitarianism; See also right(s): equal
eros  238, 250, 272, 329
eugenics  301, 302
euthanasia  See death
excellence  6, 7, 14, 15, 134, 207, 253, 255, 256, 259, 260, 261, 263, 264, 265, 266, 267, 271, 284, 285, 286, 299, 300, 303, 305, 309, 310, 311, 315, 320, 321, 326, 472
Existenz  144  See also humans: as existentially unique

### F

*The Federalist Papers*  168
Fletcher, Joseph  26
flourishing  102, 106, 113, 118, 140, 165, 261, 280, 281, 291, 299, 302, 304, 305, 306, 329, 356, 358, 359, 361, 365, 473, 476, 485, 486, 498, 514
Frankfurt, Harry  432
Franklin, Benjamin  102
freedom  12, 259, 297, 307, 311, 312, 313, 320, 324, 325, 513  See also nature: and freedom
  from natural necessity  247
  from political determination  247
  of expression  377
  of will  63, 74, 86, 92, 115, 300, 424–425, 476
  posthuman or transhuman  251

religious 88, 368
spiritual 247
to decide about treatment 511
to reason 339
Freud, Sigmund 65
Fuster, Joaquín M. 138

## G

Galef, Bennett G. 132
Galileo 45, 85
Galsworthy, John 285
*One More River* 256
Gandhi 105, 199
Garreau, Joel 159, 163
Gazzaniga, Michael
*The Ethical Brain* 117
Geach, Peter 123
*Geist* 144
George, Robert P. 248, 492, 517
*German Basic Law* (*Grundgesetz*) 12, 435, 436, 446, 448
*Gladiator,* film 8
God 26 *See also* humans: as God-like (made in God's image)
  as intelligent selector of the laws of nature 93
  as the Creator 73, 94
  Biblical 289
  fatherhood of 284, 290
  intelligent 72
  nature's 91, 230–231, 233, 248, 289
  of Israel 404
  personal 247, 248, 250, 527
Goodall, Jane 149
Gray, John 92
Gregg, Alan 162
Grisez, Germain 492
Grotius 354

## H

Habermas, Jürgen 517, 534, 535–537
Haldane, J. B. S. 160, 162

Hare, R. M. 482
Havel, Václav 249, 291
Hegel, Georg Wilhelm Friedrich 335, 339
history *See* humans: as historical; *See* nature: as historical
Hobbes, Thomas 15, 63–65, 84, 90, 237, 240, 241, 243, 245, 317, 322, 335, 472, 473, 480
  *Leviathan* 15, 63, 227, 471
Hofstadter, Douglas 46, 47
Holmes, Oliver Wendell 226
Holocaust 13, 218, 283, 301, 394, 515, 534
Homer 285
  *Odyssey* 286
humanity 15–16, 17, 26, 27, 28, 33, 66, 298, 300, 303, 307, 308, 315, 316, 323, 339, 362, 383, 384, 385, 472, 476, 523 *See also* dignity: as humanity; *See also* Kant, Immanuel: and humanity
  as an end in itself 336
  as capacity to think in terms of value 337
  as embodied rationality 334
  basic and full 261, 286
  crimes against 218, 358
humans
  as animals 44, 64, 65, 130, 161, 253, 301, 326, 329, 344, 363
  as autonomous chimps 243
  as biographical 141, 144, 145
  as embodied 130, 141, 147
  as embodied souls 62, 84, 93, 271, 313, 326
  as ethically unique 148–150
  as existentially unique 143–147
  as God-like (made in God's image) 9, 62, 73–79, 86, 94, 174, 227, 248, 262, 263, 305, 318, 323, 329, 395–396, 399, 404, 514

as heaps of chemicals 161
as historical 136–139, 145
as imitators 103
as machines 62, 63–68, 80, 90, 165, 299
as more than animals 67, 130, 131–133, 136, 240, 324, 354
as neither beasts nor gods 70, 84, 168, 259, 266
as persons 411
as rational animals 136, 272, 337, 410
as research subjects 62, 298, 300, 312
as social animals 102, 279
as tools 359
Hume, David 219, 426
Hurlbut, William 384, 386
Husserl, Edmund 207
Huxley, Aldous 303, 311
 *Brave New World* 185, 187, 303

# I
infanticide 481
informed consent 10, 15, 300, 334, 336, 348, 382
*in vitro* fertilization *See* reproduction: *in vitro* fertilization
Ishiguro, Kazuo
 *Never Let Me Go* 375

# J
James, William 534
Jefferson, Thomas 91, 167, 288–289, 386, 398
Jesus Christ 79, 318
Jewish Chronic Disease Hospital, New York City 22
Jonsen, Albert 25
 *Birth of Bioethics* 25
Judaism 8, 263, 388, 397, 399–401, 403, 470
Judeo-Christian tradition 94, 287, 388, 390, 397, 402, 405, 470

justice 23–24, 365 *See also* Rawls, John: "sense of justice"

# K
Kant, Immanuel 10–11, 12, 15, 26, 32, 33, 91, 92, 93, 168, 174, 175, 176, 178, 192, 243, 245, 246, 267, 311, 313, 353, 354, 356, 360, 361, 379, 381, 382–384, 403, 472, 473, 482, 485 *See also* dignity: Kantian notion of; *See also* embryos: and Kant; *See also* persons: Kantian
 and humanity 129
 *Anthropology from a Pragmatic Point of View* 338, 341
 as father of "autonomy" 14, 242, 312
 categorical imperative 10, 14, 312, 483
 *Groundwork of the Metaphysics of Morals* 334, 446, 472
 *Metaphysics of Morals* 337, 341
 "pure reason" 101, 116
 *Religion within the Boundaries of Bare Reason* 337
Kass, Leon R. 183, 185, 192, 249, 259–261, 262, 265, 278, 281–282, 283, 285, 286, 383, 445
 commentary on 383
Keats, John 515, 537
Kierkegaard, Søren 262, 265, 266, 287
King, Martin Luther, Jr. 482
Kolakowski, Leszek 297
Kolnai, Aurel 177–179, 180, 181, 184, 186, 198, 201, 207–212, 518, 521
Kraynak, Robert P. 247
 commentary on 83–88
Kummer, Helmut 148
Kurzweil, Raymond 159

## L

Lawler, Peter Augustine
  commentary on 291–292
Lee, Patrick 517
Lewis, C. S. 123
  *The Abolition of Man* 17, 65, 185, 217
Lewontin, Richard 53
liberalism 15, 53, 67, 360, 369
Lincoln, Abraham 105, 115, 261, 286–287, 290, 292, 391
Locke, John 12, 15, 102, 248, 287, 289, 317
Lucretius 90, 338

## M

machines *See* humans: as machines
MacIntyre, Alasdair 223
Macklin, Ruth 9, 14, 19–20, 26–27, 32, 34, 254, 276, 277, 388, 437, 469, 470, 506–508, 534
Maimonides 400
Mandela, Nelson 102, 105
Marcel, Gabriel 264, 513, 514, 516–522, 528, 529, 537
Marcus Aurelius 7
Maritain, Jacques 360, 466
Marx, Karl 357 *See also* dignity: Aristotelian/Marxian account of
Massey, Rev. Edward 109
Mather, Jennifer A. 144
*The Matrix*, film 162
McKibben, Bill 403
Meilaender, Gilbert 248, 517
  commentary on 278–283, 284–290, 292
mental retardation *See* disabilities
Merzenich, Michael 140
Mill, John Stuart 26, 106
Milton, John 403
Mirandola, Pico della 184
  *Oration on the Dignity of Man* 183, 205
mood control *See* enhancement: mood control
Moravec, Hans 197
murder *See* death

## N

Nagel, Thomas 123, 225
National Bioethics Advisory Commission 28
National Commission for the Protection of Human Subjects of Biomedical and Behavioral Research 20–33
  *Belmont Report* 20, 23–26, 28, 31, 33
National Research Act of 1974 21
natural kinds *See* dignity: through natural kind membership
natural law *See* nature: natural law
nature *See* freedom: from natural necessity; *See also* God: nature's; *See also* right(s): natural
  and convention 310
  and freedom 68, 85, 86, 92, 338
  and personhood 313
  as historical 140
  higher 314
  mastery of 8, 14, 16, 17, 66, 81, 157, 185, 204, 242, 248, 299, 300, 302, 303
  natural joints 96
  natural law 220, 346
  rhetoric of 372, 375
  state of 322, 324
neuroscience 99, 114, 115, 117, 130, 136, 137, 140, 141, 143, 145, 242
Newman, John Henry 518, 520–522
Newton, Isaac 343
Nietzsche, Friedrich 54, 90, 160, 200, 337
  "last man" 185, 305, 381
Nixon, Richard M., President 21
Nuffield Council on Bioethics 19–20
  *Genetics and Human Behavior: the*

*Ethical Context* 19
Nuremberg War Crime Trials 23
Nuremberg Code 23
Nussbaum, Martha 444, 452
  central human
    capabilities 377–378
  commentary on 381–386
  *Frontiers of Justice* 365, 454, 459
  Human Development and Capability Association 368, 373
  *Sex and Social Justice* 372
  *Women and Human Development* 456

# O

O'Donovan, Oliver 264
Ortega y Gasset, José 139
Orwell, George
  *The Road to Wigan Pier* 209

# P

pantheism 239–240
Pascal, Blaise 223
  *Pensées* 136, 318
patients 135, 260, 300, 318, 522–533 *See also* dignity: from a patient's perspective
  and autonomy 525
  and dependence 510
  and personal knowledge 510
  and privacy 509
Paul 107
Pavlov, Ivan 65
Percy, Walker 241
performance *See* enhancement: performance
persistent vegetative state 48, 363, 381, 385, 470, 496–498
persons 26, 143, 144, 145, 298, 311, 312, 340, 383, 385, 410–411, 416, 425–429 *See also* humans: as persons; *See also* nature: and personhood
  as rational and responsible 342
  being a person as criterion for moral worth 412
  Christian 244
  defined by Aquinas 412
  Kantian 245
  respect for 14, 15, 20–26, 28, 31, 302, 483, 507, 508, 517 *See also* dignity: as respect for persons
  philosophy 61, 62, 63, 68, 70, 73, 74, 79, 93, 130, 136, 158, 299, 311, 322, 342, 388, 389, 390, 399, 404
Plato 74, 93, 101, 222, 419, 451, 471
  noble lie 93
  *Phaedrus* 40, 98
  *Symposium* 327–329
Pope Benedict XVI 517, 535–537
Pope Boniface VIII 112
Pope John Paul II 226, 253, 283, 288, 291, 444, 528–529
Pope Pius XII 112
Popper, Karl 177
posthumanism 155–172, 173, 202–212, 251, 302, 303, 305 *See also* transhumanism
Potts, Richard 137
Povinelli, Daniel 133
President's Council on Bioethics 3, 19–21, 20, 27–30, 32–34, 254, 256, 257, 258, 266, 267, 274, 275, 278, 291, 292, 298, 299, 384, 387, 436, 437, 445, 494 *See also* Bush, George W., President: August 9, 2001, televised address
  *Alternative Sources of Human Pluripotent Stem Cells* 264, 441
  *Being Human* 266, 277, 330, 441
  *Beyond Therapy* 5, 271–272, 291, 330, 441
  *Human Cloning and Human Dignity* 19, 254, 268–269, 330,

441, 465
*Monitoring Stem Cell Research* 330, 441
*Reproduction and Responsibility* 264, 330
*Taking Care* 4, 255, 267, 330, 441, 464
privacy *See* patients: and privacy; *See also* right(s): to privacy

## Q

*The Queen,* film 285

## R

Ramsey, Paul 26, 27
Rand, Ayn 90
Ratzinger, Joseph *See* Pope Benedict XVI
Rawls, John 223, 358, 360, 369
"sense of justice" 460, 462, 464
*A Theory of Justice* 351, 464
reason, rationality 10–11, 12, 94, 272, 311, 313, 324, 325, 326, 352, 354, 363, 365, 409, 416, 430, 476, 513 *See also* dignity: through having a rational nature; *See also* humanity: as embodied rationality; *See also* humans: as rational animals; *See also* Kant, Immanuel: "pure reason"; *See also* persons: as rational and responsible; *See also* soul: embodied rational; *See also* soul: rational
reproduction
as an unconstitutional burden on women 374, 382
*in vitro* fertilization 40, 81, 112, 345
research subjects *See* humans: as research subjects
Richerson and Boyd
*Chimpanzee Culture* 131
Richerson, Peter 131
right(s) 12, 15, 63, 91, 108, 112, 148, 149, 208, 218, 222, 240, 243, 270, 289, 290, 298, 339, 345, 413, 414, 429, 430, 435, 498, 507, 523 *See also* dignity: through asserting rights
animal 52, 366, 413–420
civil 298
disability 356, 488
divine 106
equal 278, 286, 288, 289
human 12, 13, 91, 92, 176, 208, 218, 246, 290, 351, 381, 388, 441, 446, 536
inalienable 10, 12, 288, 386, 389, 398, 400
language of 290–292, 400–402
might makes 322
natural 12, 91, 208, 221, 283, 286, 317, 318, 485, 487
of all living things 417
property 270, 363, 366
second-generation 436, 453
to health care 485, 487
to liberty 287
to life 221, 287, 290, 317, 430
to privacy 270, 523
*Universal Declaration of Human Rights* 12, 129, 175, 218, 219, 301, 360, 448, 515
voting 361, 364, 366, 414
vs. duties 388, 396–405, 448
welfare 436
Robertson, Pat 108
*Roe v. Wade* 30, 31, 220–221, 222
Rolston, Holmes III 475
Rousseau, Jean-Jacques 65
*Emile* 65
Rowley, Janet 264
Russell, Bertrand 145

## S

Sakai, Kuniyashi L. 137
Schaub, Diana 278, 281, 283
Schiavo, Theresa 388, 402–403

Schulman, Adam 33, 215–218, 393
Searle, John 87
*Mind* 71
Sellars, Wilfrid 41
Sen, Amartya
*Development as Freedom* 54
Seneca 352–353, 471
Shakespeare, William 105, 403
*The Tempest* 211
Shaw, George Bernard 100
Shell, Susan M., commentary on 382–385
Shultziner, Doron 13
Singer, Peter 26, 220, 366, 374, 384, 413–415, 417, 418
*Ethics* 148
singularity 139
Skinner, B. F. 65, 67, 84, 90, 91
*Beyond Freedom and Dignity* 65
slavery 67, 100, 104, 112, 115, 174, 261, 287, 289, 290, 292, 297, 298, 314, 411, 515
*First Arkansas Marching Song* 307
Socrates 95, 135, 242, 311, 327–329, 422
Solzhenitsyn, Aleksandr 237, 283, 291
soul 9, 47, 62, 63, 64, 66, 80, 81, 89, 90, 92, 93, 94, 167, 192, 250, 353, 355, 360, 361, 389
animal 69, 84
Aristotelian account of 83
as genetic information 97
as silly as mermaids 279
Cartesian 96
doctrine of 44, 94
embodied rational 68–73, 84
ensoulment 40, 49, 69, 96, 346
immaterial 44, 47, 64, 85, 279
immortal 73, 79
made of lots of tiny robots 45, 84
plant 69
rational 68, 81, 85, 90, 93
species *See* dignity: through species membership
Spencer, Herbert 67
Spiegelberg, Herbert 263
sports *See* enhancement: in sports
*Star Trek* 166
Steinbeck, John 198
stem cells 9, 61, 99, 101, 108, 112, 113, 123, 225, 264, 298, 334, 374, 386, 470, 493, 514
Stockdale, Admiral James 8
Stoicism *See* dignity: Stoic account of
Straus, Erwin
*Phenomenological Psychology* 524
Sulmasy, Daniel P., OFM 517

# T

Talmud 399–401, 403
Tattersall, Ian 137
Taylor, Paul 417
Tetlock, Philip 41, 42
theology
Catholic moral 26
civil 230, 247
natural 230–233, 247
pantheism 240
personal 247
Thomas Aquinas 113, 253, 288, 412, 432, 438 *See also* persons: defined by Aquinas
Thompson, Judith 491
Thurber, James 7
Tocqueville, Alexis de 225, 237, 238, 239, 245, 248
Tolstoy, Leo 314
Tomasello, Michael 132, 142
torture 57, 161, 175, 270, 426
transhumanism 156, 170, 207, 208, 251, 292, 300, 302, 303 *See also* dignity: transhumanist; *See also* freedom: posthuman or transhuman; *See also* posthumanism
trees, dignity of 134, 196, 198, 347, 353, 359
Tuskegee Syphilis Study 21–23, 31

Twain, Mark
*Pudd'nhead Wilson's New Calendar* 135

# U

Un-Dignity 184–188 *See also* dignity: "Un-Dignity"
*Universal Declaration of Human Rights* (UN) *See* right(s): *Universal Declaration of Human Rights*
utilitarianism 22, 32, 365, 366

# V

Velleman, David 484
Venter, J. Craig 139
Vinge, Vernor 158
virtue 43, 123, 134, 167, 169, 177, 178, 181, 188, 209, 246, 282, 285, 288, 309, 310, 311, 314, 319, 355, 356, 476, 533
   Christian and classical 286

# W

de Waal, Frans 148
Weithman, Paul 267, 270
Wells, H. G. 209
White, E. B.
   *Charlotte's Web* 167
Wiggins, David 477
will *See* freedom: of will
Williams, Bernard 177
Williams, Roger 358, 359
Willowbrook State School 22
Wilson, E. O. 67, 90
wisdom 102, 107, 133, 135, 216, 246, 304, 311, 328, 329
Wojtyla, Karol *See* Pope John Paul II
Wolfe, Tom 233
   *A Man in Full* 8
Wolf, Naomi 356

Made in the USA
Middletown, DE
04 October 2017